Adelle Davis

Adelle Davis, one of the country's best-known nutri-tionists, studied at Purdue University, graduated from the University of California at Berkeley, and took postgraduate work at Columbia University and the University of California at Los Angeles before re-ceiving her Master of Science degree in biochemistry from the University of Southern California Medical School. Throughout her career she worked with phy-sicians, beginning in New York with dietetics training at Bellevue and Fordham hospitals and her first job at the Judson Health Clinic.

Later, in Oakland, California, and then in Los Angeles, she worked as a consulting nutritionist with physicians at the Alameda County Health Clinic and the William E. Branch Clinic in Hollywood, as well as seeing patients referred to her by numerous spe-cialists. After planning individual diets for more than 20,000 people suffering from almost every known disease, she gave up consulting work to devote her time to her family, writing, and lecturing.

Adelle Davis was the author of four bestselling books, Let's Cook It Right, Let's Have Healthy Children, Let's Get Well, *and* Let's Eat Right to Keep Fit. *In the light of new developments in nutritional science and the steady decline in our national health, Miss Davis revised* LET'S EAT RIGHT TO KEEP FIT. *This revised edition is also published in hardcover by Harcourt Brace Jovanovich, Inc.*

LET'S GET WELL

Adelle Davis

New Introduction by
Harriet Roth,
author of *Deliciously Low*
and *Deliciously Simple*

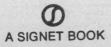

A SIGNET BOOK

*Dedicated to the hundreds
of wonderful doctors whose research
made this book possible*

SIGNET
Published by the Penguin Group
Penguin Books USA Inc., 375 Hudson Street,
New York, New York 10014, U.S.A.
Penguin Books Ltd, 27 Wrights Lane,
London W8 5TZ, England
Penguin Books Australia Ltd, Ringwood,
Victoria, Australia
Penguin Books Canada Ltd, 2801 John Street,
Markham, Ontario, Canada L3R 1B4
Penguin Books (N.Z.) Ltd, 182-190 Wairau Road,
Auckland 10, New Zealand

Penguin Books Ltd, Registered Offices:
Harmondsworth, Middlesex, England

This is an authorized reprint of a hardcover edition published by
Harcourt Brace Jovanovich, Inc.

First Signet Printing, November, 1972
33 32 31 30 29 28 27 26 25

REGISTERED TRADEMARK—MARCA REGISTRADA

Printed in the United States of America

PUBLISHER'S NOTE

FOREWORD

BY JOSEPH C. RISSER, M.D.

Miss Adelle Davis could add "and Let's Keep Well" to this her latest book, for the processes that get you well should also keep you well. The knowledge of how to keep well is most important for the layman and the professional man alike. There are three necessary rules to be observed in keeping well: 1) self-discipline, without which the other two rules are of little value; 2) proper use of the body; and 3) adequate nourishment for the body. These three rules of good living are considered so commonplace, as well as so fundamental, that each individual thinks he has the prerogative to handle these problems by himself without advice. Even the professional man assumes too often that the patient knows how to obey these rules. This book, *Let's Get Well,* is devoted to the third rule of good living, or— how adequately to nourish the body.

As we have acquired more information on this complex subject of nutrition and metabolism, it has created a greater interest among the laymen and even among some professional men. Unfortunately, the professional man is so busy diagnosing the diseases of his patients and giving the necessary medical and surgical treatment that he has little time to study the newer ideas that have developed recently in the field of nutrition. The professional man is a specialist in pathologies; he knows how to recognize the different diseases, but often pays too little attention to the standards and the requisites of good health. If more attention were paid to the problem of keeping people well by following these necessary rules, we would have less of a problem in taking care of people who succumb too readily to the degenerative diseases.

Miss Davis has compiled an excellent reference book. Her statements on how to get well and keep well are documented so well that any person may check these references for further information. It is true that many of these references are clinical observations only and need more laboratory tests on deficiencies to furnish further proof of their correctness. However, one cannot ignore repeated good clinical results from the adequate use of good nutrition as these facts come to light and it behooves all of us to be curious about the statements and to accept them as we see the good results.

Many of our big advances in medicine have come from rather commonplace beginnings—as in the case of foxglove, later known as digitalis, which was used in the treatment of heart trouble. This was first used by an herb-lady but was discredited by the medical profession until the good results made it necessary for even the profession to accept it as a remedy for heart trouble. Oftentimes patients have a disease without any known treatment, or they may even have a disease which does not allow for a ready diagnosis. It is important in these cases that we treat the patient even if we do not treat the diagnosis, and frequently in treating the patient with only these necessary rules of good health, we can bring about a great improvement. In my practice of orthopedics, I feel it is vitally important to the patient to review these true rules of good health on how to use the body and how to nourish the body—as well as to treat the patient's deformities. In so doing, we not only gain improvement in the deformity we are caring for, but also the patient will often state, "You not only cured my deformity but you have also cured my acne" or "my constipation" or some other condition.

One of the most important helps to give a patient about nutrition is some advice regarding the selection of the best foods that contain the most needed nutrients. In our country we have produced more food than we need, and to keep it from spoiling it is highly processed and refined. However, this very process of refining takes away and destroys thermolabile substances. In checking back in books on biochemistry we find that some foods contain many calories but all the nutrients have been destroyed. These foods will not allow for repair or growth of the body, but make for wear and tear—rather than wear and repair.

With recent studies, it has been found that the average daily requirement of nutrients increases remarkably under stress. Many of us are subject to unexpected and unusual stresses, and therefore to keep our good health we must increase the daily requirement of nutrients as we anticipate and experience the stresses of day-to-day living.

In reading this book the layman may be tempted to make his own diagnosis and to render his own treatment as indicated by some of the clinical examples that Miss Davis has mentioned in her book. This could be unfortunate, because the layman might go astray in his attempt at disagnosing his own condition. The patient should first see his doctor and find out his trouble. Then while talking over his problem with the doctor, he might mention the things he has gained from reading these methods of getting and keeping well.

To get the most out of Adelle Davis's book on getting well and keeping well, it must not only be read but should be studied and some of the references should even be checked for further information. There are a great number of documented statements, which makes this an excellent reference and source book on nutritional information.

July 2, 1965
Pasadena, California

INTRODUCTION

Linus Pauling, recipient of two Nobel Prizes, once remarked that "you can't have good ideas unless you have lots of ideas," an observation that I feel applies to Adelle Davis. Fifty years ago, when her voice began to be heard, attitudes toward health were so inadequate that a person interested in new nutritional concepts was dismissed as being on a health kick at best or labeled as a food faddist at worst.

The prevention of illness was the main goal of Adelle Davis's nutritional guidelines. Today proper nutrition is widely accepted as being vital to the prevention of disease as well as to its treatment.

In *Let's Get Well*, Davis compared herself to a reporter who does not make the news but simply disseminates her findings. She observed that while there is still "much to be learned . . . that is no argument against applying what is known." The book is a compilation of her ideas about nutrition and the processes she felt contributed not just to getting well but to *staying* well.

Adelle Davis wrote her book principally for the lay person, and she emphasized the importance of medical supervision where matters of health were concerned. However, she was outspoken about the inadequacy of the diets physicians frequently recommended. Davis would be delighted to learn that many doctors today refer patients to registered dietitians or qualified nutritionists, although it is still true that most medical schools do not offer physicians sufficient training in nutrition.

The connection between health and nutrition presently reflected in the guidelines of both the American Heart Association and the American Cancer Society was the main thrust of Adelle Davis's writings more than twenty-five years ago in *Let's Get Well*.

● She called attention to the dangers of atherosclerosis, which she believed was caused by eating too many saturated or hydrogenated fats, although she did not make the final connection between this fact and avoiding or limiting foods that are high in cholesterol.

● As early as 1965 she placed the optimum blood cholesterol level at no more than 180 mg. regardless of age, and she emphasized that everyone should have an *annual* blood cholesterol determination.

● She advised industry to run annual programs to test the blood cholesterol levels in employees. Many companies are now making this part of routine physicals, but more to the point, as of 1987 the National Institutes of Health plan to make cholesterol screening programs available to the public on a nationwide basis.

● She was well aware of the role that lifetime eating habits played in illness, commenting that "sudden" was a strange adjective to apply to coronary attacks that had been many years in the making.

● She warned that caffeine was a stress-inducing agent and raised cholesterol.

● She cited the soluble fiber pectin as effective in reducing cholesterol and recommended eating the pulp of citrus fruit, especially the white of orange rind. Today's research by Dr. James Anderson has expanded this to include high-fiber foods like oat bran, apples, pears, dried peas, beans and lentils, all excellent natural sources of cholesterol-lowering fiber.

● In 1965, Davis referred to the use of niacinamide to reduce blood cholesterol. Niacin is currently being used by some physicians on patients with chronic high cholesterol levels. (However, it is not without side effects and many patients cannot tolerate it. When possible, a low-fat, low-cholesterol diet high in soluble fiber is the preferred treatment.)

● Davis recognized that health and normal weight go hand in hand. She warned that obesity was dangerous to health. She cautioned dieters not to skip meals and proposed they have frequent small meals rather than three heavy ones daily. She urged them to reject reducing drugs and fasting, and simply concentrate on counting calories and watching nutrients.

● Her contention that losing weight helped diabetics was part of the medical thinking of her day, but she was ahead of her time in suggesting that a low-fat diet was as important in regulating diabetics as a low-sugar diet. Today this is accepted theory.

● She advised consulting a physician for a general checkup before starting any diet or exercise program.

● She observed that antibiotics destroyed useful intestinal bacteria and she recommended eating yogurt or acidophilus culture when taking antibiotics to prevent the occurrence of the fungus Monilia albicans.

● Adelle Davis highlighted the hereditary factor in high blood cholesterol levels and reported that improved diets could lower them, especially when this problem was detected at an early age.

● She objected to the use of mineral oil in people with elimination problems because it decreased the absorption of valuable nutrients. Mineral oil is no longer recommended as a laxative because of this effect.

● Years ago, patients with diverticulitis were given low-fiber diets. Davis disagreed with this and even then suggested foods that supplied roughage and unrefined starches—the treatment of choice today.

● She also disagreed with the traditional restricted bland diet prescribed for ulcer patients. Present practice calls for individualized diets depending on the patient's tolerance, just what Davis has suggested. (She did, however, also recommend milk as the best treatment for ulcers —we currently believe that milk actually stimulates acid secretions in the stomach.)

● Davis believed that estrogen and Vitamin D therapy played a major role in calcium absorption in women. This has recently been confirmed. (She also cautioned that large doses of Vitamin D could be toxic.) Physicians today give minimal doses of estrogen as a safeguard against osteoporosis in postmenopausal women.

● Davis suggested a dose of 1250 mg. of calcium daily as a further safeguard against osteoporosis; the Recommended Daily Allowance has just been increased to 1000 mg. daily.

● Davis addressed the important role that Vitamins A, C, and E play in cancer prevention—the American Cancer Society now says there is evidence that these vitamins may indeed be important in preventing cancer.

● Her reference to interferon as "appearing to give protection from cancer-producing viruses" has been substantiated. Today it is being used with increasing success in the treatment of cancer patients.

● She suggested using Vitamin E ointment or Vitamin E to minimize scar formation, a use frequently prescribed by surgeons today.

● Although she saw no advantage in taking natural vitamins over synthetic, Davis felt that the natural sources in food were possibly superior because they were ingested with other nutrients.

● Davis reported that an unsightly discoloration developed on the teeth of young children given the antibiotic tetracycline. Today we know it is not the antibiotic of choice for children whose teeth are forming.

● She recommended plenty of rest, a good mental outlook, and a strong desire to get well as supplements to the nutritional program for patients with multiple sclerosis—advice given by many physicians today.

● In preparing meals for the sick, Adelle Davis urged selecting the best food available and cooking it in a palatable way with the fewest possible nutritional losses. Her warnings about the presence of nitrates, pesticide residues, food additives, chemicals, and processed foods have particular meaning for the sick because of their lowered resistance.

Of course, in the light of current research, some of Adelle Davis's suggestions must be amended. Her recommendation of 60 to 80 grams of protein daily would be considered much too high now. Today low-protein diets are considered advisable because of their low-fat, low-cholesterol content. Moreover, high-protein diets have been linked to osteoporosis.

Davis quite rightly recognized that stress plays a part in worsening atherosclerosis and she suggested an anti-stress formula containing Vitamin B_2, B_6, Vitamin C, and pantothenic acid in larger-than-normal amounts. While certain vitamins may indeed assist our bodies in handling physical stress such as surgery, burns, etc., there is no hard evidence that mega-doses of vitamins bring relief for emotional stress. Moreover, current research indicates that mega-doses of vitamins are not advisable, particularly vitamins like A, D, E, and K that are not water soluble in the body. It is important to remember that while there are vitamin-deficiency diseases, toxicity from mega-doses of fat-soluble vitamins can be dangerous.

The liberal use of salt substitutes containing potassium chloride, which she suggested for patients suffering from kidney disease and high blood pressure, would not be acceptable now unless taken under a doctor's supervision. New vegetable and herb seasoning products make these possibly dangerous potassium chloride salt substitutes unnecessary.

As we approach the 21st century, further discoveries await us that may make current scientific data obsolete. To date, our knowledge has increased the average life span as well as the public awareness of each person's role in creating his or her own health.

Adelle Davis's insights and her concern for people's health and well-being laid the groundwork for today's emphasis on proper nutrition to maintain and extend life. Her clarion call that "sound nutrition stands as a fortress against disease, a fortress whose gates are open and into which all may enter who wish" is as much a rallying cry today as it was a quarter of a century ago.

—HARRIET ROTH
Author of *Deliciously Low*
and *Deliciously Simple*

CONTENTS

12 *Contents*

1

Let's Get Well

There are so many of them—the people who do not feel well. The statistics of illness in the United States are too depressing to examine for long: 40 million with allergies; 17 million with ulcers; 10 million with arthritis,[1] and so many millions whose jagged nerves have driven them to using tranquilizers or whose exhaustion has prompted the taking of pep pills that addictions to barbiturates and amphetamines have mounted into the hundreds of thousands.

Statistics of the most rapidly increasing illnesses—heart disease, diabetes, cancer, and strokes—change too quickly to be accurate. Dr. Ancel Keys, of the University of Minnesota, is quoted as saying that one no longer asks who has heart disease but merely, "How severe is your heart disease?" Is there a happily married woman free from the anxiety that a coronary attack will force her into years of unbearable loneliness? An adult who does not live in dread that cancer will strike himself or his family?

The number of ill persons, so appropriately called morbid statistics, is morbid indeed. Each figure represents the heartache and suffering of a wonderful human being longing for his birthright: health. This book would have been too depressing to write were it not that nutritional research, like a modern star of Bethlehem, brings hope that sickness need not be a part of life.

Nutritional research is being carried on at an unprecedented rate in almost every medical school, university, and pharmaceutical laboratory throughout the world. About 6,000 original scientific studies in nutrition are published annually—7,149 in 1960 alone—and summarized in *Nutrition Abstracts and Reviews*.[2] Thus the knowledge of how to build health through nutrition, which is the subject of this book, becomes greater each year. Such research has but one ultimate purpose: to alleviate the suffering of mankind. Until the findings of these investiga-

13

tors are known and applied, this goal cannot be reached, and the energies of numerous brilliant scientists are largely wasted. There is much still to be learned, but that is no argument against applying what is known.

This vast amount of research deals with 40 nutrients which cannot be made in the body: 1 essential fatty acid, 15 vitamins, 14 minerals, and 10 amino acids. Collectively these 40 nutrients are spoken of as body requirements. From them our bodies synthesize an estimated 10,000 different compounds essential to the maintenance of health. Already known are some 3,000 compounds, most of them vitamin-containing enzymes and coenzymes which, stimulated by minerals, carry on the work of the cells. All 40 nutrients work together; therefore a lack of any one might result in the underproduction of hundreds of these essential compounds. Thus nutrition is an orchestra of 40 instruments, and adding large amounts of one or two nutrients can no more render the music of health than blaring horns and pounding drums can play a Beethoven symphony.

A friend, referring to my earlier writing, complained, "But Adelle, your simplicity is so complicated." Unfortunately, the increasing knowledge of how essential compounds are produced has made nutrition far more complex than ever before. For instance, substance A, a raw material from digested food, might be changed to B, B to C, C to D, D to E, and so on, each step requiring a series of minerals, vitamins, and amino acids from digested proteins. If a deficiency makes it impossible for substance C to be changed into D, the essential compounds D and E would be lacking and so much substance C might accumulate that it could become toxic.[3] Examples of disease produced in this manner are cited later; and, while not easily remembered, they can be understood. I am all too aware, however, that the omission of certain difficult-to-comprehend details may result in a loss of accuracy.

Probably no one nutrient is ever totally lacking from an otherwise adequate diet, but partial simultaneous deficiencies of many nutrients are common. Research shows that diseases of almost every variety can be produced by an undersupply of various combinations of nutrients. Just as 52 cards can be dealt into thousands of bridge hands, no two alike, so can various combinations of partial deficiencies result in hundreds of diseases having different symptoms. The combined number of multiple deficiencies and the mildness or severity of each determine whether one disease or another will be produced. The missing nutrients which allow illnesses to develop have been discarded in processing and refining foods.

Research shows that diseases produced by combinations of deficiencies can be corrected when all nutrients are supplied, provided irreparable damage has not been done; and, still better, that these diseases can be prevented. Because information gleaned from hundreds of medical and nutrition journals can do much to prevent future illness, it is my greatest hope that persons will read this book in its entirety even though they are not interested in each disease discussed.

Nutrition is not concerned with disease, but is a study of building and maintaining health. It is essentially the same regardless of what illness may have occurred. For example, a woman for whom I had planned a diet to stimulate breast milk wrote me that when her husband's eczema had not improved after numerous ointments had been used, he had adhered to her diet. In his case, the diet failed in the purpose for which it was planned, but the eczema quickly disappeared.

It can scarcely be overemphasized that nutrition is never competitive with the practice of medicine, but is an aid to both the physician and the patient. To eat wisely is different indeed from the home treatment of disease. Because medical attention is postponed, self-doctoring can be extremely dangerous. Many a home-treated "touch of indigestion" has proved to be stomach cancer, coronary disease, or a burst appendix, and has resulted in death because a physician was not consulted soon enough. When any abnormality occurs, two steps should be taken: one should improve his nutrition, and consult a physician. Because cancer, heart disease, and many other illnesses can be treated successfully if discovered in time, a yearly physical examination has become more important now than ever before.

If a doctor recommends a diet, it should be carefully followed; he alone understands a particular case. Nutrition can often be improved, however, within the framework of any diet. A doctor may specify that bread be eaten daily but allow the patient to select a whole-grain or a refined variety. Or he may merely suggest that one eat a "well-balanced" diet. Those physicians and their patients may find this book helpful.

When improvements in nutrition do result in increased

well-being, persons frequently ask me rather belligerently, "Why didn't my doctor tell me?" Since I want no words of mine to interfere with meaningful physician-patient relationships, I feel this question should be answered fully. I bristle when doctors are criticized. For years I have been associated with them in hospitals, clinics, and private practice, known them to work all day and on throughout the night, seen them cry heartbrokenly at the death of a patient, and found much in them to admire.

During the last two decades—and since many practicing physicians have had their training—nutrition has developed into a highly technical science, a full-time specialty in itself. At first, diet seemed unimportant in treating most diseases, and by the time it proved to have a profound bearing on health, the curriculum in medical schools was overcrowded. At present, no medical school in the United States has a required course in nutrition, though a smattering of the subject is taught in biochemistry, clinical medicine, and other courses.

Numerous articles have appeared in the professional journals urging that more nutrition be taught in medical schools.[4-7] They describe the present teaching of nutrition as scattered, inadequate, "disorganized and haphazard,"[6] and "woefully weak."[7] The Council of Foods and Nutrition of the American Medical Association, after making a survey of how nutrition was taught in medical schools, found that it still centers around the now rare deficiency diseases; and that the gap is too wide between research findings and the practicing physicians' information. It reported an urgent and immediate need for improvement.[8] At present, however, the situation is tragic and causes unnecessary suffering. Furthermore, many of the magazines in which nutritional research findings are reported are unavailable except to doctors having access to a large medical library.

Often physicians themselves are upset by their lack of training in nutrition. A young pediatrician who had read my books brought his child to me for nutritional advice. He remarked sadly, "Everything you advise which I've tried on my patients works. But if what you say is true, why weren't we taught it in medical school? We had wonderful professors." And I am sure they were wonderful, but unfortunately they too were untrained in nutrition. A letter written on sixteen pages of a prescription pad came from another physician. "I've had so little training in nutrition I feel unprepared when patients ask me about diet," he wrote. "Often they know more about nutrition than I do. I try to avoid recommending diets whenever possible." He may speak for many practitioners. Excellent nutrition advice has been given to patients by their doctors, however, and all too frequently ignored.

It is literally impossible for a busy physician to keep abreast of new research on drugs, viruses, antibiotics, treatments, surgery, medical procedures, and laboratory technics. The National Library of Medicine estimates that 200,000 articles are published annually on drugs alone. A doctor attempting to keep up on all subjects related to medicine would not have time to pull a stethoscope from his pocket. Is it not grossly unfair to expect him to be an expert on nutrition?

The inadequacy of the diets physicians frequently recommend worries me far more than their failure to recommend a diet. Some commonly copy special diets listed in standard texts, which a committee of the American Medical Association and the American Dietetic Association has pointed out are based largely on tradition rather than scientific fact, and are years behind research findings.[9]

Physicians have long worked co-operatively with hospital dietitians, and a few medical groups retain dietary consultants.[10] Although I know of no one other than myself doing independent consulting work in nutrition, hundreds of dietitians have had years of excellent university and hospital training and, if persuaded to work with physicians in private practice, could fill the void that now exists.

Many physicians are doing outstanding research on one aspect or another of nutrition. The hundreds of studies used as the source material for this book have been conducted almost entirely by doctors, perhaps 95 per cent of whom are professors in medical schools; and the references on pages 349 to 404 are listed for practicing physicians who may wish to read the original articles.

That the value of nutrition is being appreciated by the medical profession is shown by such statements as one made by Dr. W. H. Sebrell, director of the Institute of Nutrition Sciences at Columbia University: "Today nutrition is finally beginning to be recognized as an important factor in the treatment of and convalescence from almost every disease."[7] Dr. Robert E. Shank, professor at the Washington University School of Medicine at St. Louis, wrote: "There is probably no other single factor so important to the achievement and maintenance of health as is nutrition."[11] Dr. W. A. Krehl, professor at the Iowa State University College of Medicine, expressed himself in these words: "No area of research in this century has yielded so much for the benefit of man as the basic science of nutrition."[12]

Dr. William B. Bean, another professor at the Iowa State University College of Medicine, speaks of nutrition as "germane to every phase of health and disease."[13] He states that if enough young doctors would take up nutritional investigation, "it [nutrition] would rise from the ashes of neglect. In the role of Cinderella it would deserve well-earned acclaim for contributing to the advancement of learning as well as the welfare of mankind." I have no doubt that nutrition, as Cinderella, will eventually marry the prince, but at present she is still a mistreated stepchild.

This book has been written because people adhere to an adequate diet in proportion to their understanding of what foods have to offer them. An individual who has ignored nutrition will often follow a diet with fanatical zeal after obtaining a knowledge of the subject. It must be understood, however, that the descriptions of diseases in the following chapters, given only to show the relationship of nutrition to the rebuilding process, are superficial indeed and are by no means intended to be comprehensive in the medical sense.

Building health through nutrition requires putting it into practice, which is often far from easy. How completely a person adheres to a nutrition program and hence how quickly he regains his health—provided irreparable damage or genetic malfunction does not exist—depends upon his determination, his will to live, and his ability to see rainbows through the rain. Every physician has seen patients miraculously recover from what appeared to be a terminal illness and others die seemingly with little cause. For some people, illness is a way of life,[14] an attempt to overcome early emotional deprivations. The vast majority of sick persons, however, if given a ray of hope, will make every effort to recover.

To encourage individuals perhaps despondent, I have included many case histories in this book. Some of these reports may, I am afraid, sound boastful. These people recovered because nutrition actually works; and it was they, not I, who ate the foods that helped them get well. The role I play is similar to that of a newspaper reporter, who certainly cannot take credit for making the news.

It is important to realize that rebuilding health through

nutrition is essentially a slow process; rarely are results as quick and dramatic as in stopping an infection with antibiotics. Yet studies in which nutrients have been made radioactive, marking them so they can be traced and observed, indicate that the entire body can be rebuilt much more rapidly than was formerly believed. For instance, calcium taken in food can be deposited in a fractured bone within half an hour.[15] When I talked to a mother understandably distraught because she had been told that her young son, who had nephritis, had only ten years to live, I said, "Isn't it wonderful that you have so long to rebuild his health?" Nutritional investigation warrants, I believe, such an attitude toward many diseases.

Every year I receive thousands of wonderful letters from wonderful people, each wanting to know how nutrition might help overcome some abnormality. Because there are not enough hours in the day to read so many letters, let alone answer them properly, I have tried to give the information the writers have requested in this book. When no research studies appear to have been done on a given subject, I have drawn on my own experience. During the past 37 years I have interviewed approximately 11,000 persons for whom I planned nutrition programs; and the progress of these individuals I have followed as best I could. In addition I have worked out more than 8,000 diets for others who live at great distances; and usually they have reported results to me. I suspect that these people have taught me far more than I taught them.

Space does not permit a detailed discussion of the value of each nutrient, the sources of supplies, and other information given in my earlier book *Let's Eat Right to Keep Fit;* hence, to prevent confusion, it should be read first. Newer findings in nutrition are reported throughout the following chapters, each of which should be read to give understanding to the next. The practical aspects of planning diets are summarized in chapters 32 and 33.

It is difficult to discuss nutrition without appearing to overestimate its value, an error as great as underestimation. Even the best nutrition can help to restore health only when a lack of nutrients has been a contributory cause of illness. Some physicians estimate that as much as 90 per cent of sickness today is partly emotional in origin. Sound nutrition may help an individual to cope with emotional problems,[16] but food cannot make a rejected person feel loved or one who undervalues himself feel worthy. It is largely because of feelings about foods and about oneself that few persons adhere to an adequate diet.

Although such abnormalities as ulcers, arthritis, allergies, and colitis, to name only a few, are undoubtedly often psychosomatic in origin, it is usually the combination of faulty nutrition and emotional problems that causes illness. In overcoming many diseases the best results can be obtained by combining adequate nutrition with good psychotherapy. People too frequently try to correct an illness unrecognized as being emotionally induced by enthusiastically improving their nutrition, and because the disease persists, feel that nutrition has little or no value.

As a child I lived with an elderly aunt, a contemporary of Pasteur's, who found it impossible to believe that anything too small to be seen could cause disease. At the mention of bacteria, she would retort angrily, "Microbes! Bah! Fiddlesticks!" Today we find it equally difficult to believe that long-forgotten anger, "stored" during a lifetime, can cause headaches or arthritis, or that the need to cry, accumulated over many years, can result in "sinus infection" or "hay fever." Because of a lack of understanding, our attitude toward psychosomatic medicine is still in the bah-fiddlesticks stage.

As I see it, every person has emotional problems, whether recognized or not, and sooner or later these problems usually cause some form of disease. We can often accept the fact that emotions may bring about other people's illnesses, yet resent the implication that our own emotions may cause abnormalities. Such an attitude, I believe, is the result of not realizing that all negative emotions are balanced by wonderful positive ones.

Because we are capable of magnificent positive emotions, I particularly dislike the statement "We are what we eat." A continuous awareness that we are very much more than what we eat, I believe, is necessary to promote health. Within each of us is an immeasurable capacity for love, understanding, compassion, creativity, joy, and all positive qualities. The tragedy of illness is that it prevents the full expression of outgoing healthy emotions and creative abilities. Instead it focuses abnormal attention inward upon one's self, causing one to retreat into a body that may become a prison with dungeons and torture chambers.

I feel that the achievement of health is worth considerable effort and expense because it can add happiness to our lives and to others, can help us to know love and warmth, song, laughter, and music, to experience the joy of creativity and the satisfaction of accomplishments well done, and to have wide interests in this age when exciting advances are being made in every field of human endeavor. It seems to me that health also can bring the oneness of understanding, the silence of meditation, and the whisper of prayer, and that it can be ventilated when need be by outbursts of justified anger and bathed now and again with tears. Such health, I believe, is in part a reward of good nutrition.

We are indeed much more than what we eat, but what we eat can nevertheless help us to be much more than what we are.

2
Meeting the Demands of Stress

To meet the nutritional demands of stress must be the first consideration in planning any diet, regardless of whom it is for, and in coping with any disease, regardless of its nature. If the body's reaction to stress is understood and the diet can be adjusted accordingly, the problem of achieving health is often largely solved. This subject, therefore, is dealt with here and in most of the following chapters.

What is stress? Any condition that harms the body or damages, breaks down, or causes the death of few or many cells is defined as stress. If the diet is adequate, repair quickly occurs, but when rebuilding fails to keep pace with destruction, illness is produced. Disease results from multiple stresses such as anxiety, overwork, perhaps bacterial or viral attack, and inadequate diet, sleep, and exercise. Unfortunately, it usually brings on numerous other stresses: poor appetite, nausea, vomiting, faulty absorption, fever, pain, diarrhea, dehydration, high urinary losses of many nutrients, exposure to x-rays, and the use of drugs.

In the same way that it requires more material for the repair of a damaged house than for the upkeep of one in good condition, every nutrient is needed in larger amounts to repair a body damaged by the multiple stresses that cause disease and result from it. For example, the stress— or damage—caused by x-raying an animal or by giving it any one of many commonly used drugs increases the need for protein, linoleic acid, several minerals, and vitamins A, C, and all the B vitamins.[1-8] Presumably the same is true of humans.

Regardless of the forms of stress, the body immediately tries to repair damage done, but it cannot unless all nutrients are generously supplied. The nutritional needs increase tremendously at the very time eating is most difficult; and a diet adequate for a healthy individual becomes markedly inadequate for an ill one.

The body's reaction to stress. The great medical genius Dr. Hans Selye, of the University of Montreal, revolutionized medical thinking with his theory, now confirmed by thousands of scientific studies, that the body reacts to every variety of stress in the same way.[4] At the onset of stress, a tiny gland at the base of the brain, the pituitary— the boss of the repair crew—starts protective action by secreting chemical messengers, or hormones, ACTH and STH. These hormones, carried in the blood to two small glands above the kidneys, the adrenals, cause the outside border of these glands, or cortex, to produce cortisone and other messengers. Although the center of these glands manufactures adrenaline, the adrenal hormones referred to throughout this book are those made by the cortex.

These adrenal cortex hormones quickly prepare the body to meet the emergency: proteins, at first drawn from the thymus and lymph glands, are broken down to form sugar necessary for immediate energy; the blood sugar soars and the remaining sugar is stored in the liver in the form of body starch, or glycogen, which can be instantly converted into sugar if needed; the blood pressure increases, minerals are drawn from the bones, fat is mobilized from storage depots, an abnormal amount of salt is retained, and many other changes take place which prepare the body for "fight or flight." These changes also make it possible to repair vital tissues by a process of robbing Peter to pay Paul. This stage, called the "alarm reaction," varies in intensity with the degree of stress.[5]

If the stress continues, the body sets up a "stage of resistance" in which it repairs itself by rebuilding with all the raw materials at hand. When the diet is adequate, a person may go for years withstanding tremendous stress with little apparent harm. Should the raw materials be insufficient to meet the needs, however, there comes a "stage of exhaustion." Disease develops, if it has not already done so, and eventually death threatens or results.

The first two stages of stress are characterized by constant damage and repair; most illnesses fall in stage three, which is reached when repair fails. Intense stress, such as drastic surgery, a serious car accident, or severe burn, may cause a person to pass through all three stages— alarm, resistance, and exhaustion—in a single day. More often we experience repeated "alarm reactions" and live through hundreds of "stages of resistance," one piled on top of the other, before pituitary and adrenal exhaustion threatens our lives. During every illness, however, we are in one of these three stages of stress, and to regain our health our diets must be planned accordingly.

If stress is prolonged after the thymus and lymph glands, whose proteins are purposely destroyed, have shriveled, proteins from the blood plasma, liver, kidneys, and other parts of the body are used.[6] Stomach ulcers may occur not only because of increased production of hydrochloric acid, but also because proteins are stolen from the stomach walls. In ulcerative colitis, the destruction of protein brought about by prolonged stress literally eats away the lining of the intestine. During a single day of severe stress, the urinary loss of nitrogen has shown that the amount of body protein destroyed equals that supplied by 4 quarts of milk.[6] Yet if such a tremendous quantity of protein can be eaten during that day, the tissues are unharmed.

In the same way that the body suffers when its proteins are necessarily stolen and not replaced, so are the bones weakened by the theft of calcium. Dozens of other destructive changes similarly occur. Increased blood pressure alone may become dangerous. It is extremely important, therefore, for each of us to learn how to protect ourselves from the ravages of stress.

Nutritional needs are increased. Experimental stress has been produced in untold thousands of animals by exposing them to loud noises, blinking lights, extreme heat or cold, rarefied air, electric shock, and x-rays and other forms of radiation; by injecting into them drugs, chemicals, bacteria, or viruses; by submitting them to surgery, burns, "accidents," fasting, immobility, or making them run on a treadmill to exhaustion; and by feeding them mineral oil, innumerable toxic substances, or diets deficient or excessive in one or more nutrients. The nutritional needs of these animals invariably skyrocket at the onset of stress and remain high in comparison with those of animals not submitted to such torments. Stress produced by forced exercise, giving excessive thyroid, or exposure to x-rays increases the need for all nutrients.[1,2] If these increased nutritional requirements are met, little harm is done; if not, damage may be severe or even fatal.

How well animals cope with stress depends to a considerable degree on their ability to produce pituitary and adrenal hormones. If the diet has been inadequate in protein, vitamin E, or the B vitamins, riboflavin (vitamin B_2), pantothenic acid, or cholin, sufficient pituitary hormones cannot be produced.[1,2,7,8] Vitamin E, which is more concentrated in the pituitary gland than in any other part of the body, is thought to be particularly essential; it prevents both the pituitary and adrenal hormones from being destroyed by oxygen.[8-11]

The adrenal cortex is even more sensitive to dietary deprivation. A pantothenic-acid deficiency causes the glands to shrivel and to become filled with blood and dead cells; cortisone and other hormones can no longer be produced, and the many protective changes characteristic of stress do not occur.[12-14] Even a slight lack of pantothenic acid causes a marked decrease in the quantity of hormones released.[15,16] The pituitary, adrenal, and sex hormones are all made from cholesterol, but without pantothenic acid, cholesterol cannot be replaced in the glands after once being used up.[17,18] If generous amounts of pantothenic acid are given and the deficiency has not been severe, adrenal hormones can be produced normally within 24 hours. When the deprivation has been prolonged, however, a period of repair is necessary and recovery is slow and uncertain.[13,17]

A slight deficiency of linoleic acid or vitamins A, B_2, or E can also limit hormone production and cause a degeneration of the adrenal cortex; hence each is as essential as pantothenic acid.[18-22] The adrenals of volunteers low in essential fatty acids produced markedly fewer hormones than when the diet was adequate.[23] Damage resulting from such deficiencies can be quickly rectified because the adrenals need these nutrients in small amounts only. Vitamin B_2 given to animals previously deficient in it immediately promotes normal adrenal function.[22] When oil supplying linoleic acid is given to rats lacking it, the production of adrenal hormones quickly increases almost 90 per cent.[24]

Although adrenal hormones can be produced without vitamin C, the need for this nutrient is tremendously increased by stress; and if undersupplied, the glands quickly hemorrhage and the output of hormones is markedly decreased.[25] This vitamin accelerates the rate of cortisone production, appears to improve its utilization and delay its breakdown, and alleviates many of the limitations resulting from a pantothenic-acid deficiency.[2,26-28] Apparently because large amounts of vitamin C are used to detoxify harmful substances formed in the body during stress, greater-than-normal quantities are lost in the urine at this time.[29,30]

Huge amounts of vitamin C appear to protect animals from every form of stress. For instance, rats exposed to severe cold died unless they received massive quantities of this vitamin.[29,30] Guinea pigs, exposed to the same low temperature, remained healthy when given 75 times their normal requirement of vitamin C; if only allowed smaller amounts, their adrenals hemorrhaged and many animals died. Translated into human terms, 75 times our normal daily requirement of vitamin C would be approximately 5,625 milligrams. Such a quantity seems startling, yet during severe stress it may not be excessive.

When 144 elderly hospitalized patients whose adrenal glands could no longer respond normally when stimulated with the pituitary hormone ACTH were given 500 milligrams of vitamin C daily, the adrenals were markedly activated.[31] Adrenal hormones in the blood and urine increased immediately. Though the patients suffered from various illnesses and their medication remained unchanged, many showed improvement.

Pantothenic-acid protection for humans. Because rats receiving adequate pantothenic acid swam twice as long in cold water as deficient animals, and those given excessive amounts swam four times as long,[32] the effect of large quantities of pantothenic acid was tested on healthy men submitted to stress. These volunteers were immersed in cold water for eight minutes before being given this vitamin and again after receiving 10,000 milligrams (10 grams) of calcium pantothenate daily for six weeks.[33] Their stress lasted only eight minutes, yet the pantothenic acid prevented destruction of protein, retention of salt, and a rise in blood sugar; and it caused the blood cholesterol to fall and gave many other "physiological advantages." There were no toxic effects even though the amount of pantothenic acid taken daily was 500 times that recommended by the National Research Council for people under the stress of illness.[34]

Such a study indicates that a nutrient that can help healthy individuals during a few minutes of stress can prove invaluable to ill persons who may have endured stress for days, months, or even years.

Experimental adrenal exhaustion in humans. Pantothenic acid is essential to every cell in the body, but its lack is so often the factor preventing the normal production of cortisone and other adrenal hormones that a deficiency causes symptoms now recognized as characteristic of adrenal exhaustion.

Physicians at the Iowa State University College of Medicine gave volunteers from the Iowa State Prison a formula diet adequate except for pantothenic acid.[35,36] Urine analyses quickly showed a decrease in adrenal hormones, which fell progressively lower as the experiment continued. The men became quarrelsome, hot-tempered, and were easily upset. They developed low blood pressure, dizziness, extreme fatigue, muscle weakness, sleepiness, stomach distress, constipation, rapid pulse on exertion, and continuous respiratory infections, especially acute pharyngitis, or sore throats. Their digestive enzymes and stomach acid were markedly reduced; and the movements of the stomach and intestine, so vital to digestion and absorption, also decreased. In 25 days these men became so seriously ill that, if it is possible for anyone to become homesick for a prison, they must have been. The investigators,' fearing permanent damage might be done, then gave cortisone and 4,000 milligrams of pantothenic acid daily. The recovery was slow, and urine analyses showed that the adrenals were not restored to normal for almost three weeks.

Yet these men were young, healthy individuals consuming a diet adequate in all other respects and presumably under no undue stress (although one took off and did not return). When the symptoms they developed—all typical of adrenal exhaustion—are superimposed on an ill person whose diet is woefully inadequate and who is enduring multiple stresses, a mild illness becomes a serious one and a serious illness may prove fatal.

Variations in nutritional requirements. Mild abnormalities may call for only a few dietary improvements, but serious illness, when stresses are piled upon stresses, causes the nutritional requirements of the entire body as well as of the pituitary and adrenal glands to be increased. Any deficiency becomes worse in proportion to the number, kind, and intensity of stresses. Often such large quantities of vitamin A are excreted in the urine that any amount stored is quickly exhausted.[37,38] Severe stress also causes the "non-essential" amino acids—those normally made in the body—to become essential because the body cannot produce them rapidly enough.[6] To meet such dietary demands is by no means easy.

How well each of us copes with stress depends on the adequacy of our diet both before and during the stress itself. Malnutrition has been compared to an iceberg, which is largely hidden until hit by the *Titanic* of stress; then its disastrous effects quickly become obvious.

The antistress factors. Certain vitamin-like substances called the antistress factors are still unidentified but have a fantastically protective action against most types of stress, though not all. For example, when rats are given strychnine, sulfanilamide, promine, atabrine, stilbestrol, excessive thyroid, cortisone, or aspirin, all cause harmful effects that cannot be overcome by increased amounts of any known vitamin, mineral, or other nutrient.[3] Yet the animals are completely protected if given foods supplying the antistress factors. These substances also prolong the survival time of rats exposed to x-rays; and wheat germ particularly causes a marked resistance in animals injected with various bacteria.[2]

The antistress factors are found in liver, especially pork liver, wheat germ, some yeasts, kidneys, and soy flour from which the oil has not been removed.[39-42] Another equally protective antistress factor, different from the one in liver, is found in the pulp of green leafy vegetables.[42] Research indicates that ill persons should work as many of these foods as possible into their daily diets.

Reaction to stress and disease. A symptom of an illness or even a disease itself is often nothing more than the body's reaction to stress.[5] An adrenal hormone, desoxycortisone, or DOC, for example, often counterbalances the effect of cortisone, keeping it in check. DOC helps the body to fight infections and protects it by setting up an inflammation around bacteria and toxic substances, preventing them from spreading to surrounding tissues; thus is a boil or tubercular lesion walled off.[5] This hormone causes blood and tissue fluids to be drawn to a damaged area and white blood cells and other defense mechanisms to be called in; although swelling, pain, and fever result, the remainder of the body is protected. Thus the reaction to stress, occurring during any inflammation, becomes the disease itself. Such a disease is given the name of the organ involved, with the ending itis. Arthritis, bursitis, colitis, nephritis, and allergies, among others, are spoken of as "stress diseases."[5]

If so little cortisone can be produced that DOC is not held in check, the inflammation can get out of hand and continue year after year, as it does in arthritis, some allergies, and many diseases. On the other hand, if too little DOC can be produced or if cortisone is given as a medication, the body becomes susceptible to infections, inflammations, and damage from toxic substances.

Another adrenal hormone, aldosterone, holds salt (sodium) and water in the body, thus preventing dehydration. When it is being produced in excessive amounts during the first two stages of stress, so much water may be retained that the hands, ankles, and eyes become puffy and too much potassium is lost in the urine.[43,44] Such a condition can be the cause of high blood pressure and may become a major problem during certain types of kidney and heart disease.[5] Restricting the salt intake at such a time causes aldosterone to be excreted and prevents the loss of potassium. Taking potassium to replace the urinary losses also rectifies this situation.[45,46]

Adrenals exhausted from prolonged stress are unable to produce sufficient amounts of aldosterone; too much salt and water are lost from the body, the blood pressure usually falls below normal, dehydration occurs, and potassium is withdrawn from the cells.[47,48] In this case salt (sodium) rather than potassium is needed. The salt intake, therefore, should be restricted during the "alarm reaction," moderate during the "stage of resistance," and high if the adrenals become exhausted. Rats under prolonged stress, allowed to select their own diet and offered separate nutrients—except vitamin C which they synthesize— will particularly increase their intake of salt and pantothenic acid.

ACTH and cortisone therapy. There are times when ACTH or cortisone must be given, and each physician carefully weighs the many advantages against the disadvantages. Either sets up a condition analogous to the onset of stress, accelerates the breakdown of body protein,[49] prevents healing, or the synthesis of new proteins,[6,50,51] causes the thymus and lymph glands to atrophy, or shrivel,[52] and water and salt may be held in the body. They decrease natural hormone production,[5] inhibit the synthesis of antibodies and white blood cells needed to fight infections,[27] and increase both the need for almost every body requirement[5,6,26,27,38,49-51,53] and the urinary losses of amino acids, calcium, phosphorus, potassium, and vitamins A, C, and all the B vitamins.[6,14,38,53,54]

Persons being given ACTH or cortisone often develop stomach ulcers and severe spontaneous bruising, nosebleeds, and hemorrhages;[55,56] and if the sugar formed from the destruction of body proteins is not used for energy, it is changed into fat, which accounts for part of the gain in weight when cortisone is taken.[57] Dr. Selye points out that while patients receiving cortisone may have an unusual feeling of well-being at first, they often develop high blood pressure, insomnia, infections, disturbances of the intestinal tract, and may become so depressed as to have suicidal tendencies.[5] Such toxicity can be markedly decreased, the period of therapy shortened, and either ACTH or cortisone made more effective if the diet is extremely adequate and especially high in protein, vitamins C and E, and all the B vitamins.[2,6,54] Much harm can be done when ACTH is given unless large amounts of pantothenic acid are taken with it; and supplements of vitamin C and potassium should accompany cortisone therapy.[45]

Recently I had letters from a man who had been given cortisone for three years for arthritis and had suffered seven broken vertebrae, which had fractured spontaneously from the pressure of his own body; and from a woman who had taken cortisone since 1952 and had developed Addison's disease, or total adrenal exhaustion. These toxic effects are unnecessary but they do occur. Because of such hazards, it is preferable to allow the body to produce its own hormones whenever possible.

Filling the demands of stress. That adrenal exhaustion has become widespread is shown both by the millions of persons suffering from "stress diseases" and by the number of illnesses for which physicians now give cortisone. Yet the person deficient in pantothenic acid—which seems to be most of our population—receives the same benefit from taking the vitamin as from being given ACTH or cortisone and with no toxic effects.[56]

To meet the demands of stress—and health can never be restored until they are met—the starting point is to obtain all nutrients necessary for the production of the pituitary and adrenal hormones. Of these, the quantities of protein, vitamin C, and pantothenic acid required are particularly large, but they vary with individuals and the severity of the stress.[17,52] It seems to me that scientists have often recommended too little, such as 20 milligrams of pantothenic acid daily for sick persons,[34] or too much, as 15,000 milligrams, which have been given daily for long periods with no toxic effects but are prohibitively expensive.[33,35,58]

A combination of vitamins which I have found to give excellent results and believe should be obtained during every illness or severe stress, we might call the antistress formula. Because these vitamins dissolve in water, they are readily lost in the urine; hence greater improvement occurs when small amounts are taken frequently rather than larger quantities at one time. Vitamin B_2 is essential for the synthesis of adrenal hormones, but if given alone, a vitamin-B_6 deficiency is produced (p. 299); therefore the amounts of these two vitamins should always be kept the same. I use a tablet containing vitamin C and several B vitamins whose need is increased by stress.

The antistress formula. During acute illness, take with each meal, between each meal, before going to sleep, and approximately every 3 hours during the night if awake, always with fortified milk (p. 329) to supply the necessary protein (p. 310), 500 milligrams of vitamin C, 100 milligrams of pantothenic acid, and at least 2 milligrams each of vitamins B_2 and B_6. These vitamins can be obtained separately or in a single tablet. They should be continued until improvement is marked. As soon as the acute stage has passed, decrease the amounts.

For mild abnormalities, half the foregoing quantities may be taken 6 times daily, although larger amounts of vitamin C would be needed during infections and/or if medication is used. A friend with a limited budget obtained excellent results in clearing up an allergy by taking only 250 milligrams of vitamin C and 10 milligrams of pantothenic acid 6 times daily, and 5 milligrams each of vitamins B_2 and B_6—she cut 10-milligram tablets in half— every morning and evening. Unless these vitamins are supplied in larger-than-normal amounts, however, recovery cannot be expected.

The antistress program. When possible, have daily in addition to the antistress formula and fortified milk: fresh and/or desiccated liver; a cooked green leafy vegetable; wheat germ as a cereal or added to some food; vitamins A, D, and especially E; and make absolutely sure that all body requirements are supplied in some form (ch. 32).

The ultimate goal. When health is once attained and further stress is recognized, the diet can be improved before serious illness occurs. If such a procedure is followed, a long and rewarding life free from disease becomes a possibility.

3

Drugs Increase Nutritional Requirements

A friend recently remarked, "Of course I know your attitude toward drugs."

"Does she?" I thought, feeling convinced she did not know that I would take an aspirin for a headache as quickly as anyone else. Pain is often a greater stress than a drug. Although our own medicine chest is a Mother Hubbard's cupboard, drugs have saved millions of lives. I do feel that too many are being used. Hospital patients now receive an average of seven different drugs and some are given as many as 35.[1] Self-medication, the refilling of prescriptions without a doctor's advice, and the demand for prescriptions against a physician's better judgment are certainly unwise.

Nutritional needs are increased. Without exception, every drug is toxic to some extent; standard tests on materia medica state that all are potential poisons.[2] The toxicity of many can be "largely if not completely counteracted" by an adequate diet containing antistress factors.[3-7] Such a diet shortens the period when drugs are needed and makes them more effective without interfering with their function, even making some 20 times more effective than when the diet is faulty.[8-11]

Drugs produce dietary deficiencies by destroying nutrients, using them up, preventing their absorption, increasing their excretion, or chemically taking their place.[12] Furthermore, since drugs are usually taken only during illness, their toxicity occurs at the very time an individual is least able to cope with it.

A scientist who tests drugs for a pharmaceutical firm told me of testing several on rats left from other experiments which were deficient in one nutrient or another. "That's when you really see damage done by toxicity!" he

32

exclaimed. His employers did not permit these results to be published. Drugs released for human use are tested on *healthy* animals suffering from no deficiencies and then given to ill persons suffering from many.

The least toxic drugs. Some drugs are highly toxic whereas others, such as aspirin, are less so. Yet aspirin interferes with digestion, the formation of body starch, the production of tissue proteins, and the ability of the cells to absorb sugar; it slows the clotting of blood, increases the need both for oxygen and for every known nutrient, and accelerates the urinary losses of calcium, potassium, vitamin C, and all the B vitamins.[7,13-16]

Aspirin poisoning causes a number of accidental deaths annually,[17] and children allergic to this drug are often harmed even by tiny amounts given for a mild cold or fever.[18] Many cases of severe toxicity have been reported, causing ulcers,[19] loss of hearing, and ringing, roaring, and hissing sounds in the ears, especially among persons given the "full aspirin treatment" for arthritis.[20-22]

It is because of its toxicity that aspirin is given for arthritis. One doctor, an authority on stress, colorfully describes this treatment as "a kick in the pants for the tired adrenals," forcing them to produce a little more cortisone. In the process, however, aspirin depletes these glands of vitamin C and pantothenic acid, causing them to hemorrhage, and unless the diet is unusually adequate, to become exhausted.[23] Many drugs similarly induce stress,[24] and exhaust the pituitary and adrenals.

Other so-called "safe" drugs are ferrous sulfate and various iron compounds, though as early as 1928 they were found to destroy vitamin E.[25] Later studies show that they tremendously increase the need for oxygen, pantothenic acid, and several nutrients, that they harm the unsaturated fatty acids, and destroy carotene and vitamins A, C, and E.[24,26-28] When little food can be eaten during illness and the protein intake is low, iron compounds can cause serious liver damage.[29] During pregnancy, taking iron salts, which increase the need for oxygen, already undersupplied the fetus, can bring about miscarriages or premature or delayed births,[30,31] and may cause the infant to be malformed, mentally defective,[32,33] or susceptible to anemia and jaundice (pp. 228-229).

Ferrous sulfate annually causes the deaths of many children, who often confuse the tablets with candy;[28] as little as 900 milligrams can be fatal.[34,35] If medical care is obtained quickly, the poisoning (or milder toxicity) can be counteracted by large amounts of protein and vitamins C, E, and the B vitamins.[36] The least toxic of the iron salts is said to be ferrous gluconate,[37] but iron that is never toxic can easily be obtained from unrefined foods.

Many drugs are relatively harmless when taken for a short period but prove toxic if continued. An example is the prolonged use of tranquilizers; a single medical article tells of 605 cases of poisoning from them.[38] Another example is the massive doses of nicotinic acid given to reduce blood cholesterol; patients taking it for more than a year have developed stomach ulcers, diabetes, severe liver damage, jaundice, and colitis; and men have reported sexual impotency.[39,40] Dozens of such examples could be cited.

The harm these mildly toxic drugs can do the body is slight in comparison to that caused by thousands of the more toxic ones. Unless the diet is unusually adequate, even though a drug has accomplished the purpose for which it is given, its toxic effects can prolong convalescence or make the outcome of the illness doubtful.

Detoxification by vitamin C. A major function of vitamin C is its "non-specific role as a detoxifying agent";[41] and for nearly 30 years it has been known to prevent the toxicity, allergic reactions, and anaphylactic shock caused by drugs.[42-44] This vitamin appears to react with any foreign substance reaching the blood,[45] and, if generously supplied, it nullifies the toxicity of fluorine,[46] saccharine and other artificial sweeteners,[37] lead,[47] benzene,[48,49] carbon tetrachloride,[50,51] and excessive vitamins A and D,[52] as well as drugs. Yet all of these substances "destroy" vitamin C, causing it to be used up and excreted in the urine and, by the same token, tremendously increasing the need for it. The more toxic the drug, the larger the amount of the vitamin required. Rats given highly toxic cancer-producing drugs excrete 50 to 75 times more vitamin C than normally.[53]

The amount of vitamin C in human blood falls drastically when drugs are taken, particularly that of people showing drug reactions, sometimes even when 800 milligrams of the vitamin are given daily with a single dose of a drug.[54] Such drugs as barbiturates, adrenaline, stilbestrol, estrogen, sulfonamides,[55-57] ammonium chloride,[58] aspirin,[57,59] the antihistamines,[60] thiouracil,[55] thyroid,[61] and atropine[62] cause a continuous destruction and high urinary loss of the vitamin as long as the drug is taken and sometimes for six weeks after it has been discontinued.

Generous amounts of vitamin C given to patients have both increased the effectiveness and decreased the toxicity of anesthetics, barbiturates,[63] benzedrine,[8] mercurial diuretics,[64] procaine, arsphenamines,[54,65,66] and dilantin.[67,68] When 300 to 800 milligrams of vitamin C were given daily with a single drug, the period of treatment was considerably shortened, and larger, more effective doses could be used when needed.[54,65,66] The vitamin also helps to prevent the liver damage known to be caused by a number of drugs.[54,69]

The amount of vitamin C needed daily to detoxify drugs is not known, but varies with the number taken, the dosage, and the toxicity of each; 100 milligrams given with a drug have been too few to protect patients from allergic reactions.[44,54] I was recently stumped when a man taking varying doses of 19 different drugs daily asked me how much vitamin C he required. Often I suggest that 250 milligrams and a whole orange or unstrained juice be taken with a single dose of any drug, but I told him to take as much vitamin C as he could afford and to watch for bruises and bleeding gums—the first signs of vitamin-C deficiency—and to increase his intake as soon as either symptom appeared.

During severe illness, the combined stresses of the disease and numerous medications often cause the vitamin-C requirement to be fantastically high. When not met, large areas of spontaneous bruising may appear, a condition physicians call purpura, which means purple; even fatal hemorrhaging can occur.[70] Other deficiencies, particularly too little vitamin E, contribute to purpura;[103,105,106] once it has appeared, huge amounts of both vitamins C and E are needed.

Other defense mechanisms. Many drugs cause severe liver damage. Mildly toxic ones can inhibit the liver's many enzyme systems and prevent vital substances from being synthesized and foodstuffs from being utilized normally.[71,72] The wide use of drugs has now caused the often fatal disease cirrhosis of the liver to become common even among children.[73]

Investigators who have studied the toxicity of drugs on animals emphasize that such damage is far greater when the diet is low in vitamin E and/or protein, especially the sulfur-containing amino acid methionine;[50,51,71] that vitamin E is some 400 times more effective in preventing such damage than the amino acid;[74] but that injury can be prevented if both vitamin E and milk proteins are generously added to the diet.[51] Eggs, the only food containing enough sulfur to tarnish silver, are the richest source of this amino acid. The time-honored practice of serving eggnogs to ill persons, therefore, should be encouraged whenever drugs are given. Jaundice caused by taking atabrine or the bromides, for instance, has been found to be prevented by a high intake of vitamin E and the sulfur-containing amino acids. Ironically, people with jaundice are usually told to avoid eggs and are rarely given vitamin E.

Adequate vitamin A is necessary for normal liver function, and its lack can contribute to drug toxicity. Drugs such as phenylbarbitol,[75] thyroid,[76] arsenicals,[3] aspirin,[77] and many others destroy vitamin A, thereby increasing the need for it.[78] Yet the amount of vitamin A necessary to prevent liver damage is unknown.

Other effects of drugs on nutrition. A number of drugs interfere with digestion and the absorption of all foodstuffs and of most vitamins and minerals, resulting in deficiencies which, in turn, cause some damage to every part of the body.[79,80,81] Several drugs, such as sulfanilamide and aminopterin, called vitamin antagonists, are effective because they replace vitamins in cells and enzyme systems without performing their functions; when these drugs are no longer needed, their toxic effects can be overcome by eating foods rich in the B vitamins. Dicumarol, given to retard blood clotting, inactivates vitamin A; and its effectiveness can be increased by giving this vitamin. The toxicity of isoniazid, used in treating tuberculosis, is prevented by vitamin B_6.[82,83] Penicillin also increases the need for vitamin B_6, and can cause brain damage[84] which this vitamin is said to prevent. Young children given the antibiotic tetracycline develop unsightly yellow pigmentation on their teeth, thought to be due to the destruction of vitamin E.[85]

Streptomycin makes manganese unavailable and keeps it from being used in many vital enzyme systems, thus causing paralysis, convulsions, blindness, and deafness in infants, and dizziness, ear noises, and loss of hearing in adults, all said to be prevented if manganese, supplied by wheat germ, is added to the diet.[86]

Oral antibiotics have brought on hemorrhages and multiple B-vitamin deficiencies by destroying valuable intestinal bacteria, which synthesize vitamin K and the B vitamins. [87,88] The fungus monilia albicans then frequently develops and may grow not only in the intestines but also in the vagina, lungs, mouth (causing thrush), or on the fingers and under the fingernails; sometimes it induces ulcers in the colon, or large intestine,[89] but severe itching around the anus is generally its most annoying symptom. Although such an infection frequently continues for years, it can be prevented or corrected by unusually large amounts of the B vitamins; and often it disappears from the intestine in a few days after bacteria have been supplied by taking yogurt or acidophilus milk or culture. Such fungus infestations can occur without antibiotics if the intake of B vitamins is low, but rarely in the intestine.

Diuretics, given to increase the flow of urine, bring about such a marked loss of potassium, magnesium, the B vitamins, and apparently all nutrients that dissolve in water[90-94] that when I am working with a person who is taking such a drug, I have learned not to expect results until after it has been discontinued. The diuretics (and also the sulfonamides and certain antiacid medications) frequently cause kidney damage[86,90] and they, benzedrine, some antibiotics, and several other drugs increase blood clotting,[95] particularly dangerous for persons susceptible to heart disease. This tendency may at times be counteracted by vitamin E,[96,97] which also prevents certain drugs from injuring the heart muscles.[98]

Too little is known. Although research indicates that drug toxicity can be largely prevented by an adequate diet, the problem is to know which nutrient or nutrients may be required in excessive amounts to meet the increased needs caused by different drugs. It may never be known how all the medications now on the market affect vitamins, minerals, enzyme systems, and other body compounds. For example, approximately 12 per cent of patients given certain drugs containing benzothiadiazines have developed diabetes,[22] but no one knows which nutrients to increase to prevent the disease. Dozens of drugs cause anemia by destroying nutrients needed for blood building and/or by breaking down red blood cells,[99] but exactly how the diet should be varied to cope with each of the drugs is not known. Approximately 1,000 promising new drugs are released each year to be tested on patients; neither the physician nor the manufacturer knows what toxic effects may appear, and the patient is usually unaware that an untested drug is being given him.

Why did the thalidomide tragedy occur? The fact that nutritional requirements increase tremendously during pregnancy undoubtedly played some role. About 60 per cent of the offspring of rats deficient in vitamin B_2 are born with foreshortened limbs,[100] but the same malformations occur less often when vitamin A, E, pantothenic acid, or folic acid is deficient.[12,101] Did thalidomide destroy vitamin B_2 or some other nutrient which, if supplied, could have prevented such lifelong grief? Many women who took the drug did not have deformed babies;[88] possibly their diets were more adequate.

Other tragedies are being caused by giving pregnant women oral synthetic progesterone, which is resulting in girls being born with overdeveloped male sex organs,[102] thus bringing untold anguish to parents and unimaginable psychological damage to the children themselves. Instead of determining sex by the time-honored method of a glance, the chromosome pattern of these babies must first be studied. Possibly vitamin E would prevent the toxicity of this drug, which is still being sold, and make its use unnecessary,[32,103] but as yet no one knows.

When a drug must be taken about which little is known, it becomes of paramount importance to see that the nutrition is improved to the utmost. The attitude is all too prevalent that a drug is safe simply because a reputable doctor has prescribed it. The reason the law requires that most drugs be sold only on prescription is that they are dangerous. Yet they are far too valuable to allow toxic effects, brought on by faulty nutrition, to defeat the purpose for which they are used.

Let your physician be the judge. Drugs have received so much publicity that patients frequently demand that one or another be given them. "I came in for a shot of penicillin, doctor," "If you won't give me reducing pills, I'll go to someone who will," and similar remarks have become commonplace in physicians' offices. Many a doctor, in order to protect his patients' health, has wisely given a placebo, an inert tablet, perhaps of milk sugar, or a somewhat expensive injection of distilled water, which, incidentally, often achieves amazingly good results.

Although the American Medical Association has long pointed out that antibiotics are ineffective in treating virus infections, last year in our community a young mother who requested penicillin for slight sniffles died minutes later in anaphylactic shock. Unfortunately, this case is far from an isolated one.[104]

The reason for consulting a doctor is to obtain the advantage of his years of experience and specialized training. Let him be the judge of the medications needed; and if a drug does prove to be toxic, realize that neither it nor the doctor may be at fault, but, rather, the inadequacy of the diet.

Drugs induce stress. All drugs, by their toxicity, induce a condition of stress, which particularly increases the need for vitamin C, pantothenic acid, the antistress factors, and perhaps for every body requirement. Because most drugs can damage the liver, the body's demands for protein and vitamin E are also especially high. The more adequate the diet can be made, therefore, the more effective the drug, and the shorter the time it need be taken.

Physicians are often criticized for writing too many prescriptions, but none has ever been written for the person who maintains good health.

4

Scars Can Be Prevented

One of the bright spots in our family life is cheerful Oleta, who comes to clean for us. One morning she brought her son, Melvin, a large, broad-shouldered athlete whose back was so dreadfully burned as to be literally cooked. Five days earlier, while working at a car-wash establishment, a pipe carrying live steam had broken directly behind him. A physician had given him only aspirin. When I saw him, his entire back was a raw, oozing mass; small scabs showed in a few areas; and the itching, drawing pain of forming scar tissue was almost driving him insane. Never have I seen such a severely burned person outside of a hospital.

I knew that vitamin E took the pain out of burns and prevented scars from forming; therefore I pierced holes in the ends of vitamin-E capsules with a sterilized needle and squeezed their contents over the boy's back. His mother repeated this procedure each morning and evening; and Melvin took 200 units of the vitamin after each meal until healing was complete. (Though I was unaware of it at that time, PABA [pp. 129-130] often soothes the pain of burns even more effectively than vitamin E.)

Later Melvin reported that the intense discomfort from the burn itself and the itching, drawing agony caused by the forming scar tissue disappeared in a few hours. Without vitamin E his back would have been a mass of scars, yet it healed rapidly and not a trace of a scar formed; three weeks later he was playing football.

The physician who had attended Melvin called in six of his colleagues to view the amazing results, particularly astonishing because colored people are notorious as "keloid formers," on whom huge tumor-like masses of tough scar tissue often grow over a minor injury. Unfortunately, none of these doctors could believe that vitamin E had prevented scars from forming. Repeatedly they have been told that this vitamin is of little value.

In my 37 years of working in nutrition, I have seen

nothing more spectacular than the role vitamin E plays in preventing ugly scars.

Seeing is believing. In 1953 I was fortunate enough to see colored slides of perhaps 100 patients treated by Drs. E. V. and W. E. Shute of London, Ontario, Canada, whose clinical work with vitamin E has been outstanding. Their pictures showed people enduring such intense agony that many viewers had to leave the room. There were slides of ulcerated amputation stubs, massive varicose ulcers, and gangrenous skin grafts, all of which had refused to heal; a young boy, run over by a bus, his entire body covered with pus-filled wounds; a steel worker piteously burned by hot slag; children horribly burned by irons or boiling water; people mangled in car accidents; and severe radiation burns resulting from cancer treatments. Yet after vitamin E, usually 600 units daily, had been given to each patient and vitamin-E ointment used generously in many cases, all had healed rapidly without contracting or disfiguring scars. I particularly remember a young man whose hands had been so severely burned that scar tissue had drawn them into inflexible, useless claws; vitamin E had given him two healthy hands.

The following day, as if guided by Providence, a woman with a horribly scarred face consulted me. My first reaction was shock because of her gruesome, startlingly red lower eyelids, turned inside out and pulled down by shiny, translucent scar tissue which stretched from her eyes to her chin like cellophane wrapped tightly around a new lamp shade. Because of blemishes, a physician had peeled her skin nine months earlier with what she described as a "roller razor blade." Since that time she had remained in miserable and lonely seclusion, her disfigurement seemingly permanent and her life ruined. Yet, thanks to the Shute brothers, 600 units of vitamin E daily, and an adequate diet, her eyelids were normal and most of the scar tissue had disappeared within a month. When I last saw her she was a happy, outgoing, and beautiful woman with no sign of a scar. Had vitamin E been taken earlier, months of suffering could have been prevented.

Persons one cannot forget. Since seeing the Shutes' pictures, I have watched dozens of individuals make spectacular recoveries without scarring. One was a young girl who had been thrown through a windshield, her face so lacerated that her physician had predicted that three years of plastic surgery would be necessary; a few weeks later not a scar marred her attractiveness. Another was a golf champion who, two days before a tournament, picked up nearly red-hot tongs while barbecuing steaks; he applied vitamin E immediately, generously, and often, and played in the tournament. Still another was a youngster with a jagged, ugly hole through his upper lip, the result of a bicycle accident; yet no blemish remained to remind him of his pain.

A friend's 11-inch incision from major surgery showed only as a tiny soft line no larger than a thread. She quoted her physician as having exclaimed, "There's not a single adhesion!" When she told him that she had taken vitamin E with the antistress program (p. 31), he had added, somewhat sadly, "We doctors should know more about nutrition."

A 26-year-old man consulted me whose face, neck, and shoulders were covered with pitted, purple masses of scars resulting from years of cruel acne. Slowly but eventually, vitamin E and an adequate diet caused them to be replaced by nearly normal fair skin.

There was the little boy who had played with matches near a can of gasoline. His brother had been killed immediately by the explosion, and the doctors had said he could not possibly live. His mother, never leaving his bedside, had pulled him through with love, prayer, good nutrition, and vitamin E. He, too, is free from disfiguring scars.

Particularly tragic, it seemed to me, was a little seven-year-old whose urethra opened at the base of his penis rather than at the end, a not uncommon birth anomaly. Repeatedly after plastic surgery, scar tissue had caused the urethra to become so constricted that the child screamed with pain each time he tried to urinate, and still more surgery had to be undergone to remove the scar tissue. When 200 units of vitamin E were given daily before and after surgery, the repair was successful. I am told that some little boys with this anomaly have had to have surgery 15 to 18 times, each attempt at correction thwarted by new scarring.

A woman whose breast had been removed because of cancer told me that her greatest suffering had been from the itching, drawing pain caused by the contraction of forming scar tissue. Recently, when her other breast was removed with far more extensive surgery, vitamin E and an improved diet allowed her convalescence to be relatively comfortable.

These are but a few of the people I have known whose

pain and disfigurement were markedly decreased by vitamin E.

Vitamin E has been undervalued. American physicians have underestimated this vitamin to the extent that most of the research on scar-tissue prevention and removal has been done in other countries.[1-19] A few Americans, however, have made outstanding contributions.[20-26]

Early food analysis indicated that vitamin E, or alpha tocopherol, was widely distributed, hence deficiencies were assumed to be rare. Later research revealed that only one of seven natural tocopherols, the alpha form, could function as a vitamin.[27] Corn and soy oils, for example, once considered to be good sources, contain only 11 and 13 units respectively of alpha tocopherol in a half cup, and the remainder proved to be inactive tocopherols.[28,29] The same was true of dozens of foods.[30] Even wheat-germ oil, the richest source, supplies only 56 units of alpha tocopherol per half cup, and this small amount is quickly destroyed when exposed to air. The vitamin E once available in oils and whole-grain breads and cereals has been lost in refining[31] until our intake has decreased from an estimated 150 units daily to a mere 8 or 15 units.[29,32]

The natural vitamin E, or d-alpha tocopherol acetate, obtained by distilling vegetable oils—usually soy oil destined to be used in paints—is customarily measured in units, and the synthetic vitamin E in milligrams. By definition 1 unit of vitamin E equals 1 milligram, although the natural vitamin, which is the only one I have used, produces better results.[4]

When reports came from other countries that vitamin E was valuable in preventing miscarriages and in treating heart disease, the mixed tocopherols available in the United States were unstable and practically worthless; hence physicians saw no improvement in patients given the almost vitaminless preparations. Although d-alpha tocopherol acetate sold today is stable, the mixed tocopherols are said not to be. Much prejudice, however, still exists, and doctors frequently make the statement that vitamin E is not needed or that deficiencies rarely occur.[24]

Research indicates that vitamin E is unique in playing a role in a wider variety of body functions than almost any other nutrient.[33,34] It has been described as a "guardian angel"[35] which protects the essential fatty acids, carotene, vitamin A, B vitamins (indirectly), and the pituitary, adrenal, and sex hormones from being destroyed by oxygen.[33,36-38] Without it blood cells break down,[39] several amino acids cannot be utilized[35] or the pituitary, adrenal, and sex hormones be produced,[36] and severe liver and kidney damage can occur.[33] Yet huge amounts have been given without toxic effects being observed.[20,40] Its outstanding functions, however, are that it reduces the need for oxygen and helps to prevent scarring.

The need for oxygen is reduced. When vitamin E is generously supplied, the need for oxygen in the tissues is markedly reduced.[33,41,42] Because scars form after blood vessels have been cut, burned, mangled, or otherwise damaged to the extent that the oxygen supply is markedly decreased, it has been suggested that scar tissue requires less oxygen than normal tissue; therefore it forms when oxygen starvation prevents healthy cells from growing.[34] Vitamin E also tremendously increases the rate at which new blood vessels develop around damaged areas.

For this reason physicians who have done research on vitamin E believe that it should be given for all conditions where the oxygen supply is limited.[28] Thus vitamin E applied locally and taken internally has repeatedly proved invaluable during skin grafting.[24]

Can old scars be removed? Facial scars, which often cause lifelong psychological damage, can be prevented by vitamin E and sometimes old scars can be removed. The more recent the scarring, the more quickly it seems to be replaced by normal tissue provided the diet is adequate. Only last week, a 65-year-old man for whom I had planned a nutrition program chanced to remark, "Strangest thing. When I was a kid I had an accident which left a scar the length of my leg. During this past year it has almost disappeared. Had it for 55 years or more."

Vitamin E has been given to colored people who form excessive amounts of scar tissue (keloids), tumor-like growths which may remain tender, painful, itching, and burning for years, making sleep all but impossible. Dramatic relief from pain, sometimes in less than 24 hours, has occurred when such persons were given 1,200 milligrams of the vitamin each day, and they remained pain-free after it was reduced to 100 milligrams daily.[24] When these growths have been removed surgically, they have returned only after the vitamin was stopped.[24] It may be that colored people have an unusually high requirement for vitamin E, which causes them to form scar tissue more readily than those of other races.

This vitamin has been used with considerable success in

removing scars from the fingers and palms which sometimes contracts them into fixed useless claws, a condition known as Dupuytren's contracture.[4,18-22,43-50] When physicians have given only 200 or 300 milligrams of vitamin E daily, within two months the leathery, puckery skin softens, further scar-tissue formation ceases, and scars on other parts of the body are replaced by normal tissue. In some cases, this abnormality has been completely corrected after it had existed for as long as 12 years,[20] although 100 milligrams must be continued daily to prevent regression.

An abnormality in which scar tissue forms on the penis, causing pain on erection and often resulting in impotency (Peyronie's disease), has been corrected, usually within two or three months, when 200 or 300 milligrams of vitamin E have been given daily.[22,23,43,49,50]

Because such results show that at least some old scars can be removed, when scar tissue interferes with health, every effort should be made to replace it with normal tissue.

Scars inside the body. Although most of us are vain enough not to want even a vaccination mark to show—my last one, anointed daily with vitamin E, completely disappeared—scars inside the body are far more dangerous than external scars. In preparing this book, I have been amazed to find that in disease after disease, scar tissue becomes a major problem because it cannot carry on the work of the tissues it replaces. When cells have been damaged or destroyed and the diet is not adequate, scar tissue is formed. It appears that any person who has frequently been ill has dozens of scars inside his body for every one showing on his skin.

For example, healthy thyroid glands in the neck produce a hormone, thyroxin, which keeps body activities at an optimum rate of speed. Thyroxin is made of nothing more than an amino acid and iodine, yet persons whose thyroids are underactive usually do not improve when adequate protein and iodine are given them, a fact that puzzled me for years. The reason is that when too little iodine is supplied, the cells in the thyroid gland break down, hemorrhage, and "appear to be virtually floating in a pool of blood."[51] Eventually they are replaced by scar tissue, which cannot possibly produce the needed hormone, and the entire body suffers accordingly. Similarly, a goiter rarely disappears when iodine alone is given because iodine has no effect upon the masses of scar tissue. A physician who recently removed a friend's underactive thyroid because of a small growth described the scarred gland as "exactly like peanut brittle." When vitamin E has been given with iodine to persons having underactive thyroids, the amount of iodine taken up by the glands and the quantity of thyroxin in the blood (protein-bound iodine) have increased almost immediately.[52]

The contraction of scar tissue formed in the urinary bladder as a result of ulcers, infections, or harm done by toxic medications sometimes causes it to shrink until almost no urine can be held. When vitamin E has been given, the capacity of the bladder has increased and pain subsided, though the condition recurs unless vitamin E is continued.[23] I worked with an attractive girl of 22 who could no longer have dates or even attend movies because of this abnormality; yet she made a rapid and complete recovery after following an adequate diet containing 600 units of vitamin E daily. Three elderly persons with the same problem also made marked improvement. Such cases show that internal scarring can be dissolved.

Scars play some role in almost every disease. In cirrhosis of the liver, the organ becomes a mass of scars, yet biopsies have shown that these scars can be replaced by normal tissue (p. 174). Scars in arterial walls prevent cholesterol from passing through, thus hastening the production of heart disease.[53] The contraction of scars on the heart valve resulting from rheumatic fever causes heart murmurs.[54,55] Scars from old ulcers are sometimes almost as troublesome as the ulcers themselves. The scar tissue formed after hemorrhoid surgery may interfere with evacuation for years. Adhesions sometimes cause such difficulty that repeated surgery is necessary to remove them, yet they are nothing more than scar tissue.

The main damage done by smoking, perhaps a forerunner of lung cancer, appears to be that non-functioning scars take the place of normal cells.[56-59] Some physicians believe that the acute pain of bursitis, arthritis, and chronic gout is in part caused by the contraction of scar tissue.[20,43,44] Doctors working with patients having Peyronie's disease and severely scarred hands observed that other forms of stiffness and inelasticity, such as bursitis, wry neck, gout, arthritis, and "frozen shoulders," also improved when vitamin E was given.[20,43] It appears that if vitamin E is undersupplied, no damage can be done inside the body without leaving scars.

Scar tissue and aging. Dr. Hans Selye has been producing in rats premature old age (p. 115), which can be prevented by giving huge amounts of vitamin E.[60,61] Since it is characteristic of scar tissue to contract, wrinkles, for instance, may be caused by the shriveling of scars which develop when healthy cells cannot be replaced. It is known that harm is continuously being done in the body by viruses, bacteria, and numerous other substances such as bacterial toxins, tars from smoking, toxic drugs, nitrites from commercial fertilizers (p. 341), and impurities in air, water, and foods. Minute damages may accumulate into the ultimate scarring known as old age, which can perhaps now be delayed.

A single nutrient cannot carry the load. Dr. Evan V. Shute stated in a letter to me: "Vitamin E often does not dissolve scars. When it will be effective or when it won't we have, unfortunately, been unable to predict. Certainly it is worth a trial, particularly when it is applied locally in ointment form to superficial scars."

My conviction is that scars will remain unless every nutrient is supplied so that healthy cells can be formed to replace them. Because vitamin E is only one of the 40 essential nutrients that work together, to expect results by adding it alone is like trying to play chess with nothing but a bishop.

In the same way that every diet should be planned to meet the needs of stress, so should each prevent the formation of both external and internal scarring regardless of the type of illness involved.

5

Those "Cholesterol" Problems

Almost everyone in America now appears to have abnormal fatty substances—of which part is cholesterol—deposited in the walls of the arteries, a condition known as atherosclerosis. These deposits, which have the same composition as the fats in the blood,[1] may narrow the channels through which blood passes to the point that circulation is markedly decreased. Such a partial blockage, limiting the blood supply in the eyes, hastens the onset of cataract and other abnormalities;[2] in the legs, feet, or hands, it causes coldness, discomfort, cramps, pain, and sometimes gangrene, making amputation necessary; in the brain it may cause confusion, forgetfulness, premature senility, or strokes; and in the heart, angina or attacks known as coronary occlusion.

These fatty deposits seriously complicate such diseases as diabetes and nephrosis and delay recovery from almost every illness. They may be localized as tumors, or atheromas, on the skin or be so generalized that they clog all arteries uniformly, the space left for the blood so decreased that high blood pressure results and becomes progressively more elevated as the atherosclerosis advances.[3] High blood pressure from other causes, however, makes atherosclerosis worse.[4]

Although atherosclerosis has been described as "universal and lifelong,"[5] it has been produced in hundreds of thousands of animals, and when the diet is made adequate, health is restored. The same is equally true of humans.

Atherosclerosis is reversible. Deposits containing cholesterol can often be seen in the skin around the eyes as yellow fatty accumulations; these tiny tumors quickly disappear after the diet is improved. A woman who consulted me had dozens of them under pendulous breasts; six weeks later none remained. On one occasion I was asked to see a ten-year-old child who had more than 200 such

deposits on her back and abdomen and a blood cholesterol above 1,000 milligrams; after her diet was made
adequate, the deposits seemed to melt away. A retired
postman, brought to see me in a wheelchair, had such
constant, severe pain in his legs because of atherosclerosis
that his physician had recommended amputation; two
months later he walked in to see me. Such cases indicate
that this problem can be corrected.

Countless experiments with healthy volunteers, survivors
of heart attacks, persons in prisons and mental institu-
tions,[6,7] and innumerable animals show that when fatty
substances are being deposited in the arterial walls, the
blood cholesterol is invariably high and in abnormally
large particles; and that the fat in the blood which is
combined with phosphorus, known as the phospholipids, or
lecithin, is too low. Yet these abnormalities are corrected
as soon as all nutrients needed to utilize fats are supplied.
Atherosclerosis and such seemingly unrelated problems as
gallstones[8] and much obesity (ch. 7) appear to be caused
by a combined undersupply of many nutrients essential
before fats can be used normally. Cholesterol is merely
the innocent little pig who got stuck in the barn door.

All tissues synthesize cholesterol but only that produced
in the liver reaches the blood.[9] Some of it is made into
pituitary, adrenal, and sex hormones; some into bile acids
which aid the absorption of foods; and some into vitamin
D if the skin is exposed to summer sunshine. Cholesterol,
however, which is particularly concentrated in the brain,
appears to have functions not yet understood. It enters the
small intestine with bile, passes into the blood, and, if all
nutrients are generously supplied, is eventually broken
down by the cells into carbon dioxide and water.

Saturated and unsaturated fats. In an attempt to correct
atherosclerosis, much attention has been focused on fats,
which, during digestion, are broken down into fatty acids.
The chemical terms saturated and unsaturated (or polyun-
saturated) refer to the hydrogen content of these acids;
and most fats are a combination of both varieties. Fats
that are solid are predominantly saturated: margarines,
hydrogenated cooling fats, tallow, butter, lard, and fats
from all meats. The unsaturated fats are liquids such as
fish oils and vegetable oils. The body and blood fat of
persons with atherosclerosis is made up largely of saturated fatty acids, whereas the storage and blood fat of
individuals free from the disease contain a high percentage
of unsaturated fatty acids.[10-12]

Three fatty acids, linoleic, linolenic, and arachidonic (a fancy word referring to peanuts), which can be obtained from vegetable oils, are essential before cholesterol and saturated fats can be utilized. If the diet furnishes sufficient linoleic acid, the other two essential acids can be synthesized from it provided a bevy of vitamins and minerals are also present,[13],[14] but several of these nutrients may be undersupplied. Though many factors are involved, when fats cannot be burned readily by the tissues, they are dammed up in the blood. Because peanut, safflower, and soy oils are among the richest sources of arachidonic, linoleic, and linolenic acids respectively, I recommend using equal parts of these three, though mixtures of other oils are also excellent.

The importance of lecithin, or phospholipids. Like cholesterol, lecithin—the phospholipids—is continuously produced by the liver, passes into the intestine with bile, and is absorbed into the blood.[15] It aids in the transportation of fats; helps the cells to remove fats and cholesterol from the blood and to utilize them; and increases the production of bile acids made from cholesterol, thereby reducing the amount in the blood.[15-18] Lecithin also serves as structural material for every cell in the body, particularly those of the brain and nerves.[18] In a healthy person, it forms 30 per cent of the dry weight of the brain and 73 per cent of the total liver fat, both of which are greatly decreased in persons dying of heart disease.[19],[20]

Lecithin is a powerful emulsifying agent and for this very reason is particularly important in preventing and correcting atherosclerosis.[21-23] Although blood is essentially water into which fats cannot dissolve, lecithin, if present in normal amounts, causes cholesterol and neutral fats to be broken into microscopic particles which can be held in suspension, pass readily through arterial walls, and be utilized by the tissues.[24-26]

All atherosclerosis is characterized by an increase of the blood cholesterol and *a decrease in lecithin*.[27] As early as 1935 it was shown that experimental heart disease, produced by feeding cholesterol, could be prevented merely by giving a small amount of lecithin;[28] and atherosclerosis has since been repeatedly produced in various species either by decreasing the blood lecithin or increasing the cholesterol.[19],[29] If enough lecithin is given, the disease does not occur regardless of how much cholesterol is fed.[30] Even when atherosclerosis is far advanced, health is restored after lecithin is supplied in the diet.[29] Further-more, animals most resistant to experimental atherosclero-sis are those with the greatest ability to produce lecithin.[30]

Under conditions of health, when a meal is eaten that is high in fat or excessive in calories which are quickly changed into fat, the production of lecithin increases tremendously; and the fat in the blood is immediately changed from large particles to smaller and smaller ones.[18,31-34] In patients with atherosclerosis, however, the blood lecithin stays disproportionately low regardless of the amount of fat entering the blood, and the fat particles re-main too large to pass readily through the arterial walls.[31,33,34] A lack of lecithin in the cells may be even more damaging.

When a solution of lecithin has been allowed to flow continuously into the arteries of animals with severe atherosclerosis and the bile duct is tied to prevent further cholesterol from entering the blood, fatty deposits in the arterial walls are quickly removed.[35] Similarly, if the cholesterol supply is cut off and injections of lecithin given, the blood cholesterol increases, showing that it is being picked up from the arterial walls.[9,10,36]

Cholesterol can be made from fat, sugar, or indirectly from protein. Lecithin, however, consists of several sub-stances (cephalin, sphingomyelin, etc.) which require es-sential fatty acids and the B vitamins cholin and inositol for their structure and numerous other nutrients to synthe-size them. Because lecithin is essential to every cell in the body, the demand for these raw materials is tremendous and an undersupply of any one limits its production.

Fortunately the identical lecithin occurs in all unrefined foods containing oil. The lecithin in vegetable oil destined to be used for paints is removed because it makes the paint smear; hence is available in a mild-flavored, granu-lar form which can be added to foods. This lecithin is used commercially as an emulsifying agent in the candy and baking industries and in heavy industry where oil must be broken into minute particles. In preparing holiday dinners I add it to gravies, where it seems to make the fat literally disappear. Its emulsifying action is apparently identical whether outside or inside the body. When lecithin from eggs, liver, nuts, wheat, and soy oil has been tested on animals with atherosclerosis, health has invariably been restored regardless of the source.[36,37]

Many physicians have successfully reduced blood cholesterol with lecithin.[38-40] For example, 4 to 6 tablespoons have been given daily to patients who had suffered heart attacks and been consistently resistant to many cholesterol-lowering medications, some for as long as ten years.[42] Although no other dietary change was made, within three months the level of blood cholesterol dropped markedly, in one case from 1,012 to 186 milligrams. These patients felt more energetic, had an increased capacity for work, and were relieved of pain and other symptoms. After the blood cholesterol has once decreased, 1 or 2 tablespoons of lecithin daily have kept the blood fats at normal levels,[43] though larger amounts have been taken over long periods with good results.[44] Supplements of lecithin have also caused the pain of angina to disappear[42,44,46] and have been especially beneficial to elderly persons who have suffered strokes or have cerebral atherosclerosis.[47]

The need for vegetable oil. Adding any nutrient to the diet which allows lecithin to be produced in normal amounts helps to alleviate atherosclerosis. Although arachidonic acid is necessary before lecithin can be synthesized, saturated animal fats, hydrogenated cooking fats, and most margarines contain little or no essential fatty acids;[48] hence they cannot increase lecithin production. The more arachidonic acid there is in the blood of animals, the more resistant they are to atherosclerosis.[50] Giving vegetable oils or arachidonic and/or linoleic acids, however, elevates low blood lecithin almost immediately.[15,42,49] Moreover, when a solid fat in an experimental diet is partly or completely replaced by vegetable oil, the blood cholesterol and fat decrease as their utilization improves; but if the vegetable oil is gradually hydrogenated and fed to groups of animals, the blood cholesterol rises with each increase in hydrogenation.[51]

Any oils, including fish oils which contain no essential fatty acids, help reduce blood cholesterol by decreasing its absorption.[42,52-54] Giving vegetable oils rich in linoleic acid, however, markedly increases the quantity of cholesterol changed into bile salts[55-57] and accelerates the breakdown of fats and cholesterol to carbon dioxide and water in the tissues.[57-59]

The amount of oil needed daily appears to be no more than 1 or 2 tablespoons, although 2 teaspoons have not decreased blood cholesterols.[54] The more solid fats eaten, the greater becomes the need for linoleic acid. If the intake of solid fats is high, a deficiency of linoleic acid can be produced even when oils are included in the diet.[61,62] It is important to understand that there is nothing wrong with natural saturated fats as long as the cells are supplied with all nutrients necessary to utilize them. The need for these nutrients is markedly decreased, of course, if the saturated fats themselves are largely avoided, which is the approach now most commonly used to combat atherosclerosis.

Practical advice is to eat the same amount of fat as usual[63] but decrease animal fat except that from fish; use oils for cooking, seasoning, and salad dressings; and avoid all hydrogenated fats—margarines, cooking fats, hydrogenated peanut butter, and processed cheeses—and foods prepared with them.

Above all else, do not go overboard in using oils. They supply 100 calories per tablespoon, and any not used are stored as a particularly soft, flabby fat. Furthermore, oils alone cannot correct atherosclerosis. For example, deposits removed from fat-plugged femoral arteries quickly returned when patients made no change in their diets except to get half of the fat from oils.[64]

Inositol and cholin are essential. If either of the B vitamins cholin or inositol is undersupplied, lecithin cannot be produced in adequate amounts. Little research has been done on inositol deficiencies, but a mild lack of cholin causes the amount of lecithin in the blood of rats to decrease,[17,65] much less cholesterol to be changed into bile salts,[66,67] and heavy fatty deposits to be laid down in the arteries.[68] A cholin deficiency also inhibits the utilization of cholesterol in the tissues,[67] the burning of fats to produce energy,[18] and the excretion of cholesterol in the feces.[69]

Cholin can be made in the body from the amino acid methionine, provided the diet is high in protein; and blood cholesterol drops when this amino acid is generously supplied.[70-74] All cells need methionine, however, and they have priority over the available supply; only when an "excess" exists is it changed into cholin; hence this vitamin is frequently deficient. Because eggs are particularly rich in methionine and lecithin itself, they should never be restricted in the diets of persons with atherosclerosis.

When patients recovering from heart attacks received daily 2,000 and 750 milligrams of cholin and inositol respectively, the size of the cholesterol particles and the amount of fat in the blood quickly decreased; two months later the blood cholesterols had dropped to normal.[75] Blood lecithin has also increased and cholesterol been reduced after cholin alone has been given.[76] Some investigators have observed similar results,[77] but in studies where multiple deficiencies have limited lecithin production, cholesterol has not been reduced by cholin and/or inositol alone.[67,78,79] Neither do a guard and a quarterback make a football team.

Liver, yeast, wheat germ, and particularly lecithin are the richest natural sources of cholin and inositol. In addition to using these foods liberally, I take daily and recommend to others B-complex tablets supplying 1,000 milligrams of both inositol and cholin.

Vitamin B$_6$ and magnesium. Lecithin cannot be synthesized in the body without enzymes containing vitamin B$_6$, or pyridoxin.[84,80] These enzymes, in turn, are active only if magnesium is present.[81] Extremely severe atherosclerosis has been produced in a variety of animals kept on diets adequate in all nutrients except vitamin B$_6$.[82] When monkeys, for example, were given such a diet, the arteries in the heart, pancreas, kidneys, abdomen, limbs, muscles, and all tissues were clogged with fatty deposits; and blood analyses showed both an extremely low lecithin and high cholesterol.[83] Though in every respect the condition was said to resemble atherosclerosis in man, monkeys given the identical diet including vitamin B$_6$ remained healthy.

Diets high in vitamin B$_6$, cholin, and inositol supplied by wheat germ, yeast, liver, or B vitamins extracted from bran have been particularly effective in reducing blood cholesterols.[84,85] Liver not only contains lecithin and all of these vitamins but also less saturated fat than any other meat.

Even when vitamin B$_6$ is adequate, a lack of magnesium prevents lecithin from being formed and thus inhibits the utilization of fats and cholesterol.[86] Patients with heart disease given 500 milligrams of magnesium daily made "dramatic improvements";[87-89] and many of the blood cholesterols fell drastically in a single month.[86]

The need for magnesium is tremendously increased when the blood cholesterol is high.[90] For example, the magnesium requirement of rats fed hydrogenated fat and cholesterol multiplied 16 times over that of normal animals.[91] Giving sufficient magnesium, however, prevented atherosclerosis from being produced despite feeding huge amounts of cholesterol and hydrogenated fat. Even after the arteries were severely plugged with fatty deposits, adequate magnesium caused the blood cholesterol to drop to normal and the arteries to become healthy.

The American diet is now extremely low in magnesium;[92,93] this mineral is readily lost in the urine;[94] and, because of the high intake of saturated fats, the magnesium requirement is apparently much greater than has been realized.[91] For these reasons, inadequate magnesium may well prove to be a major cause of our national atherosclerosis.

Vitamin E has much to offer. Numerous toxic substances such as those from cigarette smoke,[95] nitrites from fertilizers,[96] and the deposition of cholesterol itself[97] cause scars to form in the arterial walls.[98,99] Fats are first laid down over these tough scars and may accumulate quickly until the flow of blood is drastically decreased or completely cut off at certain points.[96,100] Vitamin E, therefore, is especially needed to help dissolve such scars (ch. 4). The scarring of arterial walls, however, is found in persons of every nation, many of which nations have little or no atherosclerosis.[96]

Occasionally vitamin E has elevated blood lecithin and reduced cholesterol,[52,101,102] apparently by preventing the essential fatty acids from being destroyed by oxygen.[103] Moreover, this vitamin tremendously decreases the body's need for oxygen;[104-110] hence it is particularly important to persons with atherosclerosis. Pain caused by a lack of oxygen, common in the heart, eyes, legs, feet, or any tissue where the circulation is decreased by fatty deposits, is often markedly relieved in a few days after vitamin E is added to the diet; and when patients have taken 600 units of vitamin E or more daily, the pain of angina has subsided, gangrene has cleared up, and amputation been avoided.[111,112]

Other nutritional influences. Persons suffering from atherosclerosis often have a particularly high intake of refined sugar,[113,114] which, if not burned, is quickly converted into saturated fat. Animals fed sugar instead of starch develop high blood cholesterol;[115] and the essential fatty acids in their blood and tissues decrease far more than when starch is fed.[116] The blood cholesterol of healthy volunteers fell when they ate unrefined starches, but substituting sugar caused their blood fats and cholesterol to increase markedly. In the United States the consumption of such foods as potatoes, dry beans and peas, and wholegrain bread and cereals has unfortunately decreased steadily while the sugar intake has increased and paralleled the rise in atherosclerosis.[117] If we are to combat this disease, natural starches should be appreciated and refined sugar restricted. The more deficient diets become, however, the greater is the craving for both sweets and alcohol.[118,119]

Every nutrient appears to help prevent atherosclerosis. Pectin (p. 316) effectively reduces experimental high cholesterol.[120] Vitamin B_{12} accelerates the production of bile salts, thus decreasing the cholesterol in the blood.[121,122] Lecithin increased markedly and cholesterol fell to normal when coronary patients were given large amounts of vitamin A daily for three to six months.[123-125] Adequate protein causes the blood cholesterol to fall provided it is not obtained from well-marbled steaks or roasts accompanied with rich gravies and potatoes French-fried in hydrogenated fat.[4,126] Alcohol not burned as calories and an excess of carbohydrate and/or protein are so quickly changed into saturated fat that they cause the blood fats and cholesterol to increase as readily as if saturated fats were eaten.[33]

Monkeys[33] undersupplied with vitamin C produce cholesterol six times more rapidly than do well-fed animals.[127] Severe atherosclerosis in rabbits and guinea pigs has been corrected by giving large amounts—50 times the normal requirement—of vitamin C;[128,129] and the formation of bile acids and the excretion of cholesterol both increased.[129,130] When patients with atherosclerosis and high blood pressure received large amounts of this vitamin, their blood cholesterol fell markedly and their blood pressure slowly dropped.[129] The fact that toxic substances from cigarettes destroy vitamin C may in part explain why heavy smokers are susceptible to atherosclerosis.[131-133]

Animals whose thyroid glands take up iodine readily are not susceptible to heart disease;[134] and giving iodine to rats prevents atherosclerosis produced by feeding excessive amounts of cholesterol.[135] When 12 drops of 10 per cent solution of potassium iodide were given in milk three times daily to hospitalized coronary patients, in a single month the blood lecithin increased markedly, the cholesterols dropped, sometimes as much as 125 milligrams, and the size of the fat and cholesterol particles was reduced.[136] Heart pain decreased, and the patients felt "fresh and cheerful." In cases where the basal metabolic rate had been low, or the speed with which the body utilizes energy was subnormal, it increased 11 to 28 per cent. Though adequate iodine with vitamin E (p. 46) stimulates the thyroid gland and thus accelerates the utilization of cholesterol and fats, it has been particularly neglected.

Every variety of animal allowed only two meals daily develops severe atherosclerosis, but when the identical kind and amount of food is taken in small, frequent feedings, excellent health is maintained.[137] Numerous small meals also correct atherosclerosis even after it has become severe. Similarly, coronary patients given six or more small meals daily rather than the same kind and amount of food in one to three larger meals have invariably shown marked decreases in the blood fats and cholesterol.[138,139]

Stress makes atherosclerosis worse by increasing the need for nutrients required to utilize fats; and cortisone therapy, which simulates severe stress, quickly elevates blood fat and cholesterol.[47] Stress is not necessarily destructive provided the increased requirements are met.

Though atherosclerosis is often considered to be hereditary, when 123 persons of two families, all of whom had excessively high blood cholesterols, were given improved diets, their blood fats and cholesterols readily decreased.[140] Such families undoubtedly have unusually high genetic requirements for certain nutrients needed to utilize fat.

Low-fat and low-cholesterol diets. When low-fat diets have been given to patients with atherosclerosis, appetites have usually become ravenous. Excessive calories, mostly from starches and sugars, have been consumed and quickly changed to saturated body fat, causing the blood fat and cholesterol to soar.[63,141-144] The size of fat and cholesterol particles has also become much larger;[145,146] the amount of cholesterol changed to bile acids has greatly reduced;[41,147,148] and coronary patients adhering to such a diet have become markedly worse.[45] The American Medical Association has warned physicians not to recommend such diets,[142] but they are still being used.

Diets low in cholesterol have also achieved exactly the opposite from what was hoped. Such diets throw the liver into a frenzy of cholesterol-producing activity, causing the amount in the blood to increase.[51,60,74,149] Conversely, liver biopsies showed that when volunteers were fed 3 or 4 grams of cholesterol daily—far more than would ever be obtained from foods—the production of cholesterol by the liver was "almost completely suppressed."[150]

Experimental heart disease has been produced with diets completely devoid of cholesterol.[151] Nevertheless, low-cholesterol diets have restricted so many excellent foods that the very nutrients needed to utilize fat and cholesterol have been decreased or omitted. Eggs have been condemned, their high lecithin and methionine content ignored.[152,153] Even mayonnaise has been forbidden, yet it averages 52 to 67 per cent essential fatty acids and 10 to 14 per cent lecithin.[154] Volunteers recovering from heart attacks have consumed daily for varying periods 10 eggs, 16 egg yolks, the fat from 32 eggs, and even 9 to 60 grams of pure cholesterol;[85,155-157] their blood cholesterols have not increased provided the eggs were cooked without saturated or hydrogenated fat.

Some experiments have shown that butter has increased blood cholesterol, yet persons in Denmark, Switzerland, and Finland eat far more butterfat than we and have much less heart disease.[158,159] Certain African natives obtain 60 to 65 per cent of their calories from butterfat, but all their foods are unrefined; they have no atherosclerosis, no heart disease, and their blood cholesterols average an amazingly low 125 milligrams.[14,160,161] In the days when atherosclerosis was unheard of in America, butter was slathered in or on practically every food not cooked in cream. Butterfat appears to be a problem only when nutrients needed to utilize it are undersupplied.

Lowering blood cholesterol. Though blood cholesterol varies constantly, that of persons with atherosclerosis is uniformly high, or usually above 250 milligrams in about a half cup of blood (100 cc). A group of patients with heart disease or cholesterol tumors had average blood cholesterols of 259 and 423 milligrams respectively;[162] and persons over 60 years of age with cholesterols above 260 milligrams have been found to have twice as many strokes as others with cholesterols below 200.[163] Physicians do not agree on the amount most compatible with health, but it appears to be below 180 milligrams.[162,164-166]

If a diet is adequate in every respect (ch. 32), lowering the cholesterol to 180 milligrams or less is usually not difficult. For example, one man whose cholesterol was 330 shortly after a heart attack quickly reduced it to 170 milligrams and then more gradually to 121. Almost every week someone whose cholesterol was formerly high tells me, "My doctor says my cholesterol's now the lowest he has ever taken," and quotes a figure ranging from 130 to 150 milligrams.

None of these persons has avoided eggs, liver, or butter but they did obtain magnesium, iodine, lecithin, yeast, skim or whole milk, the antistress formula (p. 31), and supplements of vitamins A, D, E, and the B vitamins. A few have taken 250 milligrams each of cholin and inositol six times daily for a short period. All were asked to reduce natural saturated fats and to avoid every form of hydrogenated fats including anything prepared with them, such as French-fried foods and package mixes; and each had 2 tablespoons of mixed vegetable oils daily. Not only did the blood cholesterols decrease, but the appearance, energy, and general well-being of these individuals can well be envied.

In correcting experimental atherosclerosis, it has been found that some fatty deposits, especially those in the arteries of the eyes and heart, remain long after the blood cholesterol is normal.[167,168] Such a finding indicates that an adequate diet should be followed for months or years after apparent recovery.

Have your cholesterol determined annually. Every person with a high blood cholesterol is a potential candidate for a heart attack, a stroke, high blood pressure, and/or various abnormalities resulting from prolonged faulty circulation. For this reason, I believe that every individual, regardless of age, should have an annual blood cholesterol determination. If this figure is above 180 milligrams, immediate steps should be taken to lower it. Untold suffering and innumerable premature deaths could be prevented were such a procedure followed.

There is no evidence that cholesterol alone causes general atherosclerosis, strokes, or heart attacks,[169] but an elevated blood cholesterol invariably accompanies these abnormalities.[144,170] Neither is a gas gauge on a car responsible when the tank is empty, but it indicates trouble ahead which can be prevented.

6

Heart Attacks, America's Most Lethal Disease

Dr. Paul Dudley White has said that heart disease has made the United States the most unhealthy country in the world. It accounts for 50 per cent of all deaths, which is ten times higher than in most civilized nations.[1,2] This disease kills more men than women under the age of 45, but during the later years more women succumb to it.[3] Although produced in thousands of experimental animals of every variety by one inadequate diet or another, always it is preventable. For animals which survive heart attacks, it is reversible.[4,5]

Types of heart attacks. The arteries supplying blood to the heart muscles are arranged somewhat like a crown, or corona; hence they are called coronary arteries. Regardless of the variety of heart disease, these coronary arteries are plugged to some degree with fatty substances. If the circulation has been so decreased that little oxygen reaches the heart, pain occurs known as angina, a cousin of the word anguish.

Should the atherosclerosis become so severe that a coronary artery is completely plugged and no oxygen reaches a given area, a heart attack known as a coronary occlusion occurs. Because fatty substances are deposited slowly, years pass before the blood supply is thus completely blocked.[6] Clots, however, form readily in the blood of persons with atherosclerosis. When a clot, or thrombus, clogs an artery and cuts off the oxygen supply, the attack is called a coronary thrombosis. A clot, which requires only minutes to form, can occur in the blood of young persons whose atherosclerosis is not advanced; hence coronary thrombosis rather than occlusion is now the major cause of heart attacks, and kills progressively younger men each year.[7-9]

In any attack, great masses of cells—perhaps even half the heart itself—are destroyed. Before health can be restored, fatty deposits must be removed from the arterial walls (ch. 5), more clots prevented from forming, and the destroyed area, known as a myocardial infarction, must be gradually filled in with normal tissue.

Blood fat and clotting. The death rate from coronary thrombosis is high whenever diets contain large amounts of saturated fats;[10-13] and the greater the quantity of saturated fat (triglycerides) in the blood, the more tendency it has to clot.[14-16] Though a clot may cause phlebitis, varicose veins, and pulmonary embolism (a clot lodged in the lungs), or a stroke as readily as a heart attack, excessive blood fat rather than high cholesterol indicates that a coronary thrombosis might occur at any time.[17-23] For example, of 100 patients who had heart attacks brought on by clots, only 18 per cent had blood cholesterols above 250 milligrams whereas almost 90 per cent had abnormally high blood fat.[21] As with excessive cholesterol, persons prone to coronary thrombosis lack the nutrients necessary to utilize fats.[24]

Fat in the blood is increased by fats eaten at the last meal; by fat formed from alcohol or an excess of carbohydrates or proteins perhaps only two hours after they have been consumed; or, if no food is eaten, by fat brought in from storage depots. When a meal is missed, so much stored fat pours into the blood that it often rises six times above normal;[25] hence missing meals, inadequate reducing diets, and fasting can be particularly dangerous for a person subject to heart attacks.[25,26] Blood fat can be decreased by judicious exercise,[27-29] but when animals are on inadequate diets, exercise can cause heart attacks.[30]

The blood fat of healthy individuals increases after a meal but drops to normal in three or four hours. In persons with or susceptible to heart disease, this amount usually stays excessively high for six hours or more;[17,19,21,23,31] and eating solid fats causes it to remain high much longer than do oils.[17,32] For instance, heart attacks and strokes frequently occur after Thanksgiving and Christmas dinners when the intake of saturated fat may be higher than at any other time during the year.

If a person with high blood fat is under stress or is given cortisone, so much additional fat from storage depots is called in that the amount in the blood soars into the danger zone.[1,33,34] Executives, for example, have higher blood fat, shorter clotting time, and seven times more heart attacks than relaxed individuals.[14,35]

Lecithin inhibits clotting. As early as 1891, lecithin was described as "the furnace in which body fats are burned."[36] It has the same effect on blood fat as on cholesterol: it causes the particles of fat, microscopic in the blood of healthy persons[37] but in giant molecules in individuals with or subject to heart disease,[38-42] to break into small molecules which pass readily through the arterial walls.[21,36] Large fat particles act as a foreign substance on which a clot may form[43] and, by inhibiting circulation, cause blood cells to clump together and initiate a clot.[44]

Persons who suffer from coronary thrombosis, particularly young men, have consistently been found to have low blood lecithin;[8,9,38,45-47] and the lower the lecithin falls, the greater becomes the danger of clotting.[43,45,47] Individuals susceptible to heart attacks often have so much fat in their blood serum that it looks milky. When lecithin is taken, however, this milkiness quickly disappears.[42] Conversely, if the normal lecithin in a sample of blood from a healthy individual is purposely destroyed, within minutes such large particles of fat form that this serum also appears milky.[16,19]

As with atherosclerosis, any deficiency that prevents lecithin from being produced in normal amounts, such as a lack of linoleic acid, indirectly allows blood fats to soar and clots to form.[48-51] The high blood fat following a rich meal has been reduced by giving magnesium.[52,53] Clots form readily if the blood magnesium is low but not when it is adequate;[54] and animals deficient in magnesium show multiple clots in the coronary arteries and large areas of destroyed heart muscle.[55] Thrombosis produced in rats by feeding saturated fat and cholesterol has also been prevented by increasing the protein content of the diet; if the protein was dropped to half, clots formed readily.[56] Similarly, heart attacks are particularly frequent in persons severely deficient in protein;[57] without adequate protein, cholin cannot be made from methionine, and lecithin production is again limited.

Giving oil alone—the present approach—does not solve the problem. When heart disease has been produced in rats by diets containing 40 per cent hydrogenated or other saturated fat, half of the animals have developed clots.[58] Rats given corn oil instead of the saturated fat developed both atherosclerosis and clots, and those receiving peanut oil had no clots but did have atherosclerosis. Other nutrients, therefore, must also be adequate.

Need for linolenic acid. The adhesiveness of blood cells known as platelets, which clump together to initiate a clot, can be markedly reduced in a few hours by giving coronary patients pure linolenic acid—less than a half teaspoon —or linseed or soy oil rich in this essential fatty acid.[59] As little as 1 tablespoon of linseed oil or 2 tablespoons of soy oil daily prevented the tendency of the blood to clot, but a half cup of corn or safflower oil, rich in linoleic acid, had little or no effect. The linolenic acid had to be continued, however, to prevent abnormal adhesiveness from returning. The oils in whole-wheat breads and cereals, peanuts, and other nuts also supply linolenic acid.

Such a finding indicates that nutrients necessary to change linoleic acid into linolenic acid may be lacking in the diets of coronary patients; and it may explain why some populations have severe atherosclerosis but no coronary thrombosis.[60]

Vitamin C and clotting. Spontaneous breaks in capillary walls are the first signs of a vitamin-C deficiency; and clots form most readily at the point where a blood vessel has been broken, severed, or mashed. An undersupply of vitamin C, therefore, is a major cause of heart attacks and strokes initiated by clots.[61-63]

As fatty substances are deposited in the arterial walls, they damage the tissues and progressively increase the danger of breaking unless vitamin C is continuously adequate.[48] Simultaneously, atherosclerosis creates a condition of stress, skyrocketing the need for vitamin C (p. 25); hence a break may occur and a disastrous clot form even when the vitamin-C intake appears sufficient. The stress of anger, fear, keen disappointment, and similar emotions can cause blood fat and cholesterol to soar in minutes,[34] but if the diet is adequate, particularly in vitamin C and pantothenic acid, this reaction to stress may do little harm (ch. 2).

Vitamin E and heart disease. Like vitamin C, a lack of vitamin E allows cells to break down because essential fatty acids, forming part of the cell structure, are destroyed by oxygen in its absence (p. 228); hence clots form readily.[64-66] Conversely, adequate vitamin E strengthens the walls of the blood vessels and thus decreases clotting.[67,68] When 100 coronary patients given only 200 milligrams of vitamin E daily were compared with an equal number not receiving the vitamin, the latter experienced four times more heart attacks caused by clots.[69] Similarly, 457 such patients had no clots while taking vitamin E compared to 23 clots suffered by 246 patients not allowed the vitamin.[55]

It is because vitamin E markedly reduces the need for oxygen[70-76] that it is particularly valuable for all persons with heart disease. In coronary insufficiency, for example, oxygen starvation is a major problem. Moreover, death from a heart attack, whether a coronary thrombosis or occlusion, results from oxygen deprivation. When ample vitamin E is obtained, so much less of the heart tissue is destroyed[75] that a patient may survive an attack which otherwise might have proved fatal.

Experiments in oxygen starvation are clearly too dangerous to be conducted on coronary patients. Healthy volunteers, however, given 300 milligrams of vitamin E daily, have been compared to persons not receiving the vitamin when all breathed an air mixture so low in oxygen that they lost consciousness.[77] Persons receiving vitamin E had more normal electrocardiograms, lost consciousness much less quickly, and had far less rapid pulse, showing that their hearts did not have to work as hard. The electrocardiograms of individuals not given the vitamin revealed drastic changes.

Animals undersupplied with vitamin E have abnormal electrocardiograms, and their hearts show degeneration of the muscles, massive scarring, and accumulations of brown pigment characteristic of this vitamin deficiency.[78-80] These same changes are found in persons with coronary disease and/or in autopsy studies of individuals who have died from heart attacks.[76,80] Analyses of their tissues show marked deficiencies of vitamin E.[81] Moreover, the death rate from heart disease is greatest among persons whose requirement for vitamin E is unusually high; men during the reproductive age,[82] women after the menopause,[83] and all obese individuals.[84]

Vitamin E strengthens the heart muscles,[85] and its action is said to be similar to that of digitalis.[86,87] Many physicians believe that its effectiveness in preventing clots from forming rivals that of the anticoagulant drugs;[88-90] and while the vitamin is never toxic,[91] such drugs have frequently caused fatal hemorrhaging.[92-95] At times vitamin E also acts as a diuretic, ridding the body of surplus water and decreasing elevated blood pressure,[96-98] probably by stimulating the output of pituitary hormones (p. 25). Patients given 600 units of vitamin E or more daily after having heart attacks have experienced marked relief, improved electrocardiograms, decrease in pain, more regular pulse, and have been able to take more exercise than before they received the vitamin.[99,100]

Because oils tremendously increase the need for vitamin E,[84,101] all types of heart disease are made worse by adding oils to the diet unless vitamin E is adequate.[80,84,102] Unfortunately, many physicians now recommend that heart patients increase their oil intake without giving vitamin E, and even believe oils to be an adequate source of this vitamin. Most oils supply only 10 units of d-alpha tocopherol per half cup,[103] 90 per cent of which may be destroyed during cooking;[104] hence 15 to 30 cups of fresh oil daily would be needed to furnish the amount of vitamin E found most helpful in restoring the health of coronary patients. The only way I know of for such patients to obtain sufficient vitamin E is from capsules.

Effect of coffee, alcohol, and diuretics. Alcohol, coffee, and diuretics, or medication given to stimulate urine production, appear to increase the urinary losses of all nutrients which dissolve in water. Of the 40 nutrients required for health, all but five—vitamins A, D, E, K, and linoleic acid—are readily lost in the urine. For example, when volunteers were given a carefully measured amount of fluid daily including orange juice (70 cc) and later 95 per cent alcohol was substituted for the juice, the magnesium excretion increased fivefold;[105] and symptoms of a magnesium deficiency—nervousness, tension, and hangover jitters —are common in social drinkers.[106]

Persons having abnormally high blood fat and cholesterols have been found to obtain almost twice as many calories daily from alcohol as normal individuals.[107] Alcohol (196 calories per ounce) readily changes into saturated fat, often causing the amount of blood fat to double.[62] It slows the blood flow, inhibits the utilization of fats, supplies no nutrients except calories, satisfies the need for food, and increases the requirement for vitamin B_1, pantothenic acid, and cholin.[108,109]

One study of 2,000 men observed over a seven-year period revealed that individuals who developed coronary disease drank five cups or more of coffee daily.[110] Even a single cup of coffee, acting as a stress, causes a prompt rise in blood fats and cholesterol; and when both coffee and benzedrine were given to patients with heart disease, their blood fat and cholesterol tripled over previous levels.[111] Strong coffee given to rats and dogs caused loss and graying of hair, convulsions, paralysis, watering eyes, and many more symptoms, none of which occurred in animals receiving decaffeinated coffee.[112,113] These abnormalities could be largely prevented by giving liver.

Diuretics frequently cause deficiencies of magnesium, potassium, the B vitamins, and many other nutrients.[114–117] Potassium and magnesium are vital in helping to prevent heart attacks,[15,54,55,118–122] and a lack allows clots to form in the heart and brain alike.[122] The loss of vitamin B_1 and pantothenic acid can result in decreased circulation (a condition conducive to clotting) and degeneration of the heart muscles;[123] and the excessive excretion of iodine and other B vitamins can be disastrous.

The only people I have worked with whose blood cholesterols have remained persistently high have been individuals who have not wished to decrease their coffee and/or alcohol intake or who were being given diuretics. In other respects these persons have followed their diets carefully. One social drinker, whose opening remark was, "Don't get any funny ideas about lowering the alcoholic content of my blood," still has a cholesterol of 330 milligrams. Another man, whose cholesterol is above 500, is being given a diuretic daily. When diuretics have been withdrawn and/or coffee or alcohol avoided, cholesterols have dropped quickly without alterations in the diet. After a heart attack, many men will give up smoking or social drinking, but not both. I have not worked with any nondrinking heavy smokers whose cholesterol was difficult to reduce.

"Sudden" heart attacks. Autopsy studies have revealed that many signs of atherosclerosis including scarring are now found in the arterial walls of the babies in this country;[124,125] that by the age of ten, half the children have coronary arterial lesions; and that 100 per cent of them have mild atherosclerosis by the age of 15.[126] I know of two boys, 17 and 19 years old, who have dropped dead of heart attacks during athletic contests. Autopsies of 300 American soldiers, the average age only 22, revealed that 77.3 per cent already had evidence of heart disease.[7]

Investigators, thinking that early heart damage may be caused by a lack of essential fatty acids, fed baby monkeys prepared infants' formulas with and without adding vegetable oil.[127] The blood cholesterols of the monkeys not receiving oil were higher than those given oil, but in both groups all arteries were severely diseased by the end of a single year. Yet such formulas invariably claim to be "identical" to breast milk.

Regardless of nationality, infants throughout the world

are born with approximately the same amount of cholesterol in their blood.[128] That coronary disease is now being produced from birth on in the majority of American children is tragic though scarcely surprising when one realizes that most diets given to babies and growing youngsters are woefully deficient in vitamin E, cholin, inositol, pantothenic acid, magnesium, essential fatty acids, iodine, and other nutrients.

The blood fat and cholesterol may be high for many, many years before heart disease manifests itself, yet little attention has been paid to these warnings. For instance, a survey—one of many—showed that almost every one of a group of executives and businessmen who considered themselves to be in excellent health had blood fat and cholesterol levels far above normal.[129] Diet analyses revealed that some executives obtained 60 per cent of their calories from saturated fats;[36] death from heart disease has been repeatedly produced in animals given only 40 per cent saturated fat and an otherwise ideal diet.

Coronary deaths are often spoken of as "sudden," a strange adjective to apply to a condition which has been perhaps 40 years in forming. The attack itself, bringing an abrupt end to ignorance concerning an abnormality of long standing, can indeed be sudden. One post-mortem study of coronary patients under 50 years of age showed that 63 per cent had died during the first hour of their first attack, 85 per cent during the first 24 hours, and only 23 per cent had lived long enough to be attended medically.[130] Nearly half had had no previous symptoms except— undoubtedly—excessive blood fat cholesterol of which they were probably unaware.

To prevent such tragic loss of life, I believe that industry should make annual tests for blood cholesterol and perhaps blood fat compulsory for all employees; that schools should require such tests for their athletes; and that each individual who values his health should know his blood cholesterol level. If either the blood fat or cholesterol is found to be high, an adequate diet, such as is outlined in chapter 33, can usually rectify the condition. A heart attack, however, is perhaps the most severe stress a human can endure; hence the antistress formula and, when possible, the entire antistress program (p. 31) should be followed until convalescence is advanced.

If your physician does not agree. The American Heart Association advises that if an individual is overweight, has heart disease in his family, runs a high blood cholesterol and high blood pressure, and leads a sedentary life full of frustrations, he should consider modifying his diet.[81] Such all-out enthusiasm about nutrition is rather like telling a person to consider trying to escape should a murderer stick a gun in his ribs.

Dr. William Dock, professor in the Medical School of the State University of New York, has pointed out that many prominent heart specialists to whom thousands of patients with coronary disease turn each year for advice completely dismiss nutrition as being unimportant, ignoring "the enormous literature" and "the vast evidence of the dietary basis of atherosclerosis."[10] He compares these men to the doctors who could not accept the fact that blood circulated throughout the body until 50 years after Harvey's death, but he fails to mention that heart specialists are dying rapidly from coronary disease themselves.

Because this situation exists, you should not be upset if your physician fails to agree with ideas you may have concerning nutrition or have gleaned from this book. Any decisions, however, should be discussed with your physician. Doctors do not necessarily agree with me or with each other any more than all housewives agree on the best way to prepare a meal. I feel it is extremely important to emphasize, however, especially to anyone who has had a coronary attack, that even if your physician is not interested in nutrition, he undoubtedly knows a tremendous amount about hearts and about your heart in particular. For this reason his advice concerning bed rest, medication, and similar problems should be followed implicitly.

After a coronary attack, the great area of destroyed heart tissue can be replaced only by slow growth. Dead cells can neither hurt nor carry on the functions of healthy tissue. If because you have improved your nutrition and feel no pain, you decide to stop digitalis, for example, given to slow down and rest a damaged heart, the resulting faster pulse coming before the heart tissue has had time to rebuild might be fatal. Your physician himself will withdraw any medication as soon as it is no longer needed; and if you build your health to the best of your ability, that time can usually be hastened.

A new disease. The first case of heart disease as it is known today was reported in 1912, the second in 1919,[131] and since then it has developed into a major killer. Stress, though often blamed, has been universal throughout all ages. The obvious changes have been the ever-increasing consumption of refined foods and hydrogenated fats.[132] The populations of the world living today on unrefined foods, in which nature packages with her fats all nutrients needed to utilize them, do not develop heart disease.

This insane process can be halted or the tragic path which has already become a form of national suicide can be continued. The choice lies with each individual.

7

Health and Normal Weight Go Hand in Hand

Egon Reich had been interested in nutrition for years but hated exercise and had been chained to a desk for so long that he described himself as "the flabbiest man alive." When I recovered from astonishment at seeing him hard-muscled, flat-abdomened, 45 pounds lighter, seemingly 15 years younger, and literally sparkling—if a middle-aged man can sparkle—I gasped, "How'd you do it?"

"Well, I'd tried every reducing diet I'd ever heard of, and all they did was make me feel lousy," he answered. "Finally I said, 'To heck with it. The only thing that matters is to build health.' I knew liver was the best food there is, so I've been eating that."

He described his diet in detail: liver, skim milk, lettuce and a little mayonnaise for breakfast; a small orange at mid-morning; a seafood salad and yeast stirred into skim milk for lunch; a tablespoon of unsalted nuts in the afternoon; liver, salad, and milk at dinner; and supplements of minerals and vitamins A, C, D, and E.

"Haven't been hungry a minute!" he exclaimed. "Never get tired any more. Got more energy and I'm more alert mentally than I've been in years. And when you feel wonderful, there's something makes you exercise. You can't help it."

In my opinion, Egon had discovered the essence of successful reducing: to increase energy production. And if you happen to enjoy liver, it would be difficult to improve on the diet he selected for himself.

Reducing is not for everyone. Physicians are realizing that not everyone should be urged to reduce.[1-5] Superficial emotional problems which prompt people to overeat can result from inadequate diets (p. 274), but obesity is often an unconscious defense mechanism for individuals who have had severe emotional deprivations early in life. Regardless of how much they may hate being overweight, they are healthier because of it.[2] When these persons force themselves to reduce, they often have emotional breakdowns, suffer from such marked depression that they develop suicidal tendencies, are overcome with guilt, disgust, and self-hatred at "being weak and gluttonous"[6] and become addicted to alcohol, cigarettes, and coffee.[2,3,5,7] If possible, such people should forget about reducing and merely strive to build health. They are usually cheerful, witty, intelligent individuals who make worth-while contributions to society.

The attitude that a slender person is somehow more acceptable than an overweight one is ridiculously immature. Unless you happen to have a husband who for ego-building purposes wishes to display you as he would a new Cadillac, there is little reason for looking like a mannequin. Overweight persons can dress attractively; and many individuals with "a lean and hungry look" are not pretty in bathing suits either.

Frequently persons use their excess weight as a scapegoat for self-hatred. Yet the very person who feels he would be more loved if slender still likes his overweight friends. His chief problem is not one of weighing too much but of failure to accept and love himself with both his strengths and weaknesses; and until we can love ourselves without egotism, none of us can love others without selfishness.

The present attitude that obesity is chiefly of psychosomatic origin[1,9-12] implies that Americans have more emotional problems now than at any other time in history and than people of any other nationality, an assumption that I find difficult to accept.

Increasing energy production. Though there are many causes of overweight, I am convinced that the one which makes this problem so prevalent now is that—like heart disease—too few nutrients are supplied in our diets to burn fat readily. Fat is lost only when energy is produced; therefore weight cannot be taken off until fat is efficiently burned, a process requiring almost every nutrient. A lack of any of the B vitamins causes a marked lag in energy production. If pantothenic acid is undersupplied, fats burn at only half their normal rate.[8] Stored fat cannot be changed to energy without vitamin B_6;[13] and rats deficient in this vitamin utilize both protein and fat so ineffectively that they become grossly obese.[14]

Similarly, proteins are needed for a host of energy-producing enzymes. Fat is burned twice as rapidly when protein is adequate rather than insufficient;[15] hence more calories are used.[16] If vitamin E is added to a diet formerly deficient in it or in protein, the utilization of fat doubles.[15,17] Protein itself cannot be used without cholin, vitamin B_6, and other nutrients, and it is quickly changed to fat if even one of them is lacking.

A principal function of lecithin is to help the cells burn fat;[15] therefore any deficiency that limits lecithin production (p. 53) causes fat to be so poorly utilized that coronary disease, high blood pressure, and overweight often occur in the same individual.[18] Overweight persons almost invariably have excessive blood fat and cholesterol,[19-21] showing that energy is not being produced normally, and unnecessary fatigue as well as obesity is the result.

Liver damage, which is now extremely common among overweight persons,[22-24] is probably a major cause of obesity. In a group of such individuals, liver biopsies showed this organ to be damaged in every case, and not one person had normal liver function.[22] Liver injury prevents energy-producing enzymes from being synthesized in adequate quantities, thus making it almost impossible to reduce until the health of the liver is restored (ch. 16).

If protein, vitamin B_2, or pantothenic acid are undersupplied, the liver is unable to produce enzymes necessary to inactivate insulin.[23-27] Excessive insulin therefore accumulates in the blood, causing fat to be formed quickly and the blood sugar to fall. This condition, known as hypoglycemia, has also become common. A person with continuous low blood sugar usually gains rapidly yet stays so ravenously hungry that it is difficult indeed to lose weight. Fortunately both liver damage and hypoglycemia are easily corrected when the diet is made adequate.

Importance of frequent meals. Every variety of animal becomes obese if forced to eat only two meals daily even though given an ideal diet; when allowed small, frequent feedings of the identical food, weight remains normal.[28] Most of the food is converted into energy when small meals are eaten, but large meals overwhelm the body's enzyme systems to the extent that much of the food cannot be utilized; hence a large portion of it is stored as fat. These obese animals, however, reduce without decreasing their food intake if again allowed small, frequent meals. Unfortunately, large meals affect humans in the same disastrous manner;[29,30] yet Americans eat 80 per cent of their food after 6:00 P.M.

A study of the eating habits of individuals who could not reduce showed that they ate little throughout the day, obtained most of their food at dinner and during the evening, and had no appetite for breakfast.[31] Anyone who has tried to reduce knows this pattern only too well. In the morning, while the blood sugar is still high from food eaten the night before, will power is strong and resolutions firm. One vows he is going to stop feeling like the anchor on the *Queen Mary* and thinking of himself as a baby blimp; hence he forgoes or merely samples breakfast and lunch. As the bright star of success begins to glitter brilliantly before him, his blood sugar drops and he becomes exhausted, irritable, and starved. His undoing was not that he ate too much but that he ate too little.

Advantages of unrefined foods. A research group wanting to study long-term effects of reducing was unable to find persons who had reduced and maintained normal weight; hence was forced to use rats.[32] The animals on a stock diet of natural foods ate all they wished and remained in excellent health without gaining. Although in some human diets 60 per cent of the calories came from saturated fats, rats given a seemingly adequate diet containing 37 per cent of the calories from hydrogenated fat became grossly obese. As soon as the rats were put back on unrefined foods, however, they quickly reduced and maintained normal weight indefinitely. When some were again given the diet containing hydrogenated fat, they gained far more rapidly than before, but they could still reduce and remain "slender" when given unrefined foods. Such research indicates that it is not entirely the amount of food eaten that causes obesity, but the lack of nutrients required to convert fat into energy.

When unrefined foods are eaten, nutrients needed for energy production are supplied with every calorie, whereas trash foods both lack these nutrients and tremendously increase the requirement for them.

The need for oil. Because the major function of lecithin is to aid in burning fats,[15] the nutrients required for lecithin production—linoleic or arachidonic acid, vitamin B_6, cholin, inositol, and magnesium (ch. 5)—are essential for reducing. Oil, for example, added to a diet lacking linoleic acid, tremendously increases energy production.[15,33-35] Too little linoleic acid can also damage the adrenals,[33,36] which then allow the blood sugar to fall and make reducing extremely difficult.

Overweight persons maintained alternately on 800-calorie diets supplying mostly oil or carbohydrate lost far more on the diet containing oil and spontaneously used an average of 400 extra calories daily.[37] Hospital patients given different diets having the same number of calories also lost the most weight while receiving one containing oil, found it easiest to adhere to, and did not regain their lost weight as long as the oil was continued.[38] Persons reducing without oil regained their weight most rapidly,[39] whereas individuals whose diets contained oil continued to lose.[40] In one investigation, overweight patients were merely asked to use oils instead of other fats and to limit their intake of starches and sugars; of their own choice they ate an average of 600 calories less than usual per day and all lost weight.[41]

When food has been marked with radioactive carbon and given in several diets containing the same number of calories, the least fat was stored on the diet containing oil but little carbohydrate.[42] Patients who lost nothing on a 500-calorie diet of carbohydrate did lose when allowed 2,600 calories daily supplied by protein and fat of which part was oil. Numerous other studies have produced similar results.[43,44] Yet as important as oils are, only a small amount is needed daily

Preventing hunger. Oils decrease hunger by retarding the emptying time of the stomach and by stimulating the burning of saturated body fat to the extent that the blood sugar remains normal for long periods.[45,46] Overweight persons develop low blood sugar faster than other individuals,[47] but even though it is low, hunger disappears after proteins are eaten.[48,49] Animals and humans on low-protein diets eat more, hence gain more, than when proteins are generously supplied.[46,50]

If too little food is eaten, a meal is missed, or the adrenals are exhausted, the blood sugar falls, causing symptoms every overweight person knows only too well: tension, irritability, headache, fatigue, hunger, and a craving for sweets.[51] The understandable result is that one overeats at the next meal or possibly goes on a candy binge. Should sweets or excessive carbohydrate be eaten, sugar absorbs so rapidly that a healthy pancreas is overstimulated and produces too much insulin. This excessive insulin causes most of the sugar in the blood to be changed immediately into storage fat;[52] the blood sugar again falls and intense hunger recurs.

As this vicious circle repeats itself, the pancreas becomes increasingly trigger-happy—actually more efficient—until the overweight person develops low blood sugar much faster than individuals of normal weight given identical food.[47] Whether one eats too little carbohydrate or too much, therefore, the invariable result is low blood sugar, hunger, overeating, and self-disgust. To lose weight successfully, tiny amounts of carbohydrate must be eaten frequently with fat and protein, neither of which can stimulate insulin production.

Low blood sugar triggers the onset of stress, causing much potassium to be lost in the urine and sodium and pounds of water to be retained; hence persons frequently follow extremely low-calorie diets yet the scales do not budge. When doctors have given 2 to 5 grams of potassium chloride to replace the urinary loss of potassium, the blood sugar has quickly increased and the unpleasant symptoms of hypoglycemia have disappeared almost immediately.[53] A drop in blood sugar cannot always be avoided, yet it can bring on a heart attack[53] and often makes it impossible to adhere to a reducing diet. Potassium chloride, sold as a salt substitute (p. 276), might be used during reducing; and 1-gram tablets (15 grains each) of potassium chloride carried and one taken when it is impossible to reach appropriate food. Taking potassium also prevents blackouts from hypoglycemia and is certainly preferable to using drugs to reduce.

Why reducing diets have failed. Though a lack of almost any nutrient causes body processes to slow down and less fat to be burned, reducing diets have become progressively more inadequate and lower in calories. In sheer desperation, starvation has been tried, but physicians who have carefully studied patients during fasts have found fasting to be exceedingly harmful.[54,55] Collectively tons have been lost by the aid of reducing drugs, which often cause liver damage.[55,57] The American Medical Association has pointed out that these drugs can be addictive and extremely dangerous.[9] Follow-up studies have shown that the lost pounds—with many additional ones—have usually been regained within a year, and often in a few months.[4,27,58-60] During the temporary period when such persons weigh less, they have been found to produce only half the amount of energy of healthy individuals.[61]

Fasting, severe calorie restriction, and reducing with the

aid of drugs are each such severe stress that the adrenals are left exhausted, a characteristic feature of which is continuous low blood sugar[62,63] and its accompanying ravenous appetite and craving for sweets. Liver damage and multiple deficiencies, induced by both the inadequacies of such regimes and the copious amounts of coffee usually drunk to ward off fatigue (p. 65), leave energy production at a low ebb.[64] The combination of the two—craving food and no energy—makes it literally impossible to keep from gaining. Yet everyone would surely agree that successful reducing means maintaining one's normal weight, once it has been reached, without undue struggle.

Much overeating may be an unconscious urge to obtain nutrients one's body needs, though most overweight persons eat far less than do their slender, energetic friends. To lose weight successfully, one must concentrate, as never before, on obtaining nutrients which increase energy production.

Your health-building program. The thyroid glands determine the speed at which energy is produced; therefore iodine, vitamin E (p. 46), and all nutrients required by these glands (p. 278) are essential to achieving normal weight and must be most carefully supplied. Sufficient iodine can be obtained daily from 1 teaspoon of granular kelp; and 600 units of vitamin E daily is desirable but under no circumstance should less than 100 units be taken.

Most human fat is saturated, yet saturated body fat cannot be burned unless approximately 2 tablespoons of oil are obtained daily to supply essential fatty acids. The body needs a continuous but extremely small amount of these acids at all times. If 2 tablespoons—6 teaspoons—of oil were to be taken at one time, much of it would be stored as flabby fat, and the free essential fatty acids needed would again be lacking. One rule that should never be broken, therefore, is to obtain some food supplying a teaspoon of vegetable oil six times daily, or about every three hours. Furthermore, that food should be enjoyable.

The following quantities furnish approximately 1 teaspoon of oil: 10 large peanuts, 3 pecan or 2 walnut halves, or 6 almonds; 1½ teaspoons mayonnaise; 2 teaspoons sunflower seeds, non-hydrogenated peanut butter, tartar sauce, or French or thousand-island dressing; 2 tablespoons avocado; or 3 tablespoons wheat germ. Oils, preferably a mixture of several (p. 50) may be used for tossing salads, cooking, and seasoning, but the amount should be carefully measured. Nuts or sunflower seeds are the easiest between-meal sources, especially for office workers, but cashews and Brazil nuts, rich in saturated fat, should be avoided. Small dinner salads with oil dressing are available at most restaurants. My at-home favorites are "breadless sandwiches," or mayonnaise between many lettuce leaves, sometimes with lean meat or low-fat cheese; mayonnaise on finger salads; or non-hydrogenated peanut butter or egg or tuna salad in celery stalks. Because oils and nuts supply 400 to 800 calories per half cup, overenthusiasm can be disastrous.

Saturated body fat is difficult enough to burn without complicating the problem by obtaining more saturated fat from food. A health-building program must be high in protein, but the only foods containing complete proteins and no saturated fats are fresh and powdered skim milk, yeast, wheat germ, soy flour, and soybeans. Liver, eggs, sweetbreads, kidneys, heart, fish, and seafoods are extremely low in saturated fats. Cold cuts, wieners, hamburger, and the lean portion of turkey, roast beef, lamb, pork, and ham average 20 to 50 per cent. Extra calories from carbohydrate or alcohol are quickly stored as saturated fat; hence the less taken the better. The so-called Air Force diet now in vogue supplies so much saturated fat that it is conducive to atherosclerosis.

Instead of counting calories or in addition to counting them, learn to count protein grams (p. 405) and obtain a minimum of 60 (women) to 80 (men) grams daily. Besides excellent protein, the B vitamins essential for energy production can be obtained with the least calories from yeast and fresh or desiccated liver, supplemented with B-vitamin tablets furnishing a daily quota of 1,000 milligrams each of cholin and inositol.

The best diet is one you plan for yourself, merely by following principles outlined in this chapter. Keep your larder well stocked with all your favorite low-calorie foods, and prepare them in the most delicious manner possible. Flavorful homemade vegetable or onion soup, broiled chicken, chow mein, sweetbreads with mushrooms, shrimp creole, steamed spinach, cabbage quick-cooked in milk, sauerkraut seasoned with oil and caraway seeds, artichokes with mayonnaise, and tossed salads can be both enjoyable and low in calories. Mayonnaise can be served on any cooked vegetable instead of butter. Many people habitually eat low-calorie foods because they prefer them to any other.

If you have only a little weight to lose, the diet outlined on pages 330-331 can be followed provided you forgo cream, butter, most fruits, cereals, and breadstuffs. When you do allow yourself an extra 100 calories, the starch in bread, a potato, or other root vegetable will give a more sustained pick-up than the sugars in fruits. All refined foods, soft drinks, processed cheese, and particularly coffee, alcohol, imitation fruit juices, and hydrogenated fats should be strictly avoided, but decaffeinized coffee may be used. Artificial sweeteners quickly destroy vitamin C[65] and probably cause liver damage, hence should be avoided.

Should you prefer a formula diet—the commercial ones are grossly inadequate nutritionally—prepare fortified milk, or pep-up (p. 329) containing 1 quart skim milk, 1 or 2 tablespoons each of oil and granular lecithin, ¼ cup fortified yeast (p. 320), ¼ teaspoon magnesium oxide, and nutmeg, a few teaspoons of frozen undiluted orange juice, or 1 teaspoon genuine vanilla. If your cholesterol is high or liver damage exists, more lecithin and protein are desirable; lecithin and kelp, which I dislike in milk, may be taken in water or juice or the kelp may be used for seasoning meat, fish, or salads. Eggs (p. 89), non-instant powdered milk, wheat germ, and/or soy flour may be added to the milk drink.

Take your choice. In case you wish both an exact regime and a particularly low-calorie diet, your schedule might be as follows:

I. Sip diet: Prepare pep-up with 2 tablespoons of oil; sip ½ cup every 2 hours or ⅔ cup every 3 hours; carry in thermos to work or, if at home, keep near a traffic lane and sip as you go by. Have decaffeinized coffee and clear bouillon as desired. Should you feel hungry, try the next suggestion.

II. Sip-and-nibble diet: Add to diet I raw vegetables such as celery, cucumbers, carrot sticks, or turnip, tomato, rutabaga, or kohlrabi wedges, and eat as much of them as you wish; or have yeast and magnesium in 2 glasses of milk, drink remainder of the quart of milk (or buttermilk) plain, take lecithin and kelp in water, and obtain a teaspoon of oil every 3 hours from nuts, mayonnaise on vegetables, or non-hydrogenated peanut butter in celery. Whenever you wish, follow the next suggestion.

III. Sip, nibble, and chew: Add to diet II a serving of liver sautéed with ½ teaspoon of oil; or 1 boiled or poached egg; or a seafood cocktail; or broiled or baked fish served with catsup or tartar sauce; and/or a tossed green salad at lunch and/or dinner. Mid-meals might be a small orange with nuts or sunflower seeds, but pep-up should be taken at breakfast, in late afternoon, and before bed. Energy output is greatest when the liver, egg, or fish is eaten at breakfast.

IV. Sip, nibble, and eat: Same as diet III except that lean fowl, lamb, veal, or beef might be eaten perhaps 3 times a week. Eggs may be fried or scrambled with ½ teaspoon of oil; a steamed green leafy vegetable, seasoned with oil and vinegar, or homemade vegetable soup could be substituted for a salad. Any vegetable that grows above the ground, such as broccoli, zucchini, or cabbage, may be steamed or added to low-fat soups.

In every case the diet should furnish a quart of milk daily and be supplemented with iodine (kelp), yeast, magnesium, vitamins A, C, D, E, the B vitamins, and, if health is below par, the antistress formula (p. 31). Six small meals daily are essential. A potassium-chloride tablet should be taken immediately if low-blood-sugar symptoms appear. Should a single nutrient be left inadequate (ch. 32) you cannot expect fat to be burned readily. The more limited the diet you wish to adhere to, the greater must be the amounts of nutrients furnished by supplements, especially pantothenic acid, vitamin C, and potassium; and salt should be temporarily restricted if water appears to be retained.

Even when your ideal weight is reached, small frequent meals high in protein and including oil and adequate amounts of all other nutrients must be continued throughout life, otherwise you will gain again.

Keys to success. With rare exceptions, any reducing diet that depends on will power—the endurance of hunger—is doomed to fail. It seems to me the key to success is not gastronomic, but mental discipline. For instance, childish impatience has rung the death knell on literally millions of might-have-been-successful reducing diets. By the end of a year, a steady loss of 5 pounds a month is far more rewarding than a 10-pound loss quickly regained after a week of crash dieting. If one disciplines himself to think of a long-term project, not of deprivation, but of intelligent progress toward a goal, success can usually be assured.

The fear of failure is a major cause of giving up and of eating foods that cannot possibly build health. The conscious mind, however, can hold only one thought at a time, and mental discipline can make that thought be one of success. The person who refuses to allow himself to think of failure feels so assured of success that no health-building regime is difficult.

Another essential discipline is to visualize yourself as you wish to be: energetic, buoyant, with radiant skin, sparkling eyes, and all other attributes of health. Keep this mental image before you at all times, never once allowing it to escape. Discipline yourself not to indulge in self-pity or to feel you are denied privileges others enjoy. Every time you are tempted by some non-health-building goodie, force yourself to answer the question, "Do I want to get fatter?"

Because the idea of reducing is associated with past failures and deprivations, avoid the word as if it were blasphemy. Think merely of following a health-building program which will bring as a secondary reward one's approximate normal weight.

The scales, too, are associated with past failures; and because weight fluctuates daily, they lead to illogical conclusions such as, "Now that I've lost, I can eat more," or "I never lose; there's no use trying." It seems to me wiser to get on the scale only once each month; persons who have adhered to a health-building diet will lose 5 pounds and often more in that time. A full-length bathroom mirror, used for frequent personal surveys, is usually far more valuable than a scale.

Every worth-while achievement requires discipline. When no weight is lost, these mental disciplines have probably been neglected and attitudes have become negative ones.

See your physician. Before a health-building regime is started, a general physical check-up should be obtained which includes a blood cholesterol determination (p. 59) and, for persons who have been on crash diets or taken appetite depressant drugs, liver function tests and/or a liver biopsy. A physician should also determine whether exercise must be limited.

Activities. Sufficient sleep and exercise are essential to a health-building program. Only during exercise are nutrients needed for maximum energy production carried to every body cell; unless sleep is adequate, no one feels like exercising.

A spontaneous urge to exercise cannot be expected until several weeks after every nutrient has been obtained, though dietary improvement quickly increases metabolism, or internal exercise. Persons who follow a health-building program carefully find that eventually they feel like swimming, hiking, bicycling, playing golf or tennis, or perhaps doing ballet or folk dancing. Some enjoyable activity should be a part of every daily regime. The one-minute static exercises worked out by Dr. Donald J. Salls, professor at Jackson State College, at Jacksonville, Alabama, are both easy and rewarding. *The Royal Canadian Air Force Exercise Plans,* sold at most newsstands and bookstores, are excellent for persons of all ages and can help tighten up flabby muscles.

Related facts. At no time in the history of the world have there been so many overweight persons in a single nation as in America today. At no time in the history of the world has a single nation consumed such a high percentage of refined foods and hydrogenated fats. These facts are closely related.

8

Learn to Live Without an Ulcer

He was a big hulk of a man, lovable, folksy, fortyish, with thick chest, thick hands, thick hair, yet he reminded one of a mistreated child. "You see, I'm a salesman," he began. "Me and a customer, we got in an argument. He got mad at me, and my boss, he got still madder when I told him." His shoulders shrugged in a helpless, what-can-you-do manner. "I was so upset I couldn't eat or sleep. Then my stomach started to hurt and got worse and worse. Two days later the doc, he said I got ulcers."

The story is familiar; only the circumstances vary.

Ulcers result from stress. The development of ulcers during the onset of stress is as characteristic of the alarm reaction as shriveled lymph tissue.[1] When rats are submitted to the psychological stress of immobilization by having a paw tied overnight, they develop deep bleeding ulcers in the stomach or duodenum. Dr. Hans Selye has pointed out the human parallel in that ulcers have developed overnight in persons during air raids, in soldiers awaiting battle, and even in students apprehensive about examinations; and in old ulcers becoming worse or new ones appearing after cortisone is given.[1]

How ulcers develop. For many years physicians at Cornell University Medical School studied a surprising number of people each of whom had a hole in his stomach, or gastric fistula, caused by a car accident, war wound, or other means; some also had ulcers.[2-5] The scientists carefully observed the appearance of the stomach walls and the movements of the stomach itself; and they measured the strength and quantity of the hydrochloric acid under a wide variety of conditions.

One man's esophagus had been permanently closed by scar tissue as a result of swallowing boiling chowder; hence a fistula had been made so that he could feed himself.[4] Whenever he became angry—for example, with his daughter for throwing her engagement ring in her fiancé's face because he had slapped her hard enough to break two teeth ("She just ain't got no brains. None of them kids has.")—his stomach walls became red, swollen, and severely inflamed, movement was markedly speeded up, and the hydrochloric acid increased in both amount and acidity. Later, when his wife became ill, worry and anxiety caused his stomach to become raw and bleeding.

Identical symptoms occurred when other individuals being studied were disgusted, worried, anxious, resentful, depressed, fearful, or were feeling insecure, hopeless, or defeated. Such changes were invariably most marked in the persons with ulcers; and their stomachs differed indeed from the pale-walled, rather quiet healthy stomach.

When a tugboat engineer who had both a fistula and an ulcer was reminded of past frustrations or disappointments, his stomach churned vigorously, the walls immediately flushed and swelled, strong acid poured out "by the cupful," his ulcer became painful, and healing stopped. This same reaction was true of all the other subjects. Nothing in the way of food, however, bothered them, although coffee, alcohol, and meat did slightly increase the stomach acid.

In all these people, heartburn was associated with the excessive production of acid and was worse when the stomach was empty; it could also result from eating too much or too rapidly or when emotionally upset, but it was not caused by indigestion. No distress occurred when the stomach walls were pinched with forceps or exposed to electric shock, strong alcohol, acid, or concentrated mustard, but stretching with an inflated balloon, comparable to gas distention, caused pain. When the natural mucus covering the stomach wall was washed from a portion of it and hydrochloric acid dropped on that area, a bleeding ulcer was produced, which became worse when exposed to normal stomach acid.[4]

A fantastic variety of foods, drugs, and chemicals had little or no effect on the stomach, even on those of people who had ulcers.[2] Frankfurters, chili, curry, pickles, vinegar, raw cabbage, anchovy paste, kippered herring, rhubarb, mustard, oil of cloves, spices, herbs, 50- to 100-proof alcohol, sugar, aspirin, digitalis, iron salts, and a wide variety of other chemicals and drugs had no effect.[2] These studies justified the conclusion that the stomach, healthy or ulcerated, "processes impartially any material classified as edible." The investigators pointed out, however, that apprehension could cause the stomach to become inflamed before a food or drug was taken, yet the food or drug would be blamed for any discomfort that followed.

Bitter materials increased the hydrochloric acid, and black pepper stimulated mucus production. Some strong drugs caused inflammation and increased the secretions and movements of the stomach, but almost the only substance that irritated the ulcers were alkalis, an ironical finding considering that the major ulcer treatment for decades had been various alkalizing powders. Ordinary baking soda, given to persons with duodenal ulcers, speeded up the emptying time of the stomach so much that the ulcers, exposed longer to corrosive acid, were made worse.[6] It also interfered with the digestion of protein to the extent that healing was delayed and at the next feeding, the stomach secreted twice as much strong acid.[56] When one subject who disliked drugs was given placebo tablets of starch that he thought to be a drug, his stomach became inflamed and he developed abdominal cramps and diarrhea; a toxic dose of medicine that he thought to be a placebo had no effect whatsoever.[4]

The Cornell doctors pointed out that ulcers are the most poignant example of how emotions can affect the digestive tract. Ulcer patients can gain an understanding of how their emotions influence their own condition by studying Dr. Hans Selye's *The Stress of Life* (McGraw-Hill, 1956) and the readable, tragic, and entertaining book, *Human Gastric Function* by Stewart Wolf and Harold G. Wolff (Oxford University Press, 1947).

Almost any deficiency can cause ulcers. Animals develop ulcers when kept on a diet too low in calories or deficient in almost any nutrient, whether protein, vitamins A, B_2, B_6, E, cholin, pantothenic acid, or folic acid.[7] Similarly, people made deficient in folic acid have developed so many ulcers on their lips and in their mouths and suffered so much abdominal pain indicative of beginning ulcers that the vitamin had to be given them;[8] and stomach ulcers have also been produced in volunteers on diets adequate except for vitamin E.[15,16]

Dogs and rats undersupplied with protein or a single sulfur-containing amino acid, cystine, develop ulcers of both the stomach and duodenum.[9] Because eggs are particularly rich in cystine, they are of great value in ulcer diets. If animals are deprived of food, or fasted, and hence no protein is given, the stress is so severe that ulcers develop within three days;[10] and they appear much sooner if the previous diet has been deficient in protein.[7] Stress causes such a rapid destruction of body protein that ulcers are also especially common in persons whose diets have been protein deficient.[9]

When little or no fat is eaten, foods leave the stomach so rapidly that the walls are exposed to strong hydrochloric acid for long periods; therefore a low-fat diet is conducive to ulcer formation.[11] Ulcers develop in six hours when rats' stomachs are tied off so that the acid is held in;[12] and ulcers caused by an excess of acid have been completely prevented by adding extra vitamin E to the diet.[13] It is therefore important for persons subject to ulcers, especially during stress, to obtain adequate vitamin E and at every meal and mid-meal some fat to prevent the stomach from being unnecessarily exposed to strong acid.

If cholin is undersupplied, bile is continuously regurgitated from the intestine back into the stomach, causing ulcers to form quickly.[7] Although the characteristic symptom of a cholin deficiency is the deposition of fat in the liver, cholin-deficient animals develop ulcers long before the liver becomes abnormal. Such ulcers heal when cholin is added to the diet, but healing is accelerated if large amounts of vitamin B_6 are given as well, although no other B vitamin has a comparable effect.

The severe stress of malnutrition itself may cause an ulcer. For example, the incidence of ulcers is said to be high among persons who, because of high blood pressure, are kept on a rice diet,[14] inadequate in almost every body requirement. It is actually doubtful whether people whose diets are continuously adequate could develop ulcers. Many nutrients that may play no role in causing ulcers are nevertheless needed in much larger quantities to promote healing (ch. 27). Although stress—the principal cause of ulcers—increases the need for all body requirements, persons and animals already deficient in various nutrients are the ones susceptible to ulcers, or most damaged by stress.[17]

Vitamin C and pantothenic acid. Monkeys and guinea pigs lacking vitamin C develop ulcers when the only stress is the single vitamin deficiency. Guinea pigs submitted to the stress of having one leg immobilized by a splint developed hemorrhaging ulcers, which could be prevented in similarly treated animals by giving them many times the normal requirement of this vitamin.[18] The need for vitamin C is so tremendously increased during stress that a deficiency can be produced in hours even though the vitamin appears to be adequate. Since blood vessels become fragile when vitamin C is lacking, too little of this vitamin allows a minor injury, such as a small ulcer, to cause a major hemorrhage.[17] The association of hemorrhage and stress is so well known that it has become part of the vernacular; my daughter's friends, for example, frequently remark, "My mother would have a hemorrhage if she knew I did that."

Ulcers cannot heal without vitamin C (p. 263). Yet repeatedly, scurvy, resulting from a total lack of this vitamin, has occurred in persons kept on ulcer diets, and is still being reported.

Adult rats develop stomach and duodenal ulcers when deficient in pantothenic acid, although none occur in similar animals given vitamin C; and as soon as pantothenic acid is added to the diet, the ulcers completely heal, leaving only scars.[17] If cortisone is given—simulating that pouring into the blood during stress—to animals mildly deficient in pantothenic acid, severe ulcers develop quickly. Conversely, no ulcers can be produced even by giving huge doses of cortisone provided the animals are on adequate diets high in pantothenic acid.[17]

Stomach or duodenal ulcers have frequently been unintentionally produced in patients when cortisone has been given as a medication.[1,11,17,19,20] Cortisone is known to destroy body protein and increase both the amount and acidity of stomach acid in the same way that stress does.[1]

When a pantothenic-acid deficiency is mild, it causes too little hydrochloric acid to be produced, but as it becomes increasingly severe, the stomach secretions grow progressively more acid until the acidity may be two or three times that of the normal stomach.[17] If anger or other emotional upset is superimposed on this situation, an ulcer can easily be induced.

Because certain strains of rats have a particularly high requirement for pantothenic acid, they are especially susceptible to ulcers.[17] For instance, one strain deficient in this vitamin developed 12 times more duodenal ulcers than another, and many were so severe that the intestinal wall was perforated.[17] The less-susceptible strain had only a few small ulcers. Individuals and families susceptible to ulcers may also have unusually high requirements for pantothenic acid, thus causing this illness to be considered hereditary.[21]

Goals of an ulcer diet. An ulcer, which is like a canker sore, is usually less than a fourth inch in diameter at first, but it may gradually become much larger. When body proteins are being broken down during the onset of stress, mucus-producing glands in the stomach walls appear to be damaged; hence they cannot secrete sufficient mucus to protect the stomach from the strong acid essential for digestion. Stress simultaneously causes the stomach to become overactive and to secrete acid which is more concentrated and in larger-than-normal amounts. With each contraction of the muscular stomach walls, the valve between the stomach and small intestine opens slightly; thus strong acid is squirted into the duodenum, or the first part of the small intestine. The corrosive action of this acid may cause an ulcer to form on any part of the stomach wall not covered with mucus. Because the intestinal wall is less well protected by mucus than the stomach, about eight times more persons have duodenal ulcers than peptic ulcers. Since the underlying conditions that bring about ulcers are identical whether they occur in the stomach or duodenum, the diet is the same for both types.

To be adequate, an ulcer diet should fulfill the following requirements: meet the demands of stress by supplying every nutrient in larger-than-usual amounts; promote healing at all possible speed (ch. 27); neutralize stomach acid until healing has occurred; and keep the stomach as quiet as possible. An ulcer can scarcely heal when strong acid pours over it or while it is being jerked, squeezed, or stretched by vigorous muscular contractions.

Tragically little has been done for the ulcer patient to meet the nutritional needs of stress. When patients whose ulcers had not healed in three years or longer were given no medication but did take 50 to 100 milligrams of pantothenic acid after each of three meals daily, all showed marked improvement within two to five days; gas distention disappeared, pain decreased, they slept more soundly, and x-rays showed some healing in all and complete healing in others.[22] In 80 per cent of another group of ulcer patients, the first 100 milligrams of calcium pantothenate markedly decreased the stomach secretions.[23]

Vitamins A, C, and E are particularly valuable for persons suffering from ulcers because respectively they stimulate the production of mucus,[24] accelerate healing, and prevent scarring (ch. 4). Yet these vitamins are rarely given in adequate amounts if at all.

The time-honored Sippy diet of hourly feedings of milk and cream[25] was originated before the science of nutrition was born. Though still used, it is too low in protein to promote healing during stress[26,27] and is deficient in iron, copper, magnesium, manganese, pantothenic acid, cholin, inositol, vitamins B_1, B_6, C, D, E, and other nutrients.[28-30] The principles of this diet, however, are sound. The protein of the milk neutralizes acid; and the fat quiets an active stomach by holding food in it for long periods, thus keeping acid from reaching the ulcer.[11,12] Milk, preferably not homogenized,[31] is still the best basis for an ulcer diet.

I learned more about ulcer diets while trying to make lemon pie than I did in college or dietetics training. If you add lemon juice to sweetened condensed milk to thicken it and then fold in whipped cream, you have a delicious lemon-pie filling. I attempted to make this recipe more nutritious by adding ½ cup powdered milk and folding in whipped evaporated milk. A lemon pie is worthless unless it is tart, however, and regardless of how much lemon juice I added, all acid was completely neutralized; it was literally impossible to make it tart. Similarly, if food high in protein is taken at frequent intervals, stomach acid can be completely neutralized and none left to irritate the ulcer.

When ulcer patients have been given test meals supplying 50 grams of protein—the amount in 6 cups of milk—and the value of each food judged by the length of time pain was alleviated and how completely stomach acidity was neutralized, ½ cup of soy flour was more effective than ¾ cup of powdered skim milk or 8 eggs; and it was almost twice as effective as huge servings of beef, chicken, or fish.[32] A single cup of milk, custard, eggnog, or milk pudding neutralized the acid as effectively as a dose of antiacid drugs. An ulcer, however, can heal while the stomach contents are still somewhat acid (pH 3.2 to 3.6). For example, orange and grapefruit juices, despite their citric-acid content, and vitamin C, which is a mild acid, hasten rather than delay healing.[33]

Ulcer diets and atherosclerosis. Persons who have adhered to a milk-and-cream ulcer regime have frequently died from heart disease, sometimes within three months after starting the diet.[34-36] Autopsy studies correlated with dietary histories have revealed that two to six times more ulcer patients given Sippy diets die of heart attacks than patients given general diets.[36-38] Both atherosclerosis and coronary thrombosis occur in rats given a Sippy diet.[36,39]

A modified Sippy diet of canned skim milk and partially hydrogenated soy oil has reduced the blood fat and cholesterol of ulcer patients and promoted satisfactory healing,[40-44] though it furnishes too little protein, pantothenic acid, and vitamin C to meet the demands of stress and too little vitamin E—32 units daily—to prevent scarring. A far more nutritious and less expensive fortified milk can be prepared at home.

A base for ulcer diets. The fortified milk described on page 329 can be used as the basis of any ulcer diet. If a high-calorie drink is desired, ¼ cup of vegetable oil, whole milk, several eggs or egg yolks, and frozen undiluted orange juice, a banana, or other fruit may be added. Fortified yeast, soy flour, and non-instant powdered milk can be increased to ½ cup each.

Any person following an ulcer regime should know what his blood cholesterol is and, if above 180 milligrams, the fortified milk and supplements should be varied accordingly (ch. 5). Acidophilus culture is especially valuable for ulcer patients because it destroys putrefactive bacteria in the intestinal tract which liberate histamine (p. 161) and increase the stomach acid.[45]

Because biotin deficiencies have been produced in volunteers by giving raw egg white,[46] I formerly recommended that eggs not be used unless cooked. Recently I was delighted to find a study in which cancer patients were fed 36 to 42 raw egg whites daily for an entire year.[47] Their general health improved and no biotin deficiency occurred. Uncooked eggs, therefore, appear to be both safe and desirable; hence I have included them in the fortified milk recipe.

Provided all materials are of high quality, fortified milk is not unpalatable, and it supplies four to five times as much adequate protein as does plain milk. If the ulcer is painful or hemorrhaging, ½ cup should be sipped slowly every hour. Later ⅔ cup might be taken at two-hour intervals throughout the day and whenever the patient awakes at night, but the greater the pain, the more frequent the feeding should be. Because unconscious anger, fear, or other emotional problems can be particularly devastating when the conscious mind is asleep, ulcer patients often secrete more hydrochloric acid at night than during the day;[60] hence night feedings are especially important until healing is complete.

For the first few days, little other food may be desired. It has been my experience that ulcers heal rapidly when the antistress formula (p. 31) is taken six times daily with fortified milk and the diet is supplemented with vitamins A, D, E, and B-complex tablets. Anyone who has had ulcers previously should continue perhaps 200 units or more of vitamin E indefinitely in hope of dissolving old scars.

Bleeding ulcers produced in human volunteers have healed in three or four days or in about the same time required to heal a canker sore.[4,5] Probably most ulcers could heal in this period provided the diet is highly adequate and the major stresses removed.

Your ulcer diet. Doctors disagree radically as to an acceptable ulcer diet. The majority still recommend the outmoded Sippy diet of milk, cream, and bland, tasteless, puréed, unseasoned foods, which makes it impossible for the patient to eat out socially, in restaurants, or even in cafeterias. As one physician puts it, "If doctors themselves were to be placed on such a program and forced to follow it, drastic changes would be quickly made."[42] They do agree, however, that all meals should be small, frequent, and taken with absolute regularity; and that the larger the meal, the more active the stomach and the stronger the acid secreted.

Ulcer patients kept in bed and on a strict diet have healed no faster than those allowed up and given a liberal diet.[48] Patients eating such formerly forbidden foods as whole-grain breads and cereals, raw fruits, sardines, coleslaw, and fresh salads have recovered more rapidly than others following a bland diet "with all its mushy variations."[49] Furthermore, ulcers have recurred less frequently when patients have been allowed unrestricted diets.[50] English investigators have even given ulcer patients a jolly diet of fried mutton and beef; healing occurred and neither the stomach acidity nor motility was affected.[51]

Cream soups, cooked fruits and vegetables, meats, eggnogs, milk toast, whole-grain breads and cereals, and puddings may be eaten as soon as pain disappears. Coffee, alcohol, and strong tea increase the amount and concentration of stomach acid, and should therefore be avoided.[31,33,52,53] Fresh citrus juices have accelerated healing,[31,54] even when given, mixed with milk, to patients with hemorrhaging ulcers.[55] Cream is no more effective in reducing the stomach acid than fried foods, oil, or fat in any other form;[31,51] hence fried, sautéed, and pan-broiled foods are acceptable as long as cooking temperatures are moderately low.

Because any worry can retard healing,[4] how quickly you should eat such foods as raw fruits and salads depends on your physician's attitude and your own feeling about them. If he is apprehensive, you are almost sure to be.

For years a man whose ulcer recurred each time the stock market fell periodically consulted me; his fear of foods was so great that he would undoubtedly have become worse had I suggested that he eat salads.

In starting any food you feel might cause distress, eat only a little at first; if no pain results, gradually increase the amount until you are eating ordinary meals. To adhere to a soft diet months after an ulcer has healed is like taking an aspirin for last year's headache.

Overneutralizing the stomach acid. Except during the alarm reaction of stress, ulcer patients usually have too little stomach acid.[17] Baking soda and various antiacids delay healing[56] and speed up the emptying time of the stomach to the extent that they can cause a healed ulcer to recur or an existing one to become more painful.[6] They should never be used as self-medication; and if frequent high-protein meals are eaten, none are needed.

Sippy powder and similar preparations, which are largely calcium carbonate, can induce a severe deficiency of magnesium (p. 207). When taken in excessive amounts over long periods, they have caused painful and dangerous deposits of calcium in the eyes, lungs, skin, kidneys, arterial walls, and other tissues.[57-59] A Mayo Clinic investigation revealed that some ulcer patients had taken more than two pounds of Sippy powder per week, and several had continued this medication for decades after a physician had recommended it.[58] Fortunately, these people recovered when the antiacid preparation was discontinued.

Learn to blow off steam. The old saying "It isn't what you eat that causes an ulcer, but what's eating you" is partially true. "What's eating you" often continues indefinitely, however, and allows the ulcer to recur repeatedly (p. 113). Until recently the effect of emotions on health has been little understood. The negative feelings of early childhood, such as anger, rejection, and fears, are long since forgotten but are unconsciously relived when a similar feeling occurs during adult life. Being forgotten, they can last a lifetime; therefore ulcers resulting from such emotional stress often become as persistent as homing pigeons. The frequently given advice "Learn to live with your ulcer" should be changed, however, to "Learn to live without an ulcer."

When large amounts of cortisone pour into the blood, preparing the body for fight or flight, the person susceptible to ulcers neither fights nor escapes. Usually he is a fine, sensitive, hard-working individual who has a need for approval, and he holds in his anger, resentment, and other negative emotions for fear of losing that approval. Yet a teakettle that blows off steam harmlessly does no damage; compressed steam is dangerous indeed. If he wishes to hold a job, of course, he cannot make a practice of telling off his employer, but there is nothing to prevent him from working out on a heavy punching bag with his boss's face painted on it the minute he arrives home. Had the salesman mentioned earlier expressed his anger in this manner, his ulcer would not have developed.

Usually the best investment a person subject to ulcers can make is good psychotherapy, which often puts an end to his illness. When such therapy is not available or one is not willing to undergo it, at the first possible moment after a frustration occurs he should do something to blow off steam: play tennis, golf, a piano, or any harmless action that uses the hitting muscles; and/or talk out his problem with an understanding friend.

The more adequate the diet, however, the less danger there is that stress will cause an ulcer. It seems to me that persons with this problem should keep nuts, protein wafers, malted-milk tablets, and vitamin C and pantothenic acid with them at all times, perhaps in a desk drawer and/or car, and take them hourly during the onset of stress. When, like the tugboat engineer, cupfuls of hydrochloric acid may be pouring into the stomach, they should get whole milk, nuts, and/or other high-protein foods with all possible speed and continue them at hourly intervals.

Some 15 years ago a university football coach came to see me; his team was losing and his ulcers were hemorrhaging. He had been hospitalized so many times by recurring ulcers that he refused to see a doctor, and I as adamantly refused to plan a diet for him until he did. We compromised, and he saw a physician who allowed him to take the fortified milk and supplements I suggested. Despite the "coffee grounds" in his stools, which indicated a substantial loss of blood, he returned to work the following week and has had no sign of ulcers since. The coach and his wife, however, became extremely interested in nutrition; and although he has had much stress and many emotional upsets, he has remained well.

Other persons with ulcer histories with whom I have

kept in close contact have had similar results. Perhaps many of the 17 million suffering from ulcers in the United States could remain well if nutrition were more carefully applied.

9

Diabetes Is Not Always Permanent

It seems to me no disease can inflict more savage cruelty than diabetes, a conviction I gained during dietetic training when my work necessitated daily visits to the diabetic ward. Invariably there were patients recovering from insulin shock and diabetic coma, and some who never recovered. Others were hemorrhaging from painful kidneys, and mere youngsters were already blinded from diabetic retinitis. Many diabetics had fatty livers, or swollen "stomachs," agonizingly tender to the touch. Arteries plugged with fatty deposits seemed an inevitable part of the disease, resulting in high blood pressure, frequent strokes, and far more heart attacks than among non-diabetics. Such deposits had caused discomfort in the legs years before the feet ulcerated, flesh rotted, and amputation could no longer be postponed. There were amputation stubs that took an eternity to heal; and tragic elderly persons pitifully learning to walk on artificial limbs.

One could not come to know and love these patients without praying that scientists would soon discover how such suffering could be prevented.

Perhaps a cause has been found. Insulin, a hormone produced by the pancreas, makes it possible for sugar (glucose) to enter the cells to be converted into energy or, if not needed immediately, to be changed into glycogen (body starch), or fat;[1] and insulin is also necessary before stored fat can be used.[2] In diabetes the insulin supply becomes inadequate, presumably the result of a damaged pancreas.

When too little vitamin B_6 (pyridoxin) is obtained, an essential amino acid from complete proteins, tryptophane, is not used normally; instead it is changed into a substance known as xanthurenic acid.[3,4,5] If animals are deficient in vitamin B_6, xanthurenic acid in the blood becomes so high that it damages the pancreas within 48 hours and diabetes is produced.[6,7] The blood sugar rises far above normal, and excessive sugar (glucose) spills into the urine. The longer animals are kept on a vitamin-B_6-deficient diet, the more extensive is the destruction of pancreatic tissue.[4] Injecting animals with xanthurenic acid also causes the pancreas to be so severely damaged that diabetes develops; again the blood sugar soars and urinary loss of sugar is heavy.[7]

As soon as vitamin B_6 is supplied, the amount of xanthurenic acid decreases; when the pancreas has not been seriously harmed, health is restored and all diabetic symptoms disappear.[3,4] If the vitamin is not given, the condition grows steadily worse until the animal dies. Magnesium decreases the need for vitamin B_6; and if it is increased in the diet, the amount of xanthurenic acid is reduced even though no vitamin B_6 is allowed.[5,8] Furthermore, magnesium is necessary to activate enzymes containing vitamin B_6; and blood magnesium is particularly low in diabetics.[9] Diabetes, therefore, may prove to be caused by the combined deficiencies of this vitamin and mineral.

Saturated fats increase the need for magnesium (p. 54) and vitamin B_6;[7,10,11] hence deficient rats given a high-fat diet excreted many times more xanthurenic acid than animals fed oils or little fat.[7] They also became grossly obese, and the urinary loss of sugar and destruction of the pancreas paralleled their gain in weight.[6] Because high-protein and high-calorie diets increase the need for vitamin B_6, they accelerate the harm done to the pancreas if this vitamin is inadequate.[5,7] Furthermore, injuries to the pancreas occur long before any other symptoms of a vitamin-B_6 deficiency appear.[7] Investigators have stated that their studies give "conclusive evidence that xanthurenic acid may cause human diabetes."[6]

Persons who are overweight are especially susceptible to diabetes; and excess calories from any source increase the vitamin-B_6 requirement.[10-12] Diabetes has been produced in cats by prolonged feeding of sugar, although control animals given starch did not develop the disease.[13] Sugar particularly increases the need for both insulin and vitamin B_6;[14] and a high incidence of diabetes occurs in persons eating excessive sugar.[15] Conversely, when food has been limited, as during wartime, diabetes has markedly decreased.

A number of drugs cause xanthurenic acid to appear in human urine, a condition that can be prevented if vitamin B_6 is taken with the drug.[8] For instance, such large amounts of xanthurenic acid are formed after penicillin is given to rats that the pancreas is quickly damaged.

Persons mildly deficient in vitamin B_6 excrete xanthurenic acid long before any other signs of the dietary insult appear.[3,16-18] In fact, the test for a vitamin-B_6 deficiency is the determination of xanthurenic acid in the urine;[16,19,20] none is found when vitamin B_6 is adequate. [3,16,17,19,21] All diabetics, however, appear to excrete large amounts of this acid,[6,22-24] which would indicate that the pancreas is being further damaged. Moreover, uncontrolled diabetics and persons with diabetic retinitis excrete far more xanthurenic acid than do individuals receiving insulin or who have no complications.[6,23]

When diabetics have been given 50 milligrams of vitamin B_6 daily, they showed a rapid and marked decrease in urinary xanthurenic acid;[22,24] in one case, the quantity dropped almost 97 per cent the first day.[22] If they continued taking 10 to 20 milligrams of this vitamin daily, none of this harmful acid was excreted,[22] showing that none was being formed in the body.

The fact that diabetics are deficient in vitamin B_6 may clarify many of the mysteries concerning this disease. The belief that diabetes is hereditary may be merely a high genetic requirement for vitamin B_6. Some infants require many times more of this vitamin than do others.[20,25] In addition, lecithin, which reduces the high blood fat and cholesterol so characteristic of diabetes,[26-28] cannot be produced unless vitamin B_6 and magnesium are adequate (p. 54); therefore deficiencies of these nutrients could in part be responsible for many serious cholesterol complications of diabetes.

Although more research must be done before conclusions can be drawn, any person with diabetes or a family history of the disease may be wise to take at least 10 milligrams of vitamin B_6 and 500 milligrams of magnesium daily.

A vitamin-B_6 deficiency can easily occur. The onset of diabetes is marked by intense thirst, the drinking of huge quantities of water, and a corresponding excessive urine output. All B vitamins including vitamin B_6—and many other nutrients—are readily lost in the urine; and the more urine excreted, the greater the losses.[29] Though vitamin B_6 may have been temporarily lacking before the onset of the disease, such a deficiency would thus immediately be made worse. Excessive urine production also rapidly induces a magnesium deficiency.[9,30]

Even after insulin is given, sugar frequently spills into the urine. To dilute this sugar, water is withdrawn from the blood, and again excessive urine is formed. Much needed vitamin B_6 and other nutrients which readily dissolve in water are therefore lost whenever the urine shows a positive test for sugar.[29] A person whose diabetes is not well controlled might thus easily have vitamin-B_6 and magnesium deficiencies even though his intake appears to be adequate.

The importance of following a physician's advice. When the pancreas has been so damaged that it can no longer produce sufficient insulin, sugar can neither enter the cells nor be changed into body starch or fat.[1,2] Sugar coming from digesting foods therefore accumulates in the blood until, when perhaps three or four times above normal, it spills into the urine. Conversely, insulin given to a person with diabetes causes the sugar to pass into the cells and the amount in the blood to fall. The quantity of insulin needed, however, varies with each individual and from time to time, depending largely on the carbohydrate intake. If too much insulin is given or too little food eaten, the symptoms of low blood sugar—weakness, nervousness, wooziness, perhaps headache, trembling hands, and loss of consciousness, or blackout—can be brought on with such lightning speed that they are spoken of as an insulin reaction, or insulin shock. To prevent such a reaction, the quantity of food prescribed by the physician must be eaten.

Whenever the blood sugar drops below normal, the alarm reaction of stress is set off. The adrenal hormones cause body protein to be broken down into fat and sugar and still more fat from storage depots to be released into the blood.[31] If insulin is still excessive, this sugar also enters the cells too quickly; the blood sugar is again reduced, and further proteins are destroyed. Simultaneously the blood fats, unusually excessive in persons with this disease,[28] soar even higher; in diabetics with atherosclerosis, the stage is set for a heart attack. To prevent insulin shock, needless destruction of body protein, and excessive blood fat, a doctor carefully balances the type and amount of food recommended against the insulin dosage.

If insufficient insulin is given, sugar cannot enter the cells. Fat alone must be used for heat and energy, yet it cannot be burned efficiently without sugar. Certain acids and acetone, formed from incompletely utilized fat, accumulate in the body and cause acetone acidosis. The acids are neutralized by combining with sodium and potassium, and the salts thus formed are excreted in the urine. Acetone, partly thrown off with exhaled air, gives a characteristic odor to the breath of patients with uncontrolled diabetes. Even mild acidosis can cause fatigue, nervousness, headache, and nausea. Severe acidosis can rob the body of so much potassium that unconsciousness, or diabetic coma, and even death can result.[32-34]

Because it is difficult for patients to adhere to strict diets, physicians have sometimes attempted to adjust the insulin dosage to the foods diabetics select for themselves. Such freedom, however, has usually proved to be disastrous. More than 90 per cent of patients allowed "free diets" have been found to develop serious complications in a relatively short time.[35]

A diabetic skis a slalom course between insulin shock on the one hand and a diabetic coma on the other. A physician, however, can largely prevent both of these reactions provided the patient follows his directions. Any changes made to improve the nutritive value of food eaten must be done within the framework of the diabetic diet he recommends.

Although diabetic specialists are expert in adjusting insulin dosage to the diet recommended, it is a tragic fact that few have become sufficiently interested in nutrition to make an all-out effort to stimulate maximum insulin production or to prevent devastating complications.

Increasing the insulin output. It has long been known that if the nutritional needs of a diabetic can be reduced, the disease sometimes disappears. When diabetic patients with overactive thyroids have been successfully treated or chronic infections have cleared up, it is not unusual for insulin to be discontinued.[36] If a diabetic has been under stress and the stress is removed—for instance, a sick child who caused worry has recovered—he may no longer need insulin.[37] Overweight diabetics can frequently stop insulin after reducing.[38,39] In each of these cases, the body requirements have decreased, and the effect is the same as if the diet were improved.

Adequate nutrition stimulates insulin production in a variety of ways. The insulin output has often increased after diabetics have taken vitamin C;[40] and guinea pigs given too little vitamin C produce insufficient insulin, have high blood sugar, and lose sugar in the urine.[41,42] This vitamin is needed before several amino acids that form insulin can be utilized.[43] Deficiencies of protein, pantothenic acid, and particularly vitamin B_2 reduce insulin synthesis in rats; and conversely, generous amounts of these nutrients stimulate insulin production,[44] as does a factor in yeast.[45-47] A lack of vitamin B_{12} or potassium causes rats to have prolonged high blood sugar.[23,48] Cortisone injections normally increase insulin production, but such an increase cannot occur if vitamins B_1, B_{12}, and pantothenic acid are deficient.[49] A wide variety of animals develop diabetic symptoms when given two meals daily but not if allowed to eat frequently.[50] Adequate nutrition also makes insulin, which exists in both active and inactive forms,[51,52] more readily usable.[51]

Diabetic patients have improved remarkably and many have been taken entirely off insulin when 300 to 600 units of vitamin E have been given daily.[53-61] Furthermore, this vitamin has been particularly helpful to persons with diabetic gangrene and other complications arising from atherosclerosis. Results have been especially striking when 3 tablespoons or more of lecithin were taken daily with vitamin E.[62] Natural insulin production has been increased by giving patients vitamin B_1,[63] vitamin C,[40] unusually large amounts of protein,[31] pantothenic acid,[64] and small, frequent meals each containing some carbohydrate.[2]

Immediately after diabetes has been diagnosed, the diet should be made so completely adequate that no possible deficiency can exist. As long as any pancreatic cells are able to produce insulin, the emphasis should be on keeping these cells healthy and on helping them to increase insulin production. The conclusion that diabetes is permanent is justified only when the insulin-producing cells have been largely or completely destroyed.

Nutritional needs are high. The dietary requirements of a diabetic are undoubtedly many times greater than those of a healthy individual. Because the urinary losses of water-soluble nutrients are unusually high, to improve health the diet must more than compensate for these losses. For example, inositol was isolated from diabetic urine over 100 years ago; and the urinary losses of this vitamin are much greater than in other persons,[65] a fact that contributes to the tragic incidence of severe atherosclerosis. Both the urinary losses and the requirements of magnesium and vitamin B_6 are markedly increased. Although the National Research Council considers 2 milligrams of vitamin B_6 adequate for adults, conscientious objectors obtaining this quantity from army rations excreted excessive amounts of xanthurenic acid.[66]

Another reason the nutritional requirements are high is that every time acidosis develops or the blood sugar falls below normal an alarm reaction to stress is set off, increasing the need for protein, vitamin C, pantothenic acid, potassium, and other nutrients.[64,67] Cortisone given as a medication, which simulates the body's reaction to stress, has caused both diabetes and inflammation of the pancreas in patients.[68,69] If pantothenic acid is undersupplied, the blood sugar drops so quickly after insulin is given that the danger of insulin shock, or a blackout, is tremendously increased.[70-73]

Certain individuals, known as "brittle" diabetics, are so unusually sensitive to insulin that their blood sugar falls rapidly from extremely high to extremely low, causing insulin shock to be common.[31] This condition appears to result largely from a deficiency of pantothenic acid,[70-73] though brittle diabetics also have unusually high requirements for potassium,[33,34] protein,[44] vitamins B_2 and C,[74] niacin amide,[75] and lecithin.[62] When these nutrients have been increased, the sensitivity to insulin has disappeared.

Dr. Kendall Emerson, Jr., of the Harvard Medical School, an outstanding authority on diabetes, emphasizes that diabetic diets should contain far more protein than they usually do.[31] He points out that when the blood sugar drops following an insulin injection or when too little food is eaten, the increased secretion of pituitary and adrenal hormones causes destruction of body proteins including those of the pancreas, thus damaging the organ still more and further decreasing insulin production. Physicians will usually increase the protein allowance if a patient requests it.

Despite a seemingly adequate intake, diabetics often show abnormally small amounts of vitamin A in the blood,[76] frequently lose this vitamin in the urine,[63] and have symptoms of a vitamin-A deficiency.[77] Marked clinical improvement has resulted when only 16,000 units of vitamin A have been given to diabetics daily.[78] Because this vitamin helps to reduce blood fat and cholesterol, it should be generously supplied at all times.

Similarly, when diabetic diets have appeared to be adequate in vitamin B_1, neuritis has developed, and was relieved as soon as larger amounts of this vitamin were given.[78-81] Vitamin B_1 is said to be especially valuable in preventing damage to the brain during diabetic acidosis.[63,82] The more insulin needed, the higher is the requirement for vitamins B_1, pantothenic acid, and biotin.[31]

Because of stress, urinary losses, and destruction by saccharine and other artificial sweeteners,[83] the vitamin-C requirement is also unusually high in diabetes,[40] and huge amounts of this vitamin sometimes bring unexpected results. An elderly attorney had taken 80 units of protamine-zinc insulin daily for ten years; after he increased his vitamin-C intake to 4,000 milligrams daily because of a prostate infection, his physican had to reduce his insulin repeatedly and finally discontinued it. A letter from his doctor states, "I have never heard of a case which made such a complete recovery." As long as the large amounts of vitamin C are continued, his urine contains no sugar. This gentleman, now in his late eighties, has repeatedly expressed almost ecstatic relief that he no longer has to take insulin.

Diabetic patients are frequently deficient in potassium,[82] which, though needed to utilize sugar,[84] drops far below normal when the blood sugar falls or acidosis develops.[33] The loss of potassium caused by salt retention during stress is especially dangerous to diabetics who suffer from high blood pressure or heart disease[85] and increases the likelihood of a heart attack.[85-87] Because a potassium deficiency can also be induced by eating too much salt,[33,34] diabetics should not eat such foods as ham, smoked fish, and salted nuts when under stress or spilling sugar unless they take potassium. During severe acidosis a lack of potassium can be fatal.[34,84] Low blood potassium also has been found to increase to normal if magnesium is given.[88]

When diabetic patients with coronary disease have been given 2 to 5 grams of potassium chloride by mouth before an insulin injection, it has prevented an excessive drop in blood sugar and an increase in blood pressure and pulse rate;[89] when given after the blood sugar fell, blood pressure and pulse have immediately decreased and the blood sugar and electrocardiograms quickly changed toward normal.[74,89] It is probably wise for diabetics to use—with their doctor's permission—potassium chloride generously as a salt substitute (p. 216) and to carry 1-gram tablets of potassium chloride to take at the first indication of insulin shock. If either stress or a pantothenic-acid deficiency has been prolonged, however, ordinary table salt (sodium) is needed rather than potassium (p. 29).

Preventing complications. Abnormalities which frequently complicate diabetes are atherosclerosis, fatty liver, overweight, cataracts, retinitis, and gangrene. The prolonged use of inadequate diets high in saturated fats often

causes the arteries of diabetics to become almost unbelievably filled with fatty deposits.[35,90-92] I was once asked to
plan a preoperative diet for a 46-year-old man who had
had diabetes for 15 years. This man's leg, in which gangrene had already set in, was tremendously swollen, purple,
and excruciatingly painful. The attending physician told me
later that it was first amputated below the knee, but the
arteries were so completely plugged that not one drop of
blood appeared and the flesh looked like cooked meat. A
second amputation near the hip was necessary to insure
healing.

Most diabetics over 50 years of age have advanced
general atherosclerosis,[31,36,91] which is far more common
in diabetics than in non-diabetics,[86,87,93] and may be as
damaging to the heart, liver, brain, kidneys, and other parts
of the body as to the legs.[26] Vegetarian diabetics, whose
diets supply B vitamins, potassium, magnesium, and vegetable oils but little saturated fat, have no atherosclerosis.
Diabetic Trappist monks, who eat eggs, whole milk, and
yogurt but no meat, have blood cholesterol levels well
under 200 milligrams regardless of age.[94]

It seems to me that all diabetic patients should have
blood cholesterol and/or fat determinations made every
six months, and if either is excessive, immediate steps
should be taken to lower it. The substitution of vegetable
oil for the saturated fats in diabetic diets has "dramatically reduced" blood cholesterol.[95,96] All nutrients needed to
utilize fats and to help prevent clotting, emphasized in
chapters 5 and 6, should be included in every diabetic
diet. Lecithin and vitamin E are particularly important,
especially if the threat of gangrene arises;[56-61] and amputation has sometimes been prevented by 600 units of vitamin
E being given daily.[53,54]

Physicians unanimously agree that overweight diabetics
—in whom atherosclerosis is markedly severe—are helped
by reducing.[14,26,97] A reducing program easily fits into the
framework of a diabetic diet, but unless it is unusually
adequate, increased blood fat brought in from storage
depots can induce heart disease or make it worse.[98] An
adequate low-calorie diet should be planned first and the
insulin dosage adjusted to it. Yeast and soy flour supply 20
and 10 grams of protein respectively in ¼ cup and contain
no starch or sugar. Because of the sugar it contains,
physicians usually allow diabetics far too little milk. If
yogurt or acidophilus is used, the sugar in milk is broken
down by intestinal bacteria to lactic acid; hence so little

sugar is absorbed that milk should be considered sugar-free.[99] As much as 6 tablespoons of lecithin have been given daily to diabetics with excellent results and without being considered part of the fat content of the diet.[62] Presumably it is not used as calories but to replace the body phospholipids. Small, frequent meals are far more important for the diabetic than the non-diabetic.[50]

Fatty liver is common in diabetes,[31,97] probably because cholin and inositol are so readily lost in the urine.[29,65] Biopsies of the livers of diabetic patients taken before and six weeks after they had adhered to a diet particularly high in protein and the B vitamins, and supplemented with cholin, inositol, and vitamin B_{12}, showed that even the more serious cases were corrected in this period.[97] Vitamins C and E and the sulfur-containing amino acids in eggs are also particularly valuable in correcting fatty liver.[96,100]

Diabetic retinitis, apparently brought on by stress,[101] is characterized by hemorrhages in the back of the eye, and sometimes occurs without diabetes when vitamin B_6 is deficient.[102] Many tiny blood-filled balloons known as aneurysms—an early and common symptom of diabetes[101]— bulge from the walls of the capillaries, are extremely fragile, break easily, and spill blood into the tissues. This condition is said to be prevented when far more protein than usual is permitted on a diabetic diet,[31,103] and improves when pantothenic acid and vitamins B_{12} and C are given.[101] Because as much as 80 per cent of the essential amino acid tryptophane is destroyed when vitamin B_6 is undersupplied,[5] this loss, coupled with the destruction of body proteins caused by stress, undoubtedly weakens the tiny bits of protein forming the capillary wall, and plays a role in causing aneurysms and hemorrhages. Since I am convinced that diabetic retinitis can be prevented, especially if the antistress formula is taken around the clock and the full antistress program followed (p. 31), I was heartbroken this year when a talented young pianist sought my help only two months after retinitis had caused him to become totally blind.

Broken aneurysms in the kidneys frequently cause blood to appear in the urine. Aneurysms can also cause multiple hemorrhages in any part of the body without the patient or physician being aware of them. They may produce local distress, troublesome scar tissue, or a clot that results in a heart attack or stroke. Both atherosclerosis and high blood pressure make them worse.[104,105]

Watch for insulin reactions. When natural insulin production is stimulated, the effect is the same as if the insulin dosage were increased. In case you improve your diet, you must be constantly alert in watching for the first symptoms of insulin shock. Carry cube sugar or small candies and possibly 1-gram tablets of potassium chloride at all times when fresh fruit is not at hand. Keeping fruit juice beside the bed and sipping a little whenever you awake can prevent insulin reaction during the night.

How quickly natural insulin production can be stimulated varies with individuals. The attorney referred to earlier had no insulin reaction for three months after adding vitamin C to his diet. On the other hand, in 1955 I was consulted by a 53-year-old woman who had taken insulin for eight years and who had angina, high blood pressure, considerable leg distress, and "was a-achin' and a-painin' all over." With her physician's permission, I suggested that she use oils instead of saturated fats, have small, frequent meals, a quart of fortified milk similar to pep-up daily (p. 329), and generous supplements of all vitamins. Symptoms of low blood sugar occurred almost immediately and were so persistent that her insulin was discontinued after ten days, when she "felt absolutely marvelous." Her blood pressure decreased, and the angina and leg distress disappeared. A letter dated January 14, 1965, states, "I have never had a recurrence of diabetes or heart disease since."

Serious cases of long standing can rarely discontinue insulin, but if their nutrition is improved sufficiently to prevent complications, insulin reactions so frequently occur that the dosage must often be decreased.

Small changes can bring large improvements. Though each individual is different, the revisions I suggested last year for a 19-year-old college athlete who was receiving 40 units of insulin daily can illustrate how nutrition may be improved and the physician's instructions still adhered to. This young man's 3,000-calorie diabetic diet allowed packaged cereals, 8 slices of white bread daily, and huge amounts of saturated fats: whole milk, 3 to 5 pats of butter per meal, hydrogenated peanut butter, bacon, sausage, ham, pork chops, hamburger, and other meats high in fat. No supplements had been given him.

I suggested that he use only whole-grain breads and cereals, avoid all hydrogenated fats, and reduce animal fats considerably; that oil, lecithin, magnesium oxide, non-instant powdered milk, and fortified yeast be blended daily with his quart of whole milk (p. 329); that eggs be cooked in oil or prepared without fat; that liver be eaten daily when possible, and fish several times a week; and that his fat quota be filled by eating modified butter (p. 312), nuts, avocados, wheat germ (the best source of .zinc, a component of insulin), oils or mayonnaise on salads and cooked vegetables, and generous amounts of mayonnaise on bread and sandwiches. Mid-meals were emphasized and consisted of unsalted nuts, oranges, and, whenever possible, fortified milk. The remainder of his diet remained unchanged.

He also took the following supplements after each meal: 10 milligrams of vitamin B_6; B-complex tablets supplying a daily total of 1,000 milligrams each of cholin and inositol; 100 units of vitamin E; and, because this boy was under tremendous stress, 100 milligrams of pantothenic acid and 500 of vitamin C. A capsule containing 25,000 units of natural vitamin A and 2,500 units of natural vitamin D was taken daily after breakfast.

He noticed insulin reactions the first week he followed his revised diet, and his insulin was discontinued a month later, a fact which his physician described as "miraculous." Although he has adhered to his diet remarkably well, he has had to take 10 to 15 units of insulin daily during periods of unusual stress.

Mild diabetes. The antidiabetic drugs given for mild diabetes are not effective unless some of the cells of the pancreas can still produce insulin. Because these drugs often cause liver damage and cannot build up the pancreas, their action is that of beating a tired horse and adding stress to stress. Unless the diet is markedly improved, more and more cells in the pancreas are gradually destroyed, until insulin must eventually be used. All the diabetics with whom I have worked have been able to discontinue these drugs after a few weeks on an adequate diet except a few who washed away nutrients with copious amounts of alcohol or coffee.

If a completely adequate diet could be given to every patient as soon as diabetes is diagnosed, this disease would be far less serious than it is today. Although diabetes is said to be the most rapidly increasing of all the degenerative diseases, it would probably be rare if our foods were unrefined.

10
Arthritis Can Often Be Relieved

For years I hated to have anyone with arthritis consult me, and I dreaded their return visits even more. It seemed to me they invariably became worse, but there were occasionally exceptions.

Mrs. Connally's hands were too gnarled to play the piano she loved so much; though in her seventies, she was soon playing several hours daily and she continued to do so to the very month of her death.

Mr. Garvey was 65 when he first consulted me. Decades of pain had misshaped his tortured body until his chin was level with his knees. Yet six weeks later he was standing nearly erect and working with hoe and shovel. For years he brought me literally basketfuls of flowers that he had grown himself.

Lovely Mrs. Watson, horribly crippled, overweight, and confined to a wheelchair, was dreadfully ashamed to have been forced to accept county aid. After she had improved, lost pounds, and established a successful business, she never failed to mention with pride that she could pay taxes. My husband claims she is the only person with the right attitude toward them.

These individuals were as puzzling as the ones who became worse. It was years before I realized that their hobbies were as important as their nutrition.

The most neglected disease. Arthritic patients have been referred to as "the most neglected segment of the medical population."[1] The fact that this disease has not been readily produced in experimental animals has been a drawback to understanding it. One strain of mice spontaneously develops an illness similar to arthritis; and a high-protein diet delays its onset and decreases its severity.[2] An abnormality simulating arthritis has been produced in rats deficient in pantothenic acid,[3] and the amount of vitamin C in the blood of these animals becomes extremely low.[4] If vitamin C is given them in huge

106

quantities, it markedly delays the onset of the "arthritis"; pantothenic acid completely prevents or corrects it.[3]

Arthritis has been produced in rats by injections of formaldehyde and in vitamin-C-deficient guinea pigs by injections of bacteria, both of which are forms of stress; the rats were protected if given massive amounts of vitamin E,[5,6] and the guinea pigs by vitamin C. Rats kept on a diet low in calcium and high in phosphorus have developed arthritis, which was corrected when twice as much calcium as phosphorus was given them.[7]

If experimental or farm animals are undersupplied with magnesium, calcium is laid down in the soft tissues, a condition that is corrected soon after magnesium is given them.[8-11] In rats deficient in vitamin E, the calcium content of the soft tissues increases as much as 500 per cent.[12,13] Both of these nutrients, therefore, may be important in helping people with osteoarthritis—osteo means bone-like—and in removing spurs.

Studies have revealed that most persons with arthritis have been under severe stress before the onset of the illness; that their diets are appallingly deficient in many respects; and that the level of vitamins in their blood, particularly vitamin C and pantothenic acid, is extremely low.[1,14-16] Human volunteers deficient in vitamin B_6 have developed sore joints similar to mild arthritis, a condition corrected soon after the vitamin was given them.[17] When several arthritic patients received 25 milligrams of pantothenic acid daily as their only dietary improvement, some experienced a decrease or disappearance of pain and stiffness within two weeks.[1]

A disease of adrenal exhaustion. Arthritis remained a mystery until it was shown that remarkable results were obtained when cortisone was given. Obviously, if the body were producing all the cortisone it needed, further cortisone could bring no improvement. Such results indicated that persons with arthritis were in the exhaustion stage of the stress reaction (p. 23); and that their pituitary and/or adrenal glands could no longer function normally. Since this knowledge became available, the arthritic individuals with whom I have worked have often improved remarkably after following a diet designed to stimulate natural cortisone production and to meet the increased nutritional needs of stress.

For example, Jimmy Fassero, a wonderful man who spent 23 years working on the 200-inch telescope and is now helping to get a closer look at the moon, had such severe arthritis in his knees and feet that every step meant excruciating pain. After he had adhered to a more-than-adequate diet for exactly one month, he told me, "I could walk the 3,000 miles from here to New York." Not a sign of arthritis remained and none has recurred.

June Gasteiro has become a crusader who is trying to get the American Arthritic Foundation to retract their statement that nutrition cannot help arthritis. She was lying on the davenport crying with agonizing pain when the postman brought her diet. At first, her improvement was rapid, then she ran into several snags and regressed, but eventually she made steady progress. Five weeks after receiving her nutrition program she wrote, "I am completely free from pain, can do all my own housework, and some of my shopping." A later letter states, "I still have to fight to keep from crying at the memory of those awful, awful days when I came so close to becoming a permanent invalid."

A recent postcard from Mrs. Grace Conroy, who had suffered from osteoarthritis for years and is now touring Europe, reads: "Gave my wheelchair to the Salvation Army. I'm walking miles through galleries every day and haven't taken an aspirin in months."

After having osteoarthritis for eight years, Mrs. Lucille P. Leisure's wheelchair is gathering dust. She states in a letter, "Before starting on the diet, I could not climb stairs and found it most uncomfortable to walk. Two doctors had recommended the removal of my knee-caps because of the arthritic spurs the x-rays showed. Now I can climb stairs with ease and walk as well as I did when I was young! I have taken no form of treatment whatsoever, but am so completely convinced of the 'magic' of good nutrition that I feel everyone should be reached."

Persons frequently believe that when arthritic spurs have formed or joints are cemented together, as are the vertebrae in spondylitis, nothing can be done. Because I have worked with many who had results similar to the ones cited, I wholeheartedly disagree.

The diet must meet the needs of prolonged stress. All nutrients that increase cortisone production (ch. 2) must be particularly emphasized in the diet of any individual with arthritis. Because stress has caused a continuous destruction of protein, necessary before ACTH can be produced,[18] the protein intake must be extremely high and obtained in small, frequent meals. Volunteers lacking essential fatty acids quickly showed a decrease in adrenal hormones.[19] Pantothenic acid can scarcely be overemphasized, and persons subject to arthritis may have an unusually high requirement for this vitamin.[20] Men deficient in pantothenic acid for only 25 days developed impaired adrenal function.[21] Prolonged stress increases the nutritional requirements so much that deficiencies of pantothenic acid and/or vitamins B_2 or C can be produced and cause the adrenals to become severely damaged;[4,22] hence several weeks may be necessary for repair before improvement can be expected.[4]

Animals under stress sometimes need 70 times the normal requirement of vitamin C to protect the adrenals;[23] and older animals—and presumably older humans of the arthritis-susceptible age—require twice as much of this vitamin as do young ones.[23] Vitamin C not only increases the production and utilization of cortisone, but also appears to prolong its effectiveness.[24,25]

People with arthritis frequently make the mistake of avoiding calcium-rich foods, yet calcium is withdrawn from the bones continuously both when under stress and when the diet is inadequate in calcium itself, in magnesium, or perhaps in vitamin E;[12,13] hence the intake of calcium should be particularly generous.[14,26] Furthermore, calcium is said to decrease the sensitivity to pain. The woman whose spurs disappeared, for example, obtained 2 grams of calcium daily from fresh and powdered milk and another gram from a mixed-mineral supplement, making a total of 3 grams daily.

The antistress factors supplied by liver, yeast, full-fat soy flour, and cooked green leafy vegetables (p. 28) should be obtained daily in as large amounts as can be well tolerated. Because stress increases the need for nutrients, probably all body requirements except calories should be supplied in considerably greater than-normal amounts.

A diet that helped arthritis. The diet used by Jimmy Fassero, the 55-year-old man whose recovery from arthritis delighted me as much as him, I believe, can illustrate the foods and supplements taken daily:

An entire quart of pep-up which contained ½ cup of non-instant powdered skim milk in addition to the other ingredients (p. 329), taken ⅔ cup with each meal, between meals, and before bed. With each serving he took 100 milligrams of pantothenic acid and 500 milligrams of vitamin C. He was told to double the vitamin C if the pain became particularly severe; and to reduce the quantities to

50 milligrams of pantothenic acid and 250 milligrams of vitamin C with each meal and mid-meal when all pain and stiffness had disappeared, but to increase them again immediately if under stress. After meals, or three times daily, he took 2 tablets of balanced B vitamins and 100 units of vitamin E; and once daily, a capsule supplying 25,000 units of natural vitamin A and 2,500 units of natural vitamin D, from fish-liver oil. He reduced all supplements to half after he improved.

To supply more antistress factors than were furnished in yeast and soy flour, he ate ¼ pound of fresh liver daily and took 1 tablespoon or more of desiccated liver or 15 liver tablets with any meal at which fresh liver was not eaten; he had wheat germ or wheat germ and middlings as a breakfast cereal on the mornings liver was not served; and at lunch or dinner he had a steamed green leafy vegetable seasoned with oil and vinegar. Because salt (sodium) is lost from the body when the adrenals are exhausted, he was asked to eat salty foods or have salted nuts daily. In other respects his diet was that outlined in chapter 33; and he was asked to forgo all refined foods, hydrogenated fats, coffee, and alcohol.

He lost 20 pounds while adhering to the diet, and reported that he found it easy to follow. Individuals with a less efficient digestive system, however, should probably take digestive enzymes and hydrochloric acid with each meal (ch. 13); people deficient in pantothenic acid have little hydrochloric acid in their stomachs.[21] Individuals with severely crippling arthritis have scar tissue around the joints,[27] and its removal is essential before recovery (ch. 4); therefore they should probably take at least 600 units of vitamin E daily.

The nutrients that must be emphasized are the same regardless of whether the diagnosis has been rheumatoid or osteoarthritis, bursitis, spondylitis, or other classifications of the disease.

When medication is given. No nutrient interferes in any way with cortisone, ACTH, or aspirin therapy. Each of these medications increases the need for vitamin C, and aspirin especially destroys huge quantities of it.[28] The "side effects" of cortisone therapy such as ulcers, pancreatitis, demineralized bones, and diabetic-like symptoms are far less severe when pantothenic acid is generously supplied;[14,29,30] and if ACTH is given without simultaneously increasing pantothenic acid, the adrenal glands can be severely damaged.[31] Since 10,000 milligrams (10 grams) of pantothenic acid have been given daily with only good results,[32] there need be no fear of taking too much. After an adequate diet has stimulated the natural hormone production, medication is rarely needed.

A diet low in salt and unusually high in protein and all the B vitamins greatly decreases the toxic effects of cortisone,[18,26,33-35] When cortisone is taken, salt (sodium and pounds of water are held in the tissues and a potassium deficiency is produced (p. 29). In rats a lack of potassium causes the adrenals to become severely damaged.[36] The retained fluid both presses against the sore joints and causes the blood pressure to increase. If several 1-gram tablets of potassium chloride (15 grains each) are taken throughout the day, sodium and water are excreted and the blood pressure usually decreases. The quantity of potassium needed varies with the amounts of cortisone taken and of water retained. A friend who was being given cortisone because of severe arthritis took 9 grams of potassium chloride daily for a week, lost 6 pounds of water, and had a marked decrease in blood pressure; later 3 grams daily prevented water retention.

A psychosomatic illness. Any variety of severe stress can exhaust the adrenals. Few stresses, however, are long-lasting—infections clear up; weather changes; quarrels are forgotten; hard work is followed by rest, ad infinitum. Arthritis, however, may appear in early adulthood and become steadily worse through each decade of life; hence the stress causing it is prolonged and unrelenting. Such stress usually comes from the bottled-up negative emotions experienced during early childhood. It is now generally accepted that severe crippling arthritis is a psychosomatic illness resulting largely from unconscious, accumulated anger.

Two books dealing with psychosomatic diseases are Flanders Dunbar's *Mind and Body: Psychosomatic Medicine*, and Arnold Hutschnecker's *The Will to Live,* but there are few others, largely I suspect because the origin of such illnesses seems too fantastic to be believed. Yet if we are to recover from such diseases, we must have some understanding of them. The following comments apply not only to arthritis, but also to all illnesses that have originated because strong emotions were not given free expression.

I learned about psychosomatic diseases and arthritis in particular from personal experience. For a number of years I was under psychoanalysis, a process by which the

emotional deprivations of early childhood can be overcome and some degree of emotional maturity attained.
Though I had rarely been sick before, during this period I
had so many psychosomatic illnesses—migraine headaches,
sinus "infections," "hay fever," skin rashes, emotionally
induced colds, arthritis, digestive disturbances, and many
others—that my unconscious mind seemed determined to
teach me there were causes of illness aside from poor nutrition. Each bout of sickness, however, lasted only a day or
two.

When a kindly woman analyst, who took the role of
loving mother to me, mentioned that I was angry because
my mother had died, I felt her remark to be utterly
ridiculous. Yet the day she told me she was going to
Europe, I developed severe arthritis; my jaws became
acutely sore and every joint in both hands grew red,
swollen, and excruciatingly painful. She helped me understand that the impending separation had unconsciously
reminded me of being taken from my ill mother when I
was ten days old, an experience which, relived later under
hypnosis to allow further understanding, had been a horri-
fying one. I learned that a tiny baby's emotions are raw
and violent and that its reaction to suffering is animalistic
and primitive anger; and I was overcome with an intense
desire to bite and claw. Next I learned that the negative
emotion I as a child had wanted to express but could not
had to be expressed before the psychosomatic illness
would clear up. My arthritis disappeared as soon as I
expressed these emotions by biting on chewing gum and
caramel corn and by clawing the eyes out of imaginary
enemies and faces made with finger paints on foolscap.

My analyst's departure caused me to "relive" my mother's death, or again to experience the feelings I had at that
time; to a 17-month-old baby, a mother's death is pure
desertion and unbelievably agonizing. Again I developed
severe arthritis, but this time it took the form of swollen,
inflamed, and intensely painful wrists, elbows, ankles, and
knees and sore, stiff shoulders and hips. An older child's
reaction to anger, I discovered, is an overpowering desire
to kick and hit. This emotion was expressed during a day
spent painfully kicking and hitting a pillow and working
out on the children's punching bag.

To understand emotionally induced illness, one must
realize that the nerves in the brain retain a detailed
permanent record of every instant of our lives; and that
this record includes all of our feelings, both our positive

and negative emotions, our convictions, and our original decisions as to how we could safely react to a given situation. The early experiences are spoken of as unconscious because they have long been forgotten. Without our awareness, however, present feelings or experiences similar to early ones cause electricity in the brain to pass instantaneously over the nerves on which the original emotions are registered. As with a tape recorder, a playback occurs, and we unconsciously relive the feeling of the earlier experience.

Young children quickly learn that negative emotions, if expressed, bring disapproval, punishment, and the temporary withdrawal of love. Unless the child is allowed some harmless way to express negative emotions, he must bottle them up and hold them in at all costs. In any form of psychosomatic illness, the "child" (who is very much alive in each of us) is doing the "thinking" rather than the logical adult mind. The unconscious mind—the mind of the child within us—purposely induces many psychosomatic illnesses to prevent the expression of negative emotions which would keep us from being loved. To the small child's way of thinking, it is better to become immobile, or to produce arthritis in one's self, than to allow bottled-up anger to explode.

Unconscious anger, which psychologists speak of as hostilities, is the accumulation or sum total of all forgotten annoyances experienced during a lifetime. It is important to realize that we need not be ashamed of anger or of expressing it harmlessly. Our race survived because we have the ability to become angry and to fight when necessary. Regardless of how kind and loving the parents, every child not a hopeless Milquetoast experiences many situations that stimulate anger; and "Don't you dare speak to me in that tone of voice" is all too familiar. It is not necessary to know the specific origin of anger, but only to recognize that it exists in all of us. Adults unconsciously express stored anger in barbed humor, malicious gossip, and a thousand petty ways, but when expressed, love, which is held back with the negative emotions, comes through to help us have warmer, closer relationships with others.

Although none of us asked for them, emotional problems stemming from early traumas and deprivations are universal and take many different forms. The person with arthritis may have had more to be angry about than other individuals, or stricter parents may have given him less freedom or mean to express his emotions harmlessly.

Because of such a background, the arthritic person usually has great difficulty in expressing anger; and since his unconscious mind prevents him from feeling it, he often denies that it could even exist. The unconscious mind also has vivid records of punishments and feelings of being unloved, and the ghosts of disapproving parents are always with us.

The patient whose arthritis is emotional in origin has three choices: to accept and express his hostilities as best he can; to find hobbies which can, with his own and social approval, drain off pent-up emotions, such as gardening, painting, sculpturing, playing a musical instrument, or working with clay; or to accept the possibility of becoming increasingly more crippled for a lifetime. Dr. Smiley Blanton, the famous New York psychiatrist, says it is not an apple a day that keeps the doctor away nearly as much as a daily "thought murder." Even the most crippled arthritic may secretly indulge in fantasies of destroying imaginary enemies.

In the past, anger was unconsciously vented at the woodpile and while gardening, wringing out clothes, and puffing up featherbeds; heads were symbolically chopped off, necks wrung, and imaginary justice meted out. The Mexican women who wash clothes by beating them against rocks probably get their husbands' pants unusually clean when they are furious with them. But alas, these outlets are not available to most of us.

The unbelievable happens. Although an injection of cortisone may bring almost immediate improvement to a severely crippled arthritic, I had no idea that expressed hostilities could accomplish the same quick results until a 64-year-old woman consulted me. The following incident is so amazing that I am certain I would never believe it had I not witnessed it. This woman crept with shuffling, agonizing steps into my office, lowered herself into a chair by painful, deliberate degrees, and told me that she had had arthritis for years but that it had suddenly become worse; that she had spent thousands on medical bills; and that she had screamed with pain all the previous night.

Because I sensed that she was writhing with anger and guessed correctly that she and her husband had quarreled on the way to see me, I placed a large pillow securely in the corner of the room, helped her walk to it, and suggested that she kick it "to improve her circulation." She amazed me by kicking with tremendous vigor. I then tucked the pillow into an arm of a davenport and asked her to hit it. She not only beat it with unbelievable rapidity but was soon swearing like a sailor's parrot. "Take this, you dirty ..." After the furious hitting and swearing had continued for a full ten minutes, she walked quickly to the chair and sat down. A moment later she realized what she had done. "Look, I can sit down!" she exclaimed excitedly. "Look, I can get up!" For another ten minutes she joyously popped up and down like a jack-in-a-box.

When she came for a second appointment three weeks later I did not recognize her. Her posture had improved, she looked years younger, and no arthritis remained. She had adhered carefully to her diet and had continued her daily hitting and kicking "exercises." Her husband was annoying her much less than before. Recently retired, he had followed her about criticizing her housekeeping, and had unconsciously reminded her of an equally domineering and fault-finding father. She even told me with great pride that after church each Sunday "people *come to me now* to talk about their troubles."

A similar case was a younger woman whose husband, a navy officer, went to sea leaving her an arthritic invalid and returned to find a glowing, outgoing woman already knee-deep in community activities. She told me that after he had heard what had happened, he had said, "I love you, darling, but right now I love Adelle more."

Such cases, of course, are rare. Sometimes it takes years of work with a psychiatrist before hostilities are sufficiently expressed for arthritis to disappear.

A possible mechanism. Years of research by Dr. Hans Selye and his co-workers have revealed a mechanism by which emotional problems may induce arthritis. When the parathyroid hormone or a toxic form of vitamin D is given to young rats, calcium is withdrawn from the bones, simulating the withdrawal of calcium during stress, and advanced old age is produced, including wrinkles, squeaky voices, cataracts, and shriveled sex glands.[27] If the soft tissues are harmed in any way, the calcium withdrawn from the bones is laid down in the damaged area.

The tissues of his animals have been harmed by being pinched, hit, scratched, or having hairs pulled out; by the animals being given a wide variety of chemicals, drugs, and organic compounds, or injections of bacteria, virus, or raw egg white, simulating an allergy. Dr. Selye emphasizes that the damage causing a specific area to be calcified may be extremely mild, that the blood calcium remains consist-

ently normal, and that the similarly harmed tissues of
other animals do not become calcified unless the bones
have been previously robbed of calcium.

By varying the type and location of the damage, Dr.
Selye has produced the counterparts of such human diseases as arthritis, hardening of the arteries, and many
other little-understood illnesses. If large amounts of vitamin E are given with the substances that cause calcium to
be withdrawn from the bones, however, the calcification
of soft tissues, the old-age changes, and the production of
disease is completely prevented.[6,37]

From this research it seems possible that the strain put
on the soft tissues near the joints when the unconscious
mind is holding back negative emotions may cause the
slight damage necessary to attract the calcium already
withdrawn from the bones by stress. An incident that
causes this slight damage may also be trivial. For example,
I was recently annoyed, when swamped with work, at
having to waste an entire afternoon going to court with
my 17-year-old son, who had ignored a stop sign. Later he
dropped me off at home with a discourteous "So long. Be
seein' ya." By evening I felt utterly exhausted, seemingly
without cause, and soon arthritic pains drove me to bed.
While wondering what had brought on this turn of events,
I realized I was furious with George for not having said
"Thank you," and that his thoughtlessness had apparently
push-buttoned earlier experiences when I had felt unap-
preciated and been angered by it. In this case, some very
unmotherly fantasies solved the problem.

Psychiatrists agree that holding back negative emotions
is a major cause of fatigue. When such emotions are
continuously held in year after year, tissues might easily
be damaged sufficiently for calcium to be laid down. It
may be that scar tissue, which forms around the joints in
arthritis[27] and is not unlike the base of bones, develops in
the absence of vitamin E before calcium can be deposited.
Certainly Dr. Selye's work indicates that people with arthritis should take generous amounts of vitamin E.[6,37]

Diets are not adhered to. The problem in attempting to
help most people with arthritis is that they can rarely
adhere to a diet. Negative feelings, even though unconscious, are difficult to hold back when one is weak; they
are doubly difficult when one becomes stronger. For this
reason, unless hostilities are expressed, the upsurge of
energy that occurs after nutrition is improved often causes
persons suffering from psychosomatic illnesses to develop

extreme anxiety, nervousness, and depression. Regardless of how much they may consciously wish to help themselves, I have learned to expect them to discard an adequate diet within three days. Even though no food is given that a six-month-old baby could not handle, the diet "doesn't agree with them," and they develop digestive upsets, headaches, or other uncomfortable symptoms. The child's mind is saying to each person, "The arthritis (or other emotionally induced disease) must be kept at all costs."

Another rapidly increasing disease. Arthritis is yet another disease that is rapidly increasing in persons of all ages. During the past few months I have planned diets for a six-month-old baby, several children four and five years old, and a 15-year-old girl, each with severe crippling arthritis, though in small children it is spoken of as Still's disease. Fortunately, all of them have responded quickly to an adequate diet, but had their nutrition been good, suffering would never have occurred.

Because the national diet becomes increasingly deficient and because it is difficult to rid oneself of stresses, particularly unconscious emotional ones, arthritis will undoubtedly always be with us. Yet stress can be relieved. Adequate diets can be followed. Tortured bodies can be rebuilt. It has been done; perhaps it can be done by you.

11
Nip Infections in the Bud

When attacked by bacteria or viruses, the healthy body mobilizes its army, navy, air force, and marines so quickly that no infection occurs. These armed forces consist of white blood cells, lymph cells, and antibodies, or globulins, which are ineffective without a co-worker, the complement. When this standing army is sufficiently large, it destroys bacteria, viruses, and their toxins by engulfing and digesting them with the aid of enzymes or by combining with them, causing them to settle out, or by other means. An adequate diet can quickly increase all of these defenses even after an infection gets a foothold provided various nutrients are given in generous amounts the minute the first symptoms appear.

The body's armed forces are identical regardless of the location of the infection or the types of viruses or bacteria involved. Because a physician is rarely consulted until illness is advanced, each individual should know the immediate steps to take to fight an infection.

The effect of stress. The adrenal hormone DOC mobilizes the body's defenses. This hormone is so completely held in check by the excessive amounts of cortisone produced during stress (p. 28) that the body often cannot protect itself, and infections may become rampant, as they frequently do when cortisone medication is given.[1] In this case, an antistress diet (p. 31) is needed to increase the production of DOC. If the adrenals are too exhausted to produce an adequate amount of cortisone, however, DOC is not sufficiently held in check, and lymph glands, such as the tonsils and adenoids, become enlarged; the white blood count soars; and inflammation at the point of the infection is marked by redness, swelling, pain, and fever.[1] To eliminate these symptoms, cortisone production must be stimulated at all possible speed. When one is under stress, therefore, whether too much or too little cortisone is being

118

produced, the body becomes susceptible to infections unless the diet is unusually adequate.

During most infections, too little aldosterone (p. 28) can be produced, salt (sodium) is lost from the body, cells become more permeable, or sievelike, and water accumulates in the inflamed area, increasing the swelling and pain. This fact has raised to scientific status our grandmothers' favorite remedy of giving ½ teaspoon each of salt and soda in hot water for colds, sore throats, intestinal flu, and any localized inflammation in which water (swelling) accumulates in a given area. After the blood sodium has thus been replaced, swelling often goes down in a few moments; a stuffy nose becomes clear and other symptoms disappear. Unless small, frequent meals are eaten, however, the blood sodium soon drops again.

The lymph glands produce antibodies and lymph cells needed to fight infections.[2] If cortisone is being synthesized normally, the proteins in these glands are broken down and the glands shrivel during the stresses that have preceded and are imposed by the bacterial or viral attack. Swollen lymph glands, such as those under the chin and behind the ears, or enlarged tonsils or adenoids always show that cortisone is not being produced in adequate amounts. Although the swollen glands are trying to fight the infection, the defense mechanisms are weak at the very time they are needed most. To recover from an infection, therefore, the first step must be to stimulate adrenal function.

Since pantothenic acid is essential for cortisone production, low resistance to spontaneous infections is the first sign of an undersupply of pantothenic acid.[3] Infections appear long before other deficiency symptoms can be detected and more quickly than if any other nutrient were missing.[4] Animals even mildly deficient in pantothenic acid or vitamin B_6 show an immediate marked reduction in antibodies, complement, and white blood cells; and if "vaccinated," immunity is not increased.[4-9] Some strains of rats—and also certain families or individuals[10]—require many times more pantothenic acid than others and are far more harmed by a deficiency.[3]

In volunteers lacking pantothenic acid and vitamin B_6, so few antibodies and white blood cells could be produced that they had continuous infections, particularly sore throats, or acute pharyngitis;[11-13] and when vaccinated for tetanus, typhoid, and polio, showed no increase in antibody production.[14] When stress has not harmed the adrenal or lymph glands too severely, giving 40 milligrams of vitamin B_6 to persons with infections increased both the white blood count and the antibody production within three hours.[15] Recovery was slow, however, even when such huge amounts as 4,000 and 600 milligrams of pantothenic acid and vitamin B_6 respectively were given daily to volunteers who had been deficient in these vitamins for several weeks.[12] In fact, 17 out of 18 patients lacking vitamin B_6 showed an "absolute decrease" in white blood cells in five days.[16]

A diet undersupplied with vitamins B_1, B_2, folic acid, biotin, or niacin inhibits the production of antibodies, white blood cells, and the complement,[5-7] though less severely than when pantothenic acid or vitamin B_6 is limited. A lack of any of these vitamins also prevents the body's defenses from being stimulated when antitoxins and other forms of immunization are given.[6,17,18]

Vitamin C can perform near miracles. A tremendous amount of research has proved that vitamin C is vitally important in overcoming infections, but the use of antibiotics—and greater profits made from their sale, I suspect—has largely kept this knowledge in mothballs. In a single year no less than 45 research projects reported that vitamin C rendered harmless a wide variety of bacterial toxins, and inhibited the growth of whatever bacteria it failed to destroy;[19-21] that its action was non-specific in that it was deadly to all types of viruses[22-27] and bacteria;[19,28] and that while small amounts could bring some immunity,[29,30] huge doses were much more effective. When large quantities were given to guinea pigs already injected with bacteria, 99 per cent of the body cells showed evidence of bacterial destruction in a single hour.[31]

Multiple protective functions are performed by vitamin C. It not only aids the adrenals,[32,33] but also stimulates the production of antibodies,[34-36] white blood cells,[37,38] and the complement,[39-41] and increases the bacteria-destroying ability of white blood cells.[42,43] A count of approximately 5,000 white blood cells is considered to be normal. A high white blood count shows that an infection exists and also that the body is fighting it; a low count indicates that the body has no resources with which to fight. When 1,000 milligrams of vitamin C have been taken daily during a cold, the white count has promptly risen from far below normal to 9,000 or more.[43,44] No amount of this vitamin or any other, however, can cause an excessive production of white cells, such as occurs in leukemia.

During the past two decades, Dr. Fred R. Klenner, of Reidsville, North Carolina, has used massive quantities of vitamin C in treating successfully patients of all ages suffering from such serious illnesses as encephalitis, meningitis, poliomyelitis, virus pneumonia, tetanus, or lockjaw, and many other infections.[22-27,45-48] Usually these patients had extremely high fever, were unconscious, and many had been given up earlier by physicians who believed them to be beyond help; some appeared to be dying, and in one case *rigor mortis* had actually set in.

To extremely ill patients Dr. Klenner gave the vitamin by injection in amounts ranging from 2 to 4 grams (2,000 to 4,000 milligrams) approximately every two to four hours around the clock, the amount and number of injections depending on the progress of each individual. Sometimes he gave antibiotics or other medications in addition to vitamin C, although these drugs had usually been given by other physicians before the patients had become so desperately ill. An amazing number of these persons regained consciousness quickly, were able to drink juices within a few hours, took further vitamin C by mouth, and were discharged from the hospital in three or four days.

Dr. Klenner has found that the vitamin is more effective when given with some form of calcium. He emphasizes that the amount of vitamin C required varies with the seriousness of the illness. Because viruses and bacteria not destroyed quickly multiply, bringing a recurrence of symptoms, and because this vitamin is not toxic,[49] he believes it is better to err by taking too much rather than too little. He has said, "Ascorbic acid in proper doses can and will save countless individuals once physicians awaken to the real value of this vitamin."[24]

Other doctors have shown that massive amounts of vitamin C compare favorably with antibiotics, but have no toxic effects;[80] and that the vitamin was particularly helpful in speeding recovery from mononucleosis[81] and infectious hepatitis[81-83] even after all medication had proved futile.[82]

Since learning of Dr. Klenner's work, I have known literally hundreds of persons who made remarkable recoveries after taking large amounts of vitamin C. One man had such severe mumps that his physician wanted to hospitalize him; he refused, knowing that vitamin C would not be allowed him. The following morning the same doctor declared the diagnosis had been wrong. The patient's wife claimed that only a computer could calculate the amount of vitamin C he took. Several children have had one-day measles; and in a single week four men with prostate infections consulted me, all of whom had taken antibiotics for weeks, yet each returned to work a few days later. Perhaps four dozen persons with mononucleosis recovered in a week when large amounts of vitamins B_6 and C and pantothenic acid were taken around the clock.

Protein cannot be overemphasized. Antibodies, the complement, white blood cells, and lymph cells are all made of complete protein; hence a lack of this nutrient can prevent recovery from infections regardless of the amounts of vitamins obtained. Of single amino acids, methionine and tryptophane, generously supplied in eggs and milk, are particularly valuable.[5,7,50-52] When a low-protein diet has been replaced by one high in protein, the production of antibodies has increased a hundredfold within a few hours. Of single proteins tested for their ability to build body defenses, liver, yeast, and especially wheat germ proved most valuable.[53,54] Egg yolk, meat, milk, and full-fat soy flour, in this order, particularly increased the production of white blood cells.[50]

Although the stress of the infection itself tremendously increases the need for protein, the protein requirements are made even higher during many infections because albumin from the blood is lost in the feces.[55-57]

Physicians frequently give injections of gamma globulin —one form of antibodies—to persons suffering from infections, but unless the patient is too ill to eat or has severe diarrhea, his own body can produce far more gamma globulin than can be given by injection provided he obtains adequate protein.[14,58] When the nutrition is improved, the production of all defense mechanisms increases simultaneously.

Vitamin A and infections. Deficiencies of vitamin A are far more widespread in America than we like to believe.[59] This vitamin plays a particularly important role in preventing or clearing up infections of the skin, the cornea of the eye, and the mucous membranes which line all body cavities, although it is also necessary for the production of antibodies and white blood cells.[5,7] When vitamin A is undersupplied, millions of cells in the lower layers of the skin and the surface of the mucous membranes die quickly and accumulate; cells lining the body cavities can no longer secrete mucus, which normally washes the tissues and carries the white blood cells.[60] Whether in the skin or the mucous membranes, the accumulation of dead cells serves as food for bacteria.

A five-year study of 1,100 people revealed that individuals whose blood was consistently low in vitamins A and C contracted by far the most infections.[61] The blood vitamin A drops sharply during infections,[62-64] is often lost in the urine,[65] and may disappear completely during measles and high fever.[66] Moreover, cortisone and a number of drugs rapidly deplete the body of its vitamin-A stores and tremendously increase the need for it.[4] Unless vitamin A is generously supplied, the body is left susceptible to more serious infections. Well-known examples are kidney infections following rheumatic fever, encephalitis following measles, and endocarditis following a strep throat.

Vitamin A given to groups of patients has shortened the duration of such infections as measles, scarlet fever, pneumonia, and infections of the eyes, middle ear, sinuses, kidneys, intestines, ovaries, uterus, and vagina.[67-70] The vitamin has proved valuable, too, in clearing up impetigo, boils, carbuncles, and open ulcers, particularly when applied locally.[15,71,72]

Though vitamin A is usually well absorbed during infections,[65] a water-dispersed preparation is preferable to that dissolved in oil when an illness is acute or diarrhea occurs.[73] Physicians have given 200,000 units daily to adults for six months[17,72] with no signs of toxicity being recognized, though rarely are more than 25,000 units needed daily.[74] Unless vitamin E is amply supplied, however, the vitamin A obtained from foods or supplements, the vitamin A already in the blood, and that stored in the liver and other body tissues is quickly destroyed by oxygen;[75] therefore, what appears to be a lack of vitamin A may in fact be a deficiency of vitamin E.

Prevent acidosis. If a person feels too ill to eat, the blood sugar quickly drops and acidosis develops (p. 97), causing irritability, headache, nausea, and vomiting, often mistakenly considered to be symptoms of the illness itself. Acidosis can be completely prevented if, immediately at the onset of any infection, some food containing sugar is taken every hour or two: sections of orange, bits of cooked fruit, sips of fruit juice, eggnog, milk sweetened with honey, or any food containing starch or natural sugar.

If vomiting has already set in, it can usually be stopped if a few tablespoons of sweetened orange juice or teaspoons of honey are taken every 15 minutes and continued even though the vomiting persists for a time. As soon as vomiting has stopped, milk, juices, and other liquids should be given to replace the fluids lost. Feverish children can sometimes be tempted by popsicles made of undiluted frozen orange juice and yogurt. Because the nutritional needs at this time are so great, a patient should not be given soft drinks.

Diet during an infection. Aside from preventing acidosis, the diet should meet the increased nutritional demands of stress, mobilize all defense mechanisms, detoxify any drugs used, and, if antibiotics are taken by mouth (p. 145), replace the intestinal bacteria destroyed by them. When these requirements are met, recovery is often remarkably rapid.

For example, a 19-year-old girl with mononucleosis— she wished to remain anonymous because it is called the kissing disease—was heartbroken last spring when her physician told her she could not finish the college semester. In addition to the medication he was giving her, she started on Tuesday to take every two hours she was awake a half cup of highly fortified milk (p. 329) with the antistress formula (p. 31) and 500 extra milligrams of vitamin C. Because she soon felt better, she took the vitamins only haphazardly the two following days. By Thursday night, however, her sore throat had become worse and she could scarcely talk or breathe, an experience which, according to her mother, "made a Christian out of her." For the next three days she obtained the full quart of pep-up with the supplements; and her physician permitted her to return to college Monday morning.

An almost identical report came recently from a young man who had taken the antistress formula, extra vitamin C, and fortified milk every two hours during an attack of rheumatic fever. Although previous attacks had lasted six months, he too returned to college in a week.

When the throat is sore or if a child is too young to swallow tablets, supplements should be obtained in powder form or the tablets dissolved in water (p. 326).

The amounts of vitamin C needed. The severity of an infection should determine the quantity of vitamin C to take; and unless huge amounts are obtained, a deficiency can quickly occur, causing bruises, bleeding gums, nosebleeds, and hemorrhages even when the intake seems adequate.[33] The largest amount of vitamin C I have ever known a person to use over a prolonged period was that taken by a Texas attorney who had such severe phlebitis that his doctor wanted to amputate his leg at the hip. Later he wrote me, "Instead, I took 25 grams of vitamin C a la Dr. Klenner, and the swelling was very much less the following afternoon. I got completely well in 3 weeks and in fact only lost 2 weeks from my office. I had 2 other attacks of phlebitis, and commenced taking vitamin C in 5 gram doses and continued taking it until I had taken 1,600 grams; and I am well aware that a gram is 1,000 milligrams. I finally broke out in a rash from too much C but this did not come until I had taken 1,600 grams at the rate of 15 to 40 grams a day."

A woman in Maryland had much the same experience when she took approximately 25 grams (25,000 milligrams) of vitamin C daily for phlebitis, although half that quantity had not brought improvement. She wrote, "In 5 days the pink stripe and the terrible looking bumps and discoloration between my knee and ankle disappeared and my leg is as beautiful as when I was 17. My doctor, who had wanted to operate, says it was bed rest and not vitamin C which did it, but when I asked him why 4 months of bed rest earlier had not cleared it up, he had no answer."

Massive amounts of vitamin C have been used without toxicity in a wide variety of illnesses, including certain mental conditions. One physician gave a 45-year-old woman with schizophrenia 1,000 milligrams of vitamin C every hour, and at the end of 48 hours, by which time she had taken 45 grams, she was mentally well and remained so until she died some time later of cancer.[84]

The largest quantity of vitamin C I have known to be given in a short period was to an eight-year-old girl who had been unconscious from encephalitis for 36 hours and whose physician had been unable to get her into a hospital. Because vitamin-C solution spilled when her mother and I tried to give it, we froze it in an ice tray; almost continuously throughout an afternoon we slipped tiny bits of this "sherbet" into the child's slightly opened mouth. That evening she was admitted to the hospital and put in a ward with other children who had been unconscious from ten days to five weeks. The following morning, however, this child was alert, free from fever, and ate a hearty breakfast. She was permitted to go home at noon after tests showed that her brain had not been damaged. Her mother and I had each dissolved 100 tablets of 250 milligrams each, a total of 50 grams—50,000 milligrams—and we had given her this amount in a single afternoon.

Far less vitamin C is needed when pantothenic acid and vitamin B_6 are given simultaneously, but this fact was not known at that time.

In general, the more serious the illness, the larger should be the quantity of vitamins obtained, particularly at first, and the more frequently they should be taken. For example, at the onset of an infection, one might take 2,000 to 3,000 milligrams of vitamin C, 100 to 300 milligrams of pantothenic acid, and 10 to 30 milligrams of vitamin B_6, and then take half these quantities every two or three hours thereafter. If the infection is acute, the vitamins should be given every three hours during the first night, always with fortified milk. As the symptoms subside, smaller amounts can be taken, but if a relapse occurs, the quantities should be immediately increased. When recovery is complete, the antistress formula (p. 31) may be discontinued.

Provided the vitamins are consistently taken with a highly fortified drink, the quantities suggested here have brought excellent results to persons suffering from such a wide variety of infections as sore throats, pancreatitis, shingles, rheumatic fever, flu, infections of the sinuses, eyes, ears, or kidneys, and any of the respiratory infections. I have yet to know of a child whose tonsils or adenoids had to be removed after he was given the antistress formula with an adequate diet. Unless the illness is extremely mild, however, each individual should be under the care of a physician, and the vitamins and milk drink taken with whatever medication is prescribed.

The rashes that occasionally occur when vitamins are taken are apparently caused by the filler holding the tablets together and usually disappear when a different brand is purchased. Extremely large amounts of vitamin C will sometimes cause diarrhea, indicating that more is being taken than is needed; if this tendency is noticed, the amounts should be immediately decreased. When not under stress, 75 milligrams of vitamin C daily is considered to be ample.

Special problems of particular infections. Some infections cause the requirements for certain nutrients to be unusually high. Thus, during and after rheumatic fever, nephritis, and many other infections, vitamin E should be generously supplied to prevent the formation of scar tissue, which may be more damaging than the illness itself. Measles cause the need for vitamin A to skyrocket, and if not supplied, the eyes or kidneys may be permanently harmed. In polio, which still exists, the requirement for all the B vitamins is markedly increased; and paralysis can apparently be prevented if these vitamins are taken in generous amounts. Undulant fever is said to clear up if above-adequate amounts of magnesium and manganese are given. All nutrients helpful in stopping infections and rebuilding bones (ch. 26) are needed when pyorrhea exists. Vincent's disease, or trench mouth, and canker sores are often corrected when 100 milligrams of niacin amide are taken at each meal.[76,77] The need for vitamin B_6 appears to be particularly high during any infection of the alimentary tract, and a lack of it even causes rampant tooth decay.[78]

If the adrenals can produce cortisone, the lymph glands immediately decrease in size when the body is under stress; therefore enlarged lymph glands, whether tonsils, swollen adenoids, the lymph glands in the neck, or anywhere in the body invariably show adrenal exhaustion and an increased need for all body requirements. Pantothenic acid and vitamins B_6 and C particularly should be given until all swelling has subsided.

During prolonged infections, such as tuberculosis, undulant fever, or subacute bacterial endocarditis, no fewer than 500, 50, and 2 milligrams of vitamin C, pantothenic acid, and vitamin B_6 respectively should be taken with each meal and between each meal, or six times each day. When stress is unrelenting, it becomes vitally important to see that every body requirement is amply supplied (ch. 32); and a full quart of fortified milk should be obtained daily. When the nutritional needs are met, recovery can sometimes be unbelievably shortened.

Once I planned a diet—essentially that outlined on pages 330 331—for a young woman suffering from severe tuberculosis. She asked me how long it would be before any healing could be expected. My estimation was four months. She then told her physician that I said she would be well in four months. He answered that such a thing was impossible. I not only agreed with him but was annoyed at being misquoted. Yet exactly four months after starting her nutrition program, she insisted on a thorough examination and was indeed pronounced well. When we were building a new home some time later, the chief carpenter turned out to be this woman's husband; and because he was deeply grateful, probably no nails have ever been driven with more tender loving care.

Some "infections" are psychosomatic. A number of so-called infections, which include some—but certainly not all—colds, postnasal drips, hay fever, sinus "infections" and puffiness around the eyes, are psychosomatic in origin and stem from an unconscious need to cry. Literally hundreds of times during early childhood when the desire to cry may have been intense, many of us heard such expressions as "Don't be a crybaby" or a harsh "If you don't shut up, I'll give you something to cry about." Such experiences, though forgotten, are permanently recorded in the brain. When current happenings unconsciously remind us of similar earlier experiences and tears are still held back, the need to cry seeks a socially acceptable form of expression. For this reason the common cold will probably never be conquered. In our culture we prefer that a man writhe with hemorrhaging ulcers rather than shed a tear.

Lucy Freeman in her book *Fight Against Fears* tells how her chronic sinus "infection" cleared up when she was given the freedom of tears while under psychoanalysis. I was repeatedly embarrassed during my own psychotherapy by developing what appeared to be extremely severe colds, which no amount of good nutrition would budge; and persons who consulted me at that time understandably lifted a heal-thyself eyebrow. Yet invariably all symptoms dsappeared immediately after I permitted myself to cry or the analyst pointed out why I was "crying." Such "infections" are impossible to distinguish from those induced by viruses or bacteria, but obviously cannot be helped by the best of nutrition.

An elderly unmarried woman who had had a lifelong stuffy nose and postnasal drip once consulted me. She assured me she could not cry, but she was so eager to co-operate when I suggested that she cry freely that she peeled onions daily, which of course was of no value. Eventually, after reading about some children who had been frozen to death while lost in the mountains, tears flowed copiously; she herself had been "frozen" from lack of love early in life. When she could once cry without shame, her postnasal drip disappeared.

Every nutrient is important. In attempting to overcome infections, it is particularly important not to overemphasize any one nutrient to the exclusion of others. Even during illness it is best not to put all your eggs in one basket, nutritious eggs though they may be.

12
Skin Problems Are More Than Skin Deep

When nutrition is less than adequate, the skin is subject to an amazing number of abnormalities; and the synthetic beauty fostered by the cosmetic industry is poor counterfeit for genuine attributes of health.

Oily or dry skin. When volunteers have been kept on diets mildly lacking in vitamin B_2, the first symptoms were whiteheads and oily hair and skin.[1] This condition cleared up soon after 5 to 15 milligrams of vitamin B_2 were given daily. To my knowledge, this abnormality has not been produced by any other deficiency.

Dryness of the skin has resulted in volunteers lacking vitamins A, C, linoleic acid, or any one of several B vitamins.[2,3] The oils of the skin are unsaturated and appear to be made almost wholly of the essential fatty acids; therefore unless vegetable oils are consumed, the skin is invariably dry. One young woman who consulted me had adhered to a fat-free diet for five years and described herself as looking like a mummy, a statement one could not dispute; and her friend said she was as flaky as a strudel. When the diet is adequate, however, both oiliness and dryness are usually corrected in a few weeks.

Susceptibility to sunburn. Persons especially prone to sunburn have tolerated 50 to 100 times more exposure than previously when taking 1,000 milligrams daily of the B vitamin PABA (para aminobenzoic acid); and applying a salve containing this vitamin has been equally effective.[4] Other individuals normally susceptible to sunburn but using a PABA ointment have remained eight or more hours in Florida sun without burning.[5] My secretary's three redheaded sons speak of PABA ointment as "weird" or "neat"; formerly their sore peeling skin, diagnosed as

129

precancerous, had interfered with their favorite sport, surfing. Their mother and many friends who used to sunburn quickly declare it to be "fabulous" and "miraculous."

Individuals previously unable to tolerate sun because of skin cancers have found PABA ointment to be particularly beneficial. Furthermore, this ointment takes the pain out of severe sunburns and other burns almost immediately. It has also been shown that the changes in aging skin are "practically identical" to those in the skin of young people overexposed to sun.[55-57] This finding indicates that PABA ointment, used as a cold cream, might delay old-age skin changes. Because PABA makes sulfanilamide ineffective, it cannot be purchased for internal use without a prescription, but preparations for external application are available.

Stretch marks. Although healthy skin is amazingly elastic, previously overweight persons and most women who have had children retain stretch marks. This abnormality appears to result from the stress of inadequate reducing and pregnancy diets, which have allowed body proteins to be destroyed to the extent that scars have taken the place of weakened tissues.

A friend who developed severe stretch marks during her first pregnancy stayed on an unusually adequate high-protein diet supplemented with 600 units of vitamin E and 300 milligrams of panthothenic acid daily throughout a subsequent pregnancy. Although she gave birth to full-term twins, the stretch marks from the first pregnancy completely disappeared and none formed during the second.

Wrinkles. In Dr. Selye's experiments in premature aging (p. 115), wrinkles could be prevented by giving large amounts of vitamin E.[6] It may be that the multiple stresses that induce aging cause cells in the lower layers of skin to be destroyed and bits of scar tissue to take their place; and that wrinkles form when such scar tissue contracts.

At times wrinkles do seem to disappear, and a few women of my acquaintance are taking vitamin E in hopes that theirs will. I am convinced, however, that scars remain unless the diet is so completely adequate that healthy tissue can be built to replace them.

Pigmentation of the skin. When the adrenals are exhausted, as in Addison's disease, the skin may become so deeply pigmented that formerly fair individuals are assumed to be of Mexican or Negro blood. Such people sometimes literally change beyond recognition after a few weeks of adhering to an adequate diet. Minor pigmentation, which appears first across the forehead and occurs so frequently during the stress of pregnancy that it is spoken of as pregnancy cap, is also common among undernourished persons[7] and probably always indicates a deficiency of pantothenic acid. This pigmentation quickly disappears when an antistress program is adhered to (p. 31).

People deficient in either of the B vitamins folic acid or niacin amide develop pigmentation of the skin, particularly in exposed areas.[8] Such pigmentation has cleared up when 5 milligrams of folic acid or 100 milligrams of niacin amide have been taken with each meal.[9]

Lack of pigmentation. In a condition known as vitiligo, areas of skin lose their pigmentation while other areas become darker. This increasingly common abnormality is another symptom of malnutrition,[4] and has been corrected by giving 150 to 300 milligrams of pantothenic acid daily[10] or 1,000 milligrams or more of PABA.[4,11] Applying PABA ointment to the depigmented areas sometimes brings marked improvement. This condition generally clears up after the diet is unusually high in all the natural sources of B vitamins. I once told a 30-year-old woman with severe vitiligo that liver would probably help her more than any other food. A week later she joyously returned to show me that not a trace of it remained but she had eaten ¼ pound of raw liver, frozen, diced, and covered with catsup, at each meal. Several other such persons have had the condition clear up slowly on a more appetizing diet.

Psoriasis and fatty tumors. The eczema-like skin condition psoriasis appears to result from the faulty utilization of fats. People with this abnormality usually have excessive amounts of cholesterol in their skin and blood,[12] and by the time their blood cholesterol has been reduced to normal, their psoriasis has cleared up. When 254 patients with psoriasis were given 4 to 8 tablespoons of lecithin daily, no new eruptions occurred after the first week and even the most severe cases recovered within five months.[12] Psoriasis has also been helped by vitamins A and B₆.[3,13] I recommend only 3 tablespoons of granular lecithin daily with every nutrient needed to help the liver produce its own lecithin (ch. 5).

Fatty tumors and cholesterol deposits, or atheromas, on or under the skin are also associated with low blood lecithin,[14] have been produced in animals by diets containing hydrogenated fat,[15] and are reduced by giving oil, lecithin, or unusually large amounts of vitamin C.[14,16] These tumors contain cholesterol, saturated fats, and a large percentage of peroxides, or toxic substances formed from fats in the absence of vitamin E,[17] a finding that indicates that vitamin E has been deficient and should be obtained in generous amounts.

Lip problems. Sore lips, whistle marks, and cracks at the angles of the mouth (or the eyes or around the base of the nose) have been produced in humans undersupplied with linoleic acid, folic acid, pantothenic acid, or vitamins B_2 or B_6.[1,18,19] When the diet is improved, the cracks and soreness usually clear up rapidly, but the whistle marks disappear with maddening slowness. Cold sores, or fever blisters, are discussed on page 135.

Eczemas result from many deficiencies. Various types of skin rashes and eczemas have been produced in humans and animals by deficiencies of essential fatty acids or almost any one of the B vitamins. The eczema resulting from too little linoleic acid starts as dry, scaly skin (pityriasis) and can become worse until the body is encrusted with heavy, itching scabs.[20] It is common in babies, small children, and adults who avoid oils, but usually clears up quickly when 1 to 3 tablespoons of safflower oil or other pressed oils are made part of the daily diet. Giving vitamin B_6 helps to alleviate this eczema, and conversely, oils help to correct eczemas occurring when vitamin B_6 is undersupplied.[21] Every mother unable to nurse her baby should give him a half teaspoon of oil daily; breast milk, although often low in vitamin B_6,[22] does contain linoleic acid whereas most formulas do not.

A dry, scaly, itching eczema occurs when a deficiency of the B vitamin biotin is brought on by taking oral antibiotics, which destroy the intestinal bacteria synthesizing this vitamin. The condition is corrected when the intestinal bacteria are replaced by taking acidophilus culture or eating generous amounts of yogurt.

A lack of PABA causes dermatitis in animals,[8] and this vitamin has been used successfully in clearing up a wide variety of human eczemas.[4] Another eczema, or dermatitis, which most frequently appears on the face, hands, and arms, and is usually associated with diarrhea and mental depression, clears quickly when 300 milligrams of niacin amide are added to the daily diet.

Deficiencies of vitamin B_2, or riboflavin, repeatedly produced in humans, result in a seborrheic dermatitis characterized by extreme itching and the oozing of a waxlike substance which dries into a hard, yellow crust.[3] In men this eczema first appears on the scrotum, or skin covering the testicles, and the red, scaly, raw, and weeping areas may surround the anus and extend onto the thighs; later it spreads to the face, scalp, and chest.[23] Although unaffected by numerous medications, it and a similar itching rash that occurs in and around the vagina "respond dramatically" after 15 milligrams of vitamin B_2 are taken daily.[23,24] Yeast, however, often clears up such eczemas more quickly than separate B vitamins.[3]

Vitamin-B_6 deficiencies produced in men have resulted in scaliness of the skin and "showers of dandruff"; and an itching, red rash on the skin over the testicles appeared during the first week.[25] This condition became steadily worse and more troublesome; and by the fourth week, the face, scalp, and arms were also covered by a dry, scaly, red, and itching eczema which did not clear up for two weeks after 600 milligrams of vitamin B_6 were given daily. Because magnesium decreases the need for vitamin B_6,[26,27] such skin problems can be helped by taking this mineral.

Other investigators, working with volunteers more mildly deficient in vitamin B_6, found that a scaly, oily eczema first appeared in the eyebrows, behind the ears, and around the nose and mouth;[13,28] and that it cleared up in two or three days as readily when 5 milligrams of vitamin B_6 were given as when 100 to 200 milligrams were used.[28,29] Because all the B vitamins mixed with salve absorb readily through the skin, a salve containing vitamin B_6 quickly corrected the eczema.[13] Often such salve takes away itching almost immediately.

A surprising number of patients living on hospital diets have been found to have eczemas identical to those produced by deficiencies of vitamin B_2 or B_6, and as much as 1,000 milligrams of vitamin B_6 have been given them for one to three weeks without improvement.[23,29] When a salve containing vitamin B_6 has been applied to the skin, however, all recovered.[29] Vitamin B_6 and magnesium are needed before certain enzymes containing vitamin B_6 can be made and activated.

When simultaneous deficiencies of vitamin B_6 and pantothenic acid have been produced in volunteers, the skin pained as if from sunburn.[30] Again dandruff was severe, and eczema appeared on the face, arms, and scrotum; this soreness and scaling became worse, the skin on the hands cracked, and a dry, scaly dermatitis eventually covered most of the body. Even after 600 and 2,000 milligrams of vitamin B_6 and pantothenic acid respectively were given daily, the skin did not become normal for three weeks.

Because eczemas can occur from a lack of so many separate B vitamins, spontaneous eczemas of unknown origin can be most successfully corrected by obtaining generous amounts of yeast, liver, and wheat germ.[3]

A young man once consulted me whose face, hands, and arms had been thickly encrusted with angry sores for years; and he told me, "It's also on my body," meaning scrotum. He was planning to be married, but, too sensitive to mention his condition to his bride-to-be, had puzzled her no end by repeatedly postponing the wedding date. He was convinced that his eczema was highly contagious, that he would infect her, and that the only solution was simply to disappear, deserting her, as it were, at the altar. Fortunately, an adequate diet quickly corrected the condition without further postponement of the wedding.

Because eczema around the testicles appears to be extremely common in men,[23,29] this case caused me to suspect that many marriages are damaged and full sexual expression thwarted by it.

Warts and skin infections. Various medications have been used with some success in alleviating warts. I have seen several unusually severe cases in adults permanently corrected within a few weeks when 50,000 units of vitamin A and 500 units of vitamin E were taken daily in addition to an adequate diet; after one month the vitamin A was reduced to 25,000 units daily. One of these cases was a boy with warts which were prying loose his fingernails, and several had already been painfully removed by an electric needle only to return. Recently a woman wrote me that a 100-unit vitamin-E capsule emptied onto a Band-Aid and placed over each wart caused hers to disappear in three days. I have heard of nothing, however, which prevents or removes moles.

The diet for anyone with boils, abscesses, carbuncles, impetigo, or virus infections such as shingles should be essentially the same as for other infections (ch. 11). Vitamins A and E should be particularly emphasized during such infection and for three or four months afterward. Impetigo often disappears rapidly when vitamins A and E are applied directly to the infected areas.[3]

The virus infections classified as herpes simplex, which appear as water blisters on the skin and may occur on the face, hands, abdomen, genitals, lips (cold sores or fever blisters), inside the mouth, and as shingles (herpes zoster), usually respond quickly if vitamins B_6 and C and pantothenic acid are taken with highly fortified milk (p. 329) around the clock.

Adolescent acne. Generous amounts of vitamin A have been reported to help adolescent acne, and while I have seen many stubborn cases clear up when the nutrition has been made adequate and vitamin A emphasized, numerous others have not. It is now my conviction that adolescent acne results from the combined stresses of rapid growth, inadequate diet, school and social pressures, and emotional problems; and that only when the nutrients required to fight an infection and meet the needs of severe stress are generously supplied will this condition consistently clear up.

Some time ago I planned a diet for a girl acutely ill with rheumatic fever and asked her to take the full antistress program (p. 31). Although her acne had been a problem for years, it cleared up almost immediately and has not recurred. Several youngsters whose diets were already fair found that their acne disappeared after they took yeast, oil, vitamins A and D, and 300 milligrams of pantothenic acid daily. Taking vitamin B_6 has also helped to clear up acne,[19] and increasing the intake of nuts, unhydrogenated peanut butter, mayonnaise, and safflower oil has caused the skin to improve markedly.[31]

Vitamin E is vitally important to prevent scarring from acne and in removing old scars, especially if x-ray treatments have been given. Because nine out of every ten cases of acne treated with x-ray have been found to develop skin cancers later, these scars should be removed as quickly as possible.

Acne rosacea. This abnormality is caused by tiny blood vessels forming in the outer layers of the skin, which normally obtain oxygen from the air; vitamin B_2, if adequate, carries oxygen to these cells much as hemoglobin does in the blood.[32] Sometimes acne rosacea is corrected in two to four weeks after 5 milligrams of vitamin B_2 are taken at each meal, but I have seen it persist in spite of a seemingly adequate diet.

Skin ulcers. Considerable amounts of all nutrients can be lost through open sores; hence far larger than normal quantities should be supplied when a skin ulcer occurs. The loss of nutrients can even cause death when bedsores are severe; and to obtain satisfactory healing, as much as

250 to 400 grams of protein daily have been given.[33] Because oxygen rarely reaches a bedsore, healing is increased when 5 milligrams of vitamin B_2 have been taken with each meal.

Varicose ulcers are said to heal in a fraction of the time usually required if 400 milligrams of vitamin E are taken daily;[34,35] and generous amounts of this vitamin may be equally effective in healing other skin ulcers, especially when vitamin-E ointment is applied locally.[36-39] Unusually large quantities of vitamin C and pantothenic acid are particularly needed to stimulate healing,[40] although they are perhaps no more valuable than folic acid, essential fatty acids, and other nutrients. Every nutrient should be adequate (ch. 32).

Fungus infestations. A number of fungus infestations can develop on the fingers, under the fingernails, on and around the genitals and anus, and especially on the toes, where it is spoken of as athlete's foot; and ringworm, which may appear on any part of the body, is usually caused by a fungus. These conditions, especially itching around the anus, become particularly severe after antibiotics taken by mouth have destroyed the intestinal bacteria that produce B vitamins. They often clear up quickly if the diet is made unusually high in these vitamins and large amounts of yogurt and/or acidophilus milk or culture are taken to insure the normal growth of intestinal bacteria (p. 144).

Two years ago our daughter, Barbara, whose need for the B vitamins appears to be extremely high, developed athlete's foot. Because she was in an antinutrition mood and is fond of our handsome doctor, she visited him frequently and smeared numerous salves on her feet without improvement. After two weeks of this fruitless procedure, I lowered the boom; as a friend says, "We have a democracy in our house and I run it." A week of eating liver, wheat germ, and yogurt and taking 3 tablespoons of yeast daily caused all signs of athlete's foot to disappear and none has been evident since.

When the diets have been grossly inadequate, large amounts of B vitamins must be obtained for a prolonged period before some fungus infestations, like those around the fingernails, clear up.

Bites, stings, and poisons. Dr. Fred R. Klenner has reported successfully treating black widow spider bites and bites of highland moccasins and rattlesnakes with 4,000 milligrams of vitamin C given every few hours around the clock with small amounts of calcium gluconate.[41,42] Calcium appears both to increase the value of vitamin C and to decrease the sensitivity to pain. Although his patients were extremely ill, they made complete recoveries, some in as short a time as 38 hours after being bitten.

A woman wrote me that while weeding ivy she had been bitten simultaneously on the arm and leg by black widow spiders. At the time she was taking vitamin C because of a sore throat, which "fortunately had not improved." The bites resulted in little more than a slight swelling, whereas a black widow bite on the foot of an acquaintance had caused his leg to be excruciatingly painful and swollen to the hip for a month or more.

Many persons are extremely allergic to bites of almost every variety, and more such persons die each year from bee stings than from bites of poisonous insects. Individuals with known allergies of this type might carry the antistress formula or 500-milligram tablets of vitamin C with them, and if they are stung, take large amounts immediately and frequently thereafter.

Calcium and huge quantities of vitamin C help to alleviate poison oak, poison ivy, and any allergy which causes a skin manifestation (ch. 15). Probably the poison from all forms of stings, or bites, whether from Portuguese men-of-war, sting rays, scorpions, or from other animals or insects could be detoxified if sufficient vitamin C were taken. Pantothenic acid, however, should be immediately increased; and local applications of vitamin E or vitamin-E ointment often reduces pain. When life is at stake, vitamin C and pantothenic acid should be given by injection.

Fingernails are made of protein. Fingernails that split, break off, are extremely thin, or fail to grow indicate a lack of protein or vitamin A;[43] and the rate of nail growth has been used as a measure of protein adequacy.[44] Many drugs stop nail growth, and the degree to which the nails are affected indicates the toxicity of the drug.[44] Such stresses as cold weather, illness, and inadequate reducing diets retard nail growth.[45-47] Transverse ridges are formed during menstruation and longitudinal ones occur when anemia is present.[18,48]

If the nails are abnormal in any way, both vitamin A and protein should be markedly increased. Of the single amino acids, the sulfur-containing ones rich in egg yolk stimulate nail growth most.[44,49] Neither gelatin (p. 310) nor calcium helps nails.

Felons around or under fingernails are virus infections

(ch 11). Frequent hangnails usually indicate that vitamin C, protein, or folic acid is undersupplied. Fungus growth under and around the nails is discussed on page 136. Abnormalities of the nails always indicate that the diet is not adequate, and when the nutrition is sufficiently improved, the nails quickly become strong.

Hair problems. Even a partial lack of almost any nutrient causes hair to fall out. To rectify such a condition the diet must be completely adequate.

The hair of animals becomes thin if any of the essential amino acids is undersupplied. Rats have a marked loss of hair when magnesium is inadequate,[50] and become hairless if kept on diets low in the B vitamins biotin or inositol.[51] Large amounts of B vitamins have stimulated human hair growth in some cases.[52] Persons lacking vitamin B_6 lose their hair;[53] and those made deficient in folic acid often become completely bald, but the hair grows in normally after the vitamin is given.[54] Men who become bald early may have unusually high requirements for several of these nutrients.

Increasing the intake of protein, particularly of liver, wheat germ, and yeast, and supplementing the diet with a teaspoon of inositol daily usually stops a man's hair from falling; and I have seen three or four persons whose hair became thick after these improvements were made.

Hair falls out during periods of stress, as after pregnancy or a severe illness. When typhoid was common, it was not unusual for persons to become bald following the disease. Several months ago, after nearly two years of working on this manuscript and missing far too much sleep, I discovered that my own hair was falling out and was receding at the temples, an alarming experience. I immediately attempted to get more sleep, followed the antistress program (p. 31), and in addition supplemented my daily diet with ½ teaspoon of inositol, 5 milligrams of folic acid, 50 micrograms of biotin, and 300 milligrams of PABA. Not only did new hair, now 4 to 6 inches long, start growing with a vengeance, but the natural color is gradually returning.

Falling hair, dry skin, and nails which break easily are often symptoms of an underactive thyroid. Every effort should be made to restore the health of the gland (p. 278), but at times irreparable damage has been done and thyroid medication is needed.

The graying of hair has been produced experimentally by a lack of copper, folic acid, pantothenic acid, and

PABA; and hair has been restored to its natural color in some cases when PABA alone was given daily.[11] Unfortunately, the two vitamins which appear to be most important, folic acid and PABA, are now sold only on prescription. I have seen many instances of gray hair which returned temporarily to its original color, but it quickly becomes gray again unless one continues to eat yogurt, liver, yeast, and wheat germ. Persons who take 5 milligrams of folic acid and 300 milligrams of both PABA and pantothenic acid daily with some B vitamins from natural sources can usually prevent hair from graying and often restore its color.

Recently I noticed a magazine article entitled "Your Malnutrition Is Showing." In no instance does it show more vividly than in abnormalities of the skin, hair, and nails. Fortunately, however, the rewards of good nutrition are equally obvious.

13
Problems of the Digestive System

Unless digestion and absorption are efficient, the most carefully planned diet fails to accomplish its purpose, and recovery from any illness is inhibited. Yet of hundreds of letters reaching me each month, fully 95 per cent tell of digestive disturbances and of nutritious food being avoided because it "disagrees." Although some foods digest more completely than others, none are "hard to digest." When the diet has been inadequate, however, both digestion and absorption become faulty. Inability to gain weight is frequently caused by nothing more than faulty digestion.

Bad breath. Diseased gums or tonsils can cause halitosis, but more often putrefactive bacteria, living on undigested food, form foul-smelling gases which are thrown off in exhaled air. Any deficiency that impairs digestion is a contributing factor. Volunteers lacking vitamin B_6 developed foul breath, which disappeared after the vitamin was given them.[1] When there is an odor to the stools, halitosis invariably occurs simultaneously. The condition is rectified by improving the digestion and destroying the putrefactive bacteria by taking yogurt or acidophilus milk or culture.[2,3]

Sore mouth and tongue. Normal tongues are an even red color, smooth but not shiny, and without cracks, fissures, or indentations. A prolonged lack of the B vitamins, however, causes the taste buds to clump together, forming grooves and ridges spoken of as a geographic tongue. A purplish or magenta tongue usually indicates a vitamin-B_2 deficiency; a smooth shiny one, an undersupply of vitamin B_{12} or folic acid; a brilliantly red tongue occurs when niacin amide is lacking; and one that is enlarged and beefy results if a pantothenic-acid deficiency predominates.[4] A coated tongue is caused by bacteria growing on it and reflects a corresponding growth of putrefactive organisms in the intestine.

Burning sensations in the mouth may be the first symp-

140

tom of a vitamin-B$_6$ deficiency.[5] Persons severely lacking in folic acid develop ulcerated lips, sore mouths and throats, and an inflamed esophagus (esophagitis).[6] Too little niacin amide causes the gums to be sore and the mouth, tongue, throat, and esophagus to be inflamed. Inadequate vitamin C allows the gums to become puffy, tender, and to bleed easily. An undersupply of either vitamin C or niacin amide causes the oral membranes to be susceptible to canker sores.

These deficiencies make it difficult to wear dentures, and "nervousness" resulting from an inadequate calcium and/or magnesium intake can make the wearing of dentures sheer torture. Such discomfort can quickly lead to more serious malnutrition; and the diet should be improved rather than the dentist blamed.

Nausea and vomiting. Food poisoning, an infected appendix, the onset of many diseases, and even low blood sugar are marked by vomiting. If persistent or particularly violent, a physician should be immediately consulted.

Both nausea and vomiting have been produced in persons deficient in magnesium[7] or vitamin B$_6$; and the latter deficiency is accompanied by butterflies and burning pain in the stomach, bloating, abdominal soreness and cramps, and the passing of excessive amounts of gas both orally and rectally.[1,5] Conversely, vitamin B$_6$ has been used successfully to stop the vomiting of pregnancy and of car, sea, air, and radiation sickness.

Mothers are usually too unconcerned when babies vomit, yet much throwing up can be prevented merely by adding a little magnesium oxide—¼ teaspoon daily—and 2 or 3 teaspoons of yeast to the formula or drinking water and/or by giving wheat germ as a cereal. Even pyloric stenosis, a violent form of vomiting not uncommon in infants, can sometimes be stopped in a few hours. Years ago a pediatrician asked me to go into a home and feed a seven-month-old baby with pyloric stenosis a refined cooked cereal so thick that presumably it could not be thrown up; if the child did vomit again, I was instructed to repeat the feeding immediately. The unbelievable violence with which this hungry baby repeatedly threw up, the exhaustion of the distraught mother—the vomiting had gone on for days—and the mess to be cleaned up caused me to suggest that we soften wheat germ in warm milk and feed him a few teaspoons each hour. Although the pediatrician was furious with me, the baby stopped vomiting and remained healthy thereafter.

Need for stomach acid. I once heard a doctor, lecturing on nutrition, state that the hydrochloric acid of the stomach was so valuable that the sale of every antiacid preparation should be prohibited by law. Too little hydrochloric acid impairs protein digestion and vitamin-C absorption,[8] allows the B vitamins to be destroyed, and prevents minerals from reaching the blood to the extent that anemia can develop and bones crumble.[9]

One physician, reporting in a medical journal, told of a woman who had been miserably ill and depressed for 17 years.[10] She had consulted doctor after doctor, all of whom had recognized that she suffered from multiple deficiencies of the B vitamins, and one after another had given her individual B vitamins, B-complex preparations, liver, and liver extracts. Nothing had helped her. When she was finally given hydrochloric acid with each meal, she made a "rapid and dramatic recovery" in a single week and remained well afterward.

An orthopedic specialist told me recently that he had gastric-juice analyses run on all of his patients and found them consistently deficient in hydrochloric acid; that he asked them to take a teaspoon of dilute hydrochloric acid (10 per cent solution) in a half glass of buttermilk with each meal, and that without this acid supplement, so little calcium was retained that the knitting of broken bones or healing after bone surgery was slow or impossible. Unless hydrochloric acid is taken through a straw and the mouth rinsed immediately, it can harm the tooth enamel; therefore most physicians recommend tablets of glutamic acid hydrochloride. This bone specialist, however, stated that 4 or 5 tablets are required to supply the acidity of a single teaspoon of the diluted acid, and that patients would not take enough tablets to insure healing.

An insufficiency of hydrochloric acid can result from a low intake of protein, vitamins A,[11] B$_1$,[12,13] B$_2$,[14] B$_6$,[1] pantothenic acid,[15-17] niacin amide,[4] cholin,[18] and other B vitamins; and this lack is usually accompanied by a decrease in digestive enzymes and stomach movements necessary to mix food with the enzymes. Volunteers deficient in pantothenic acid showed a simultaneous decrease in hydrochloric acid, digestive enzymes, total digestive secretions, and motility;[15,17] and recovery required approximately three weeks after tremendous quantities of pantothenic acid were given them.

When the digestion is below par, especially during illness, hydrochloric-acid tablets or liquid and digestive enzymes are necessary as temporary crutches. Recovery cannot be expected unless digestion and absorption are efficient. If the diet is kept adequate, normal quantities of hydrochloric acid can usually be produced within three or four weeks[19] and the crutches discontinued.

Importance of bile. Another factor vital to digestion is normal bile flow. This subject, discussed in detail elsewhere (ch. 17), should be studied carefully by anyone suffering from digestive disturbances and/or faulty absorption.

Importance of enzyme production. Digestive enzymes are necessary before proteins can be converted to amino acids, starches and complex sugars to simple sugars, and fats to fatty acids and glycerol (glycerin). These changes must take place before the nutrients can enter the blood without causing allergies (ch.15).

The stomach, the small intestine, and the pancreas normally produce liberal amounts of digestive enzymes, but a wide variety of nutritional deficiencies can decrease or prevent the synthesis of these enzymes. In this case, foods can be neither digested nor absorbed efficiently; and bacteria, living on food left undigested, form tremendous amounts of gas. For example, dry beans, notorious for their gas-forming talents, contain a substance that inactivates a single protein-digesting enzyme, trypsin.[20] Fat-splitting enzymes are essential not only for the digestion of fats but for the absorption of carotene and vitamins A, D, E, and K.[21-23]

When digestive disturbances prevent an adequate diet from being eaten, enzyme tablets with bile should be taken temporarily, the number depending on the amount of gas formed. Sometimes 4 or 5 per meal and 1 or 2 per mid-meal are needed at first. As soon as no digestive disturbances are noticeable, the number may be gradually decreased; if the diet is adequate, such tablets can usually be discontinued within a month.

Importance of intestinal motility. Normally rhythmical contractions of the muscles in the walls of the stomach and small intestines continue for hours after eating, mixing the food mass with digestive juices, enzymes, and bile and bringing the already digested food into contact with the absorbing surface of the intestinal walls. Without such contractions, foods cannot be well digested or absorbed.

A potassium deficiency causes the contractions of the intestinal muscles to slow down markedly or these muscles to become partially or completely paralyzed.[16,24,25] Such a deficiency occurs following surgery, diarrhea, and other forms of stress; the taking of cortisone or diuretics; and the consumption of highly refined foods or too much salt. This condition, which allows gas pains to become excruciating, is usually associated with constipation. For instance, a study of 655 colicky infants—probably enduring the combined stresses of having no pantothenic acid and nervous, overanxious mothers—revealed that the lower the blood potassium dropped, the worse the colic became.[16] When 1 gram of potassium chloride was given them by injection, the colic quickly disappeared. Pantothenic acid, added to formula or drinking water, would probably have been equally effective.

Relatively normal individuals can obtain ample potassium by eating fruits and vegetables, especially cooked green leafy ones, and by avoiding refined foods. Potassium chloride can also be mixed with table salt (p. 216). Severely ill adults often require much larger amounts of potassium. Although physicians frequently give 10 grams or more of potassium chloride daily, it is rarely used to relieve digestive disturbances.

The movements of the stomach and intestine also slow down or become intermittent when the diet has been deficient in protein, vitamin B_1, pantothenic acid, or other B vitamins;[15,26] again undigested food stagnates for hours or days and so much gas forms that acute suffering may result. Giving the missing nutrients usually increases the motility of the intestine within a day or two.[26] "Relaxing" drugs interfere with the movements of the intestines and increase gas pain.[27]

The value of intestinal bacteria. Vitamin K and apparently all the B vitamins can be synthesized by certain intestinal bacteria such as those obtained from yogurt and acidophilus milk or, in far greater concentration, from pure acidophilus culture. If any of these products are taken daily, the entire bacteria population of the intestine, which make up 80 per cent of the solid material of the stools, become exclusively lactic-acid organisms which destroy the gas-forming and disease- and odor-producing bacteria.[2,3,28] The desirable bacteria live only on milk sugar and can die within five days unless milk in some form or milk sugar is supplied them.[29] Powdered milk is an excellent concentrated source of milk sugar, but if milk is avoided, 1 teaspoon of milk sugar (lactose) should be taken with each tablespoon of acidophilus culture. When given a continuous supply of food, the lactic-acid bacteria may grow for weeks or months after yogurt or acidophilus has been discontinued.[29]

Antibiotics taken by mouth kill the intestinal bacteria, thus causing severe vitamin-K deficiencies, which often result in internal hemorrhages,[4] and deficiencies of folic acid and many other B vitamins.[30] Conversely, when attempts have been made to produce vitamin-B_6 deficiencies in volunteers, a few individuals showed no signs of a deficiency for an entire year, presumably because the vitamin was amply supplied by the intestinal bacteria.[5] Some persons remaining on diets lacking vitamin B_2 or other B vitamins have developed no symptoms until oral antibiotics were given.[31,32] Frequently ten times more B vitamins have been excreted in urine than was obtained in food.[33] Under many circumstances, therefore, health can depend on the amount of vitamins produced in the intestines.

The growth of these valuable bacteria also depends on the general diet. Rats have remained healthy without vitamin B_1 when allowed starch or pectin, which supported the growth of desirable organisms, but have developed a severe deficiency when honey or sugar (glucose) was given instead.[34,35] A pantothenic-acid deficiency in rats can be relieved by giving vitamin C, which stimulates the growth of the intestinal bacteria capable of producing the B vitamins.[36] If the diet supports vigorous bacterial growth, animals can remain healthy and their tissues and blood contain high levels of B vitamins in spite of none being given in the diet.[37-40]

Carrots, cabbage, and other vegetables containing "roughage" (cellulose) markedly increase both the growth of the valuable organisms and the amount of B vitamins, particularly pantothenic acid, in the blood, urine, and feces.[41] Conversely, the number of intestinal bacteria and the amount of B vitamins in the blood and urine drastically decrease when animals are kept on a "smooth" diet lacking fibers. Even mixing filter paper with smooth foods causes improvement. Such findings explain in part why vegetarians rarely have heart disease, high blood pressure, digestive disturbances, constipation, and many problems common among non-vegetarians.[42]

When putrefactive bacteria are allowed to grow, they produce histamine, causing allergies (p. 161), and liberate quantities of ammonia, which irritate the delicate intestinal membranes, pass into the blood, and cause nausea, vomiting, decreased appetite, and other manifestations of toxicity.[3] In many disease conditions, the toxicity of ammonia from this source imposes serious problems.[2] Because yogurt and acidophilus milk or culture destroy putrefactive bacteria,[2,3] they should be used liberally during all illnesses.

Some individuals harbor intestinal bacteria that produce a vitamin-B_1-destroying enzyme, common in the feces of persons suffering from constipation;[43] and people eating raw fish and shellfish, which contain this same enzyme, often develop vitamin-B_1 deficiencies.[44] The bacteria producing this enzyme, however, are themselves destroyed by yogurt or acidophilus organisms.[43,45]

Food is not vengeful. When digestive disturbances occur, some innocuous food is almost invariably blamed, yet the digestive system processes all food impartially (p. 83). The problem, which lies with the eater and not with the eaten, has many causes. So-called "sour" or "acid stomach" is usually the result of eating too fast or when exhausted or emotionally upset. Foods often have symbolic meanings which cause individuals to become unconsciously tense and fearful. Adults also swallow air during meals, particularly when anxious or high-strung, in the same way that infants gulp air while nursing. This air expands as it heats to body temperature and may be belched with sufficient force to carry the strong stomach acid into the esophagus, irritating delicate membranes and resulting in the discomfort spoken of as heartburn. The problem is that no one tucks such an adult over a kindly shoulder and pats his back. Taking antacid tablets and alkalizers—which are said to cost Americans 90 million dollars per year—or baking soda neutralizes the valuable stomach acid, interferes with digestion, decreases mineral absorption, causes vitamins to be destroyed, and can even harm the kidneys; thus temporary relief may cause permanent damage.

The obvious remedy is to eat slowly only small, frequent meals; prevent air-swallowing by sipping cold liquids through a straw temporarily; avoid eating when exhausted or emotionally upset; search out the symbolic meanings of foods; get additional rest; and improve your nutrition. If the problem persists, ask your doctor for a thorough physical examination.

Bloating and gas pain. The most common digestive disturbance is gas in the intestines. This gas includes both swallowed air, which if not expelled orally continues to expand and can cause considerable discomfort before reaching the rectum; and gas liberated by putrefactive bacteria living on undigested food. Often both occur simultaneously. Swallowed air, passed rectally, however, has no odor whereas gases from undigested food have a foul odor. A stool passed by a healthy individual is odorless.

The person who eats too much overwhelms his digestive enzymes.[28] If the amount of food eaten at one time can be efficiently digested and absorbed, none remains to support the growth of undesirable bacteria, and no gas is formed.

Unfortunately, when the digestion is so below par that much food remains undigested, improving the nutrition also improves the diet of the putrefactive bacteria; hence these bacteria may multiply especially rapidly, causing much gas to be formed. Excellent food is then forgone and recovery is defeated. Efficient digestion and freedom from gas depend on the production of hydrochloric acid, bile, and digestive secretions and enzymes; on the type of intestinal bacteria; and the motility of the stomach and intestines. These problems can usually be corrected by an adequate diet taken in small, frequent meals with temporary supplements of enzymes, bile, and hydrochloric acid.

Some well-nourished adults on excellent diets nevertheless suffer severely from digestive disturbances, yet repeated medical examinations reveal nothing wrong. On questioning, I have found that these persons feel unloved or are lonely and have had severe colic as babies. In such cases, the unconscious mind allows one to feel loved by reliving infant colic, when attention was showered on the child. Indigestion is but the price paid to regain this wonderful feeling.

Constipation. Because the purpose of the large intestine is to conserve water, any deficiency that decreases the motility of the intestinal muscles allows too much water to be reabsorbed; hence the stools become dry and firm. Constipation, which is defined as a hard stool rather than an infrequent one, can be relieved by increasing the intake of fruits and vegetables, the natural sources of B vitamins, especially of B_1 and pantothenic acid,[1,15] and of yogurt or acidophilus milk or culture. Acidophilus culture taken with milk sugar is particularly laxative.

Inadequate bile flow frequently causes constipation by allowing undigested fats to react with calcium and/or iron to form hard soaps. Lecithin, oils, and the use of bile tablets rectify the condition temporarily, but permanent correction lies in increasing bile production (ch. 17).

Spastic constipation, characterized by spasms in the large bowel, occurs when deficiencies of calcium, magnesium, potassium, and/or vitamin B_6 are superimposed on other deficiencies which result in faulty elimination.

Constipation in itself is not harmful or "autointoxicating." Far more harmful is the use of laxatives and cathartics which irritate delicate intestinal membranes and interfere with digestion and absorption. Mineral oil, probably the most damaging of all laxatives, decreases the absorption of calcium and phosphorus,[46] and itself absorbs vitamins A, D, E, K, and carotene from the foods in the intestine; it passes into the lymph and blood,[47,48] picks up more fat-soluble vitamins from liquids and tissues throughout the body,[49,50] and is then excreted in the feces.[47,51-57] The persons for whom mineral oil is most often recommended are ill ones, who can least afford this drastic loss of vitamins. Though for more than 20 years the American Medical Association has urged physicians to discontinue its use,[58] it is still prescribed.

Much constipation is psychological in origin. Branches of the same nerve go to both the rectum and the sex organs; hence when sexual expression is so unsatisfactory as to cause anxiety, general inhibitions and Puritanical background often force this concern to be diverted to worry about elimination. Constipation is also at times an unconscious "holding back" characteristic of frigidity.

Hemorrhoids. Bleeding hemorrhoids (piles) have been produced in volunteers deficient in vitamin B_6 and corrected when the vitamin was given.[1] Every person with whom I have worked who has had hemorrhoids has reported a "miraculous recovery" after adhering to an adequate diet supplemented with 10 milligrams of B_6 after each meal. Since pregnant women are notoriously deficient in vitamin B_6, a lack of this vitamin may prove to be the cause of the hemorrhoids so common during this period.

In cases where surgical removal of hemorrhoids is necessary, particular attention should be given to the prevention of scar tissue (ch. 2). The shriveling and inelasticity of such tissue can cause serious problems in elimination for years afterward.

Diarrhea. The main problem in diarrhea is that food is forced through the body so rapidly that few nutrients can be absorbed. Not infrequently, diarrhea occurs when we are unconsciously trying to get rid of something we do not like about ourselves. A variety of nutritional deficiencies can result in diarrhea, however, particularly a lack of niacin amide. I have known of dozens of persons, many of whom had had diarrhea for years, whose problem cleared up in a day or two after natural sources of the B vitamins and 100 milligrams of niacin amide were taken at each meal. This vitamin is sold both as niacin amide, which causes no reaction, and as niacin, which causes the skin to flush and prickle and the blood vessels to dilate, a harmless but frightening reaction. Unless niacin is prescribed by a physician, only niacin amide should be used.

A lack of folic acid, vitamin B_6, or magnesium also results in diarrhea, which can be quickly overcome when the missing nutrient is supplied.[1,6,28] Because a high calcium intake causes magnesium to be excreted, diarrhea brought on by a magnesium deficiency is common in bottle-fed babies, persons on conventional ulcer diets, and individuals who take an excess of calcium.[59,60] As little as ¼ teaspoon of magnesium oxide daily added to milk, prevents or corrects such diarrhea, and should probably be given to all bottle-fed infants, particularly if they are wakeful or irritable.

By forcing food through the body so quickly that digestion and absorption cannot take place, persistent diarrhea can cause deficiencies of almost every nutrient. An acute potassium deficiency is a frequent result, which physicians rectify by giving tablets of potassium chloride several times daily.[62,63] A magnesium deficiency is also often produced and may bring on tremors, muscle spasms of the arms, hands, legs, feet, and eyes, or epileptic-like convulsions; and fluids given to relieve dehydration dilute the already undersupplied magnesium, thus making these symptoms worse.[59] Such a condition has been corrected in a few hours by giving 500 milligrams of magnesium, or about ½ teaspoon of a magnesium salt.

The diet taken during severe diarrhea should be unusually adequate. When the amounts of nutrients absorbed by persons with diarrhea have been compared with the losses in the urine and feces, it has been found that far greater quantities of all nutrients are retained if large, frequent meals are eaten instead of small ones, even though hearty meals may make the diarrhea temporarily worse. The foods need not be smooth or low in residue, but merely as rich as possible in vitamins, minerals, oils, and proteins.[28] Diets high in fats slow down the passage of foods through the body.[60] When different fats have been radioactively labeled and given to persons with severe diarrhea, the absorption of oils has been virtually complete whereas solid fats have not been digested.[61]

The starting point. Recovery from no disease can be rapid until both digestion and absorption are efficient. At first vitamin and mineral supplements, which need no digesting, and yogurt or acidophilus, largely digested during the culturing process, should be heavily relied upon. Digestive enzymes with bile, hydrochloric acid, and lecithin should be used temporarily, and the amounts increased if bloating is noticeable. Gas distention indicates that putrefactive bacteria are being fed rather than one's own body.

When a completely adequate diet can be taken without difficulty, digestion and absorption usually become efficient in approximately a month.

14

Diseases of the Digestive Tract

Most illnesses increase the need for practically every body requirement. Diseases of the digestive tract, however, so often interfere with digestion and absorption that super-nutrition is called for.

Gastritis. Inflammation of the stomach, or gastritis, is usually a forerunner of ulcers and can be brought on by almost any variety of stress including fungi, alkalis, poisons, and corrosives. It is produced experimentally by any deficiency which induces ulcers (p. 84). Studies of persons with stomach fistulas show that gastritis is not caused by irritation from foods or aggravated by them, but most often results from worry, anxiety, grief, and similar emotions.[1,2]

Nutritionally, an antistress diet is needed (p. 31), and the antistress formula should be taken with fortified milk every three hours until recovery is assured. Because abscesses sometimes form on the stomach walls or parts of the mucous membrane may shred off, vitamins A, E, and lecithin are particularly beneficial.

Colitis, enteritis, and ileitis. Inflammation of the large bowel, or colon, is spoken of as colitis. Enteritis may mean an inflammation of only the small intestine or of the entire intestinal tract. An inflammation confined to the last section of the small intestine (the ileum) is referred to as ileitis. In these conditions diarrhea may become severe and ulcers, similar to canker sores, form on the intestinal walls and at times bleed or hemorrhage.

Psychotherapy can usually do more to correct such conditions than various diets or medication.[1] A group of patients with colitis was given a carefully planned diet, medications, and antibiotics. A second group, consisting of more severe cases, received no diet or medication, but had

151

three months of superficial psychotherapy, during which each individual met frequently with a sympathetic physician who listened to his worries and emotional problems concerning housing, marriage, sex life, children, income, social status, and other complications; fewer had to be treated surgically, and fewer died.

During any form of severe stress, the outpouring of adrenal hormones causes such destruction of body protein that at times parts of the walls lining the intestines are literally eaten away. Such stress quickly depletes the body of pantothenic acid. Enteritis and ulcerative colitis have been produced in pigs kept on pantothenic-acid-deficient diets.[3] The intestinal walls of these animals became highly inflamed, produced excessive amounts of mucus, and showed ulcerated areas which bled or hemorrhaged. Severe diarrhea occurred, and blood albumin passed into the intestinal tract, causing dropsy or retention of water, a condition common in human ulcerative colitis.[3] Such experimental enteritis could be entirely prevented or corrected by pantothenic acid.

Barium given to persons with colitis often passes from glass to toilet in 20 minutes.[4] There is so little time for digestion and absorption to take place that colitis patients have been found to be severely deficient in vitamins A, C, E, all the B vitamins, potassium, magnesium fat, protein, and practically every nutrient;[4-6] hence no nutritious food should be forgone because of the diarrhea.

The more severe the diarrhea, the larger should be the amounts of food eaten and the higher its fat content. When colitis patients have been given 1 cup every two hours of fortified milk furnishing 3,600 calories daily and their diet supplemented with vitamins, they improved far more rapidly, felt stronger, and had fewer liquid stools than similar patients given smaller amounts of food.[7]

The nutrients to be emphasized in any inflammation of the intestines should be those suggested for severe stress (p. 31) and for diarrhea (p. 149). The diet should temporarily contain daily 4 to 6 tablespoons of oil, which holds food in the stomach and is well absorbed;[8] and be high in vitamin B_6, folic acid, niacin amide, and proteins including eggs or egg yolks and all varieties of cheese. In severe cases, the antistress formula (p. 31) might be taken every two hours with a cup of fortified milk (p. 329) to which frozen undiluted fruit juices, bananas, and/or other fruits may be added for extra calories and flavor. Digestive enzymes and lecithin are extremely important, but hydrochloric acid, usually excessive during stress, and bile are not needed.

When the blood pressure is low, indicating adrenal exhaustion and loss of salt from the body, salty foods should be eaten temporarily or ½ teaspoon of salt taken one or two times daily in water. If the pressure is above normal, however, potassium-chloride tablets are needed instead (p. 216).

Because the first sign of a folic-acid deficiency is damage to the intestinal walls,[9] it is well to have fresh or desiccated liver and/or a 5-milligram tablet of folic acid daily. The diet should be supplemented with magnesium and all vitamins. A smooth diet need not be adhered to;[10] any favorite foods may be eaten provided they build health. Because scarring can be severe, a high-protein diet and generous amounts of vitamin E should be continued long after recovery appears to be complete.

The best nutrition possible combined with good psychotherapy undoubtedly yields the speediest recovery. If psychotherapy is not available, try to find a sympathetic ear, perhaps a minister, social worker, or understanding friend. Tears should be allowed to flow freely and some means found to blow off steam harmlessly (p. 114). When feelings such as worry, anger, and resentment have caused the inflammation, good results cannot be expected until these emotions have been expressed.

Sprue. Another intestinal disease, sprue, characterized by sore mouth and tongue, anemia, severe diarrhea, and large amounts of fat in the stools, is caused by the lack of the B vitamin folic acid.[9,11-14] The tiny fingerlike villi that normally cover the walls of the small intestine become shortened, fuse together, or may be absent, thus decreasing the absorption of food to only a fraction of that of a healthy individual.

Sprue can be corrected by daily injections of 25 micrograms of folic acid, but because food is so poorly absorbed, a diet containing 60 times that amount brings no improvement.[11] After an injection is given, patients may improve in a single day[9] and absorb the vitamin well by mouth within a few days.[13] A physician will give injections and/or tablets of folic acid, but the diet for sprue must make up for the multiple severe deficiencies brought on by the diarrhea.[6,13-16] Although oils rather than solid fats should be used, fats need not be restricted nor a smooth diet adhered to.[10] Two tablespoons of lecithin daily tremendously increases the absorption of fats and fat-soluble vitamins.[16]

Without folic acid, persons with sprue have improved when given cortisone or ACTH;[17] therefore the antistress program (p. 31) should be followed to stimulate the natural production of these hormones. A regime similar to that suggested for colitis might be ahdered to until recovery is complete (p. 151–152). Because the problem is one of absorption rather than digestion, enzymes, hydrochloric acid, and bile are usually not needed.

Celiac disease. This disease, which occurs mostly in infants and small children but is said to be increasing among adults,[18,19] is also called idiopathic steatorrhea, gluten enteropathy, and non-tropical sprue. It appears to result from difficulty in digesting gluten, a protein found mostly in wheat,[18,20-26] but may prove to be largely a deficiency of vitamin B_6.[27,28]

When gluten is eaten by persons with celiac disease, diarrhea becomes severe, most of the fat intake is lost in the feces, the appetite decreases, vomiting may occur, and eczema, or seborrheic dermatitis, is common. Gas distention and abdominal pain is usually acute, and the stools often contain so much gas that they are frothy. The tiny fingerlike protuberances on the walls of the small intestine clump together, become sore and inflamed, or may completely disappear, making the absorption of food practically impossible.[24,29-34] Before gluten-free diets were used, a large percentage of the children with celiac disease died, chiefly because fats and fat-soluble vitamins could not be absorbed.[18,20] If wheat protein is strictly avoided, however, dramatic improvement is made and the symptoms disappear.[18,30-35] Mild symptoms of this disease have been produced in volunteers who ate large amounts of gluten (100 grams) daily for ten weeks.[36]

Fat-free diets were formerly used and, although harmful, are sometimes still recommended. Oils but not solid fats are well absorbed by persons with celiac disease,[8] especially when taken with lecithin.[16,37] At the present time, however, the entire dietary emphasis is being placed on avoiding all foods containing gluten: wheat, rye, barley, oats, buckwheat, and prepared foods containing these grains. Even wheat starch is highly toxic to some people with celiac disease. After gluten has been avoided for months or years, some patients can eat foods containing this protein,[18,31-33,35] but in others the symptoms quickly recur, and biopsies of their intestinal walls show them to have become abnormal again.[30,34]

A diet can be made adequate without gluten, but it is a nuisance. The finding that celiac patients are severely deficient in vitamin B_6—the lack of which causes vomiting, eczema, much gas, and diarrhea—has been reported so recently that it is not yet known if this vitamin can clear up the disease.[27,28] Probably no less than 5 milligrams of this vitamin should be given daily to infants with celiac disease and 30 milligrams or more to adults. Magnesium, necessary to utilize vitamin B_6, is also severely deficient in persons with celiac,[38] and may play a causative role.[39]

As with other kinds of diarrhea, deficiencies of magnesium, potassium, proteins, fats, calories, and practically all vitamins quickly develop.[6,15,21,40] Many symptoms of patients with celiac disease, including changes in the intestinal walls, are identical to those of persons with folic-acid deficiencies.[9,21] Furthermore, the body's reaction to the diarrhea is similar to that of any stress. At first too much salt is retained, potassium is lost, and dropsy may develop;[21] when prolonged, too much salt is lost and salty foods should be eaten. For many reasons, therefore, the diets should not only be gluten-free but extremely high in all nutrients.

The problem, of course, is not gluten itself; grains are excellent foods, which have sustained nations for centuries. Probably persons with this disease have unusually high requirements for certain nutrients necessary to utilize gluten. It is known that celiac disease is triggered by nutritional deficiencies, intestinal infections or parasites, and psychological trauma,[25,26,41] facts that have been summarized in an article with the delightful title of "Bread and Tears, Naughtiness, Depression, and Fits."[42] During World War II, celiac disease increased tremendously in Holland where malnutrition and psychological trauma were both severe.[23] Furthermore, this disease is common in bottle-fed babies but does not occur in breast-fed infants until after they are put on inadequate diets.[26]

Through the years I have seen a number of children with celiac disease who, according to the physicians who referred them to me, later made spectacular recoveries; yet in no diet were grains restricted. In fact I particularly specified that wheat germ as well as liver and yeast be taken daily. In every case the diet was unusually high in each nutrient; and powdered digestive enzymes were mixed with all foods immediately before they were eaten. I am, therefore, convinced that correction may be attained without the prolonged use of gluten-free diets provided the B vitamins are generously supplied.

Ameba, worms, and other intestinal parasites. Animals kept on diets deficient in protein or vitamins A, B_1, B_2, biotin, folic acid, or other nutrients have been infested with many types of parasites, including trichinae, obtained from undercooked pork, and trichomonas, which can grow in the lungs or intestines as readily as in and around the vagina.[43-46] When these same parasites have been repeatedly implanted in healthy animals, however, infestations have not occurred as long as the diet has been adequate.

If a deficient diet is not improved and the parasites are killed by medication, reinfestation quickly occurs, but they gradually die out when the diet is made highly nutritious. Both parasites and worms infest animals deficient in vitamin A, whereas well-fed controls remain free of infestation.[43,45,46] The entire intestines may also be filled with worms when animals are allowed to eat too little of an excellent diet to obtain the nutrients they need; and if the worms are destroyed by medication, the animals died of infections in the intestines.[47]

Although intestinal parasites are surprisingly common, I have seen no studies showing the effect of dietary improvement on humans infested with them. It is known that a high intake of refined foods, particularly sweets, which supply little or no nutrients yet satisfy the appetite, causes individuals to become susceptible to pinworms which thrive on sugar. Research indicates that in any type of parasitic infestation, however, the diet should be unusually adequate and refined foods strictly avoided. Yogurt or acidophilus milk or culture appears to be especially helpful in cases of amebic dysentery and perhaps all intestinal infestations; and every effort should be made to maintain normal stomach acid (p. 142) which destroys many parasites obtained from food. A physician must determine when vermifuges should be used, but often such medication imposes severe stress and is unsuccessful.

Diverticulosis. When tension is so great that gas cannot be expelled normally but is forced—or diverted—against the intestinal walls, it sometimes forms small balloon-like protuberances known as diverticula. A person with these little uninvited guests, usually ranging from the size of a pea to that of a thimble, is said to have diverticulosis or, if they become inflamed, diverticulitis. He should quickly find harmless ways of blowing off steam (p. 91) so that his frustrations cannot cause such severe tensions in a normally elastic tissue.

People apparently have diverticula for years without knowing it until a chance x-ray reveals them; hence they are not necessarily troublemakers. Stagnant food or fecal matter, however, held in these thin-walled "balloons" can become a breeding place for putrefactive bacteria; inflammation, discomfort, and pain may result. Although diverticula can be removed surgically, others soon form unless a preventive campaign is undertaken.

Individuals with diverticulosis frequently develop anemia; and when loops simulating diverticula are formed in the intestines of animals, anemia is produced even though the diet is adequate.[48] The bacteria in the diverticula appear to grab all the folic acid from the food and prevent it from reaching the blood. When these putrefactive bacteria are destroyed by a generous intake of yogurt or acidophilus milk or culture, the anemia is corrected provided the diet contains folic acid.[48,49] Because foods supplying cellulose, or roughage, and unrefined starches support the growth of valuable bacteria, whereas smooth and refined foods cannot (p. 145), the diet generally recommended for diverticulosis appears to be the very one that should be avoided.

A nutrition program designed to improve digestion, decrease gas formation, bring maximum relaxation (p. 220), build strong intestinal walls which can resist ballooning, meet the needs of stress, and promote bacterial growth readily relieves diverticulosis. If inflammation has occurred, an antistress diet should be followed (p. 31).

Whether or not diverticula, once formed, can be replaced by normal, healthy tissue is not known. Given a chance, however, the body has an amazing ability to rebuild itself.

Pancreatitis. The pancreas, a long, slender organ that secretes insulin and digestive enzymes, lies below and to the left of the stomach. An inflammation of this organ, or pancreatitis, has been produced by diets deficient in vitamin B_6, protein, or certain amino acids,[50] and by giving various drugs or chemicals.[51] Human pancreatitis also occurs when the diet has been inadequate,[52-54] and has resulted from cortisone or ACTH therapy.[51] This fact indicates that stress, which causes an excessive production of these hormones, plays a major role in bringing about such an inflammation. Persons with pancreatitis also absorb and store abnormally large amounts of iron, a phenomenon characteristic of a vitamin B_6 deficiency (p. 227); and a lack of vitamin B_6 quickly damages the pancreas (p. 94).

During a mild inflammation, the tiny canal, or duct, leading from the pancreas to the small intestine becomes so swollen that fluid carrying digestive enzymes cannot pass through it. When acutely inflamed, the pancreas loses its ability to produce these enzymes. Digestion, therefore, is incomplete and so few nutrients can be absorbed that recovery is markedly delayed. Tremendous quantities of gas are formed, and fat is lost in the feces. When the illness is prolonged, hemorrhages often occur in the pancreas itself, the kidneys, and the retina of the eyes, as they do in diabetes when vitamin B_6 is undersupplied (p. 103). The damaged cells in the pancreas are replaced by scar tissue which shrivels and may become calcified.[55]

The person with pancreatitis need not restrict fats or other health-building foods,[10] but oils and lecithin should be used liberally, solid fats temporarily avoided, and enzyme tablets or powdered enzymes added to every bite of food eaten; if gas occurs, the amount of enzymes should be immediately increased. For the first few days, the antistress formula (p. 31) should be taken every three hours with highly fortified milk (p. 329); and no fewer than 60 milligrams of vitamin B_6 and 300 units of vitamin E should be obtained daily. Yogurt and acidophilus milk, largely predigested during the culturing process, may be emphasized. Because there is always danger that the insulin-producing cells may be damaged, a highly adequate diet should be continued for many months.

Replacing of emphasis. In the past, diets for persons with digestive diseases have emphasized smoothness rather than nutritive value; yet a smooth diet does not necessarily build health. If maximum nutrition is obtained and every step taken to assure efficient absorption, recovery can be tremendously speeded up.

15
Allergies Are Stress Diseases

Allergies, said to affect 20 per cent of our children, result when foreign substances, usually protein particles, gain access to the blood. They enter as injections of drugs, vaccines, and serums;[1] through the skin, as do cosmetics, insect venoms, and poison oak or ivy; by way of the mucous membranes of the nasal passages (pollens, dust, dandruff); and from the intestinal tract, as do foods, bacteria, molds, histamine, and drugs. The reaction to these substances may be a skin rash, eczema, hives, hay fever, asthma, headache, running or stuffy nose, sinus "infections," and/or digestive disturbances.

Healthy individuals remain unaffected when exposed to allergens; hence the emphasis must be placed on building health rather than on avoiding an offending substance.

Allergies are stress diseases. Dr. Hans Selye has pointed out that allergic symptoms are often nothing more than the body's reaction to stress.[2] If animals' adrenal glands are removed to prevent cortisone from reaching the blood—simulating adrenal exhaustion in humans—the allergic reaction to an injection of a foreign substance is extremely severe or fatal; identical injections affect animals with healthy adrenals but little.[2,3] All types of human allergies have been treated with temporary success by ACTH and cortisone,[2,4,5] which obviously could not alleviate symptoms were the body producing sufficient amounts of these hormones. Such stresses as inadequate diet, emotional upsets, insufficient sleep, infections, or the use of drugs usually precede the onset of allergies, and the added stress of a toxic allergen is the straw that breaks the camel's back.

Though stress increases the need for practically all nutrients, persons suffering from allergies have been found to be woefully deficient in every body requirement except carbohydrate;[6-9] and when the missing nutrients are supplied, the allergies often disappear. For example, children

159

suffering from asthma, hives, or eczema markedly improved when the only change in their diets was the addition of liver daily[10-12] and/or they were given vitamin B_{12}.[10,13]

Despite the need for improved nutrition, I can find one study of a mere 32 allergic children in which an attempt was made to give an adequate diet.[9] These youngsters, who suffered from bronchial asthma and allergic eczema, were given generous amounts of protein, no refined carbohydrates, adequate essential fatty acids, and a daily supplement of 600 milligrams of vitamin C, 32 milligrams of vitamin E, 20,000 and 800 units respectively of vitamins A and D, and moderate amounts of the B vitamins. Most of these children recovered in a single month and all within two months.

Are allergies pantothenic-acid-deficiency diseases? Allergies have been repeatedly produced in animals by injections of numerous foreign substances, and invariably the allergic reaction is particularly severe or fatal when pantothenic acid is deficient; the lack of no other nutrient has a comparable effect.[2,14,15] Because cortisone cannot be produced without pantothenic acid, injections of raw egg white, for instance, cause severe hay-fever-like symptoms and are fatal to animals deficient in this vitamin.[3,14] If the diet is adequate in all respects or if cortisone is given, injected animals have few or no allergic reactions. Similarly, if persons subject to severe hay fever when exposed to pollens are given cortisone before exposure, they do not develop the disease.[2]

The symptoms that accompany allergies[16-18] and those produced in volunteers deficient in pantothenic acid[19-21] are strikingly similar: fatigue, listlessness, poor appetite, digestive disturbances, headache, irritability, nervousness, mental depression, quarrelsomeness, increased need for sleep, recurrent respiratory infections, and abnormally large numbers of cells known as eosinophils in the blood and lymph.[2,22] Often the addition of pantothenic acid alone brings relief to allergy sufferers. One physician severely allergic to house dust and pollens noted marked relief soon after taking pantothenic acid, and he could keep symptom-free as long as he continued the vitamin.[23]

Some strains of animals and certain human families require four to 20 times more pantothenic acid to maintain health than do others.[23,24] Because allergies sometimes occur in four generations of a single family,[16,25] it has been suggested that allergic persons have unusually high hereditary requirements for this vitamin.[23] The average daily intake of pantothenic acid in America is 4.5 milligrams, yet such individuals may require 40 to 200 millgrams daily to maintain health. Because of rapid growth, children, especially babies, have unusually high requirements for pantothenic acid, yet this vitamin is rarely given them, a fact that probably explains why allergies are so common among infants. Many children "outgrow" their allergies when their need for pantothenic acid decreases.

It must be remembered, however, that many nutrients are required to produce pituitary and adrenal hormones (ch. 2); and that adrenals damaged by a lack of pantothenic acid do not recover for several weeks after the diet is improved.[20]

The importance of efficient digestion. Food allergies cannot occur when foods are completely digested; simple sugars, amino acids, fatty acids, and glycerin, the products of normal digestion, are never toxic. Only when digestion is below par can undigested or partially digested food enter the blood, act as a foreign irritant, and cause allergies. Emotional upsets as well as many forms of malnutrition prevent digestion from being efficient (ch. 13).

When proteins remain undigested, the amino acid histidine can be changed by putrefactive intestinal bacteria into a toxic substance, histamine.[26-29] This substance is found in abnormally large amounts in the blood of many allergic persons.[2,4] Vitamins B_6, C, and pantothenic acid each have an antihistamine action;[30] and a lack of any one allows certain blood cells, the eosinophils, to increase abnormally, which is a characteristic feature of allergies.[31] Major emphasis in overcoming food allergies, therefore, must be on supplying these vitamins, improving the digestion, and destroying undesirable intestinal bacteria (p. 145).

Liver damage may play a role. When under stress, the body itself forms histamine from the breakdown of tissue proteins.[32] Histamine thus formed is thought to be a cause of allergic reactions in persons emotionally upset and in people allergic to intense cold, heat, or sunshine.[1] The liver of a healthy individual, however, quickly destroys histamine by means of an enzyme, histaminase,[26,27,33] whereas a damaged liver cannot.[26,34]

Although people with allergies are often unable to produce sufficient amounts of histaminase,[26] a number of investigators have questioned the indiscriminate use of antihistamine drugs.[35-37] They point out that these drugs are toxic and can easily harm the liver, thus causing the amount of blood histamine to increase;[4,26,27,38] and that in cases where they have been used with success,[2,4] their very toxicity, by causing stress, has forced the tired adrenals into producing more cortisone.

When an adequate diet is followed, liver function becomes normal (ch. 16) and histamine, regardless of its source, is readily destroyed.

How allergens enter the body. Healthy cells can prevent harmful substances from entering them. A lack of almost any nutrient, however, increases cell permeability, as if a fine sieve were replaced by a coarse one; therefore valuable nutrients can leak from such cells and toxic materials pass into them. If the protein intake is low, for example, injected dyes can enter cells which they cannot penetrate when the diet is excellent.[7]

Too little vitamin C increases permeability by allowing connective tissue to break down. Similarly, if the essential fatty acids are undersupplied or damaged by oxygen because vitamin E is inadequate (p. 55), the cells become so permeable that harmful substances readily enter them;[39] thus vitamin E is particularly important in preventing such permeability.[40,41] The fact that bottle-fed babies and growing children are deficient in vitamin E[42] undoubtedly plays a role in the tragic early onset of allergies. Only 0.3 to 0.7 unit of vitamin E is supplied in a 24-ounce formula, a fraction of the amount furnished by breast milk[43] and perhaps a twentieth of an infant's requirement.[42]

Vitamin A decreases the permeability of cells both in the skin and mucous membranes.[1] When large amounts of vitamin A and vitamin E were given daily to adults for only a short time, their cells showed a rapid and marked increase in the ability to prevent foreign substances from penetrating them.[30] Many years ago a physician told me that he gave large amounts of vitamin A with vitamin E daily for four months before the expected hay-fever season to all his patients who suffered annually from this allergy, and that 98 per cent of them remained symptom-free. Since that time I have found the same supplementation to be effective for dozens of hay-fever sufferers.

In one way or another, each nutrient helps to prevent foreign substances from entering the cells.

Vitamin C and allergies. Abnormally small amounts of vitamin C are found in the blood of persons with allergies[6,9] and of animals in which allergies have been produced;[15,44] and individuals become particularly susceptible to allergens when vitamin C is undersupplied.[45] This vitamin makes cortisone more effective, decreases the permeability of cells, has an antihistamine action,[30,46] and detoxifies foreign substances entering the body.[45,47,48] Because vitamin C is used up during the detoxifying process, the quantity needed is in proportion to the amount of toxic material entering the body. Substances that cause acute allergies in some persons have been found in the blood of normal individuals,[25] indicating that detoxification has taken place.

Many early studies showed vitamin C to be tremendously effective in relieving allergic conditions, but interest was lost with the advent of cortisone and the antihistamine drugs. When 300 milligrams of vitamin C were given every 15 minutes to a group of patients during asthma attacks, some experienced relief almost immediately, and the remainder within an hour; further attacks were prevented when 1,500 milligrams of the vitamin were taken daily.[30] Hay-fever sufferers showed marked improvement when they took 250 milligrams of vitamin C four times daily,[49] and many improved on a daily intake of only 200 to 500 milligrams.[50] Because the diet was not otherwise changed and such small amounts of the vitamin were given, these results are all the more remarkable.

As few as 300 to 700 milligrams of vitamin C daily have proved valuable in preventing allergies to a number of drugs,[30,51,52] simultaneously shortening the time the drugs were needed.[53] The vitamin was most effective when taken daily, but still prevented allergies if given only with the drug[55] or two hours before it was administered.[54] In some cases even 100 milligrams of vitamin C daily effectively prevented allergies[56] but usually this amount was far too small.[57] Because allergies which have at times proved fatal are often brought on by mothers giving children aspirin or other drugs,[25,58] vitamin C should be taken with any medication.

On several occasions I have seen persons with severe hay fever whose streams of tears ceased flowing within minutes after 2,000 to 3,000 milligrams of vitamin C were given them. Such suffering can usually be prevented if large amounts of vitamin C are taken before an allergic person goes into a "danger zone." A friend so allergic to dog dandruff that his social life was curtailed can now accept invitations to homes of dog owners by taking vitamin C before leaving his house. One woman who consulted me could not attend church because she was allergic to face powder, but taking additional vitamin C every Sunday morning corrected the problem. Persons with hay fever should take additional vitamin C before driving into the country during pollen season; individuals allergic to horse dandruff, before going near a stable; housewives allergic to dust, before starting to clean; and children allergic to chocolate, eggs, or milk, before attending a birthday party, If allergy symptoms should appear, several 500-milligram tablets of the vitamin swallowed immediately usually bring quick relief.

The amount of vitamin C needed by the allergic person depends on the quantity of allergen reaching the blood; hence it varies with each allergic attack. Such a person must watch carefully for any signs of a vitamin-C deficiency—bleeding gums, nosebleeds, or even the slightest bruise. Medical dictionaries list purpura (which literally means purple and refers to severe bruising or hemorrhaging) as being brought on by allergies and injections of foreign substances. Since vitamin C is not toxic, it seems wise to err on the side of taking too much rather than too little.

The need for salt. When stress has been so prolonged that the exhausted adrenals allow allergies to occur, too little of the hormone aldosterone is produced; and large amounts of sodium are lost in the urine, causing that in the blood to drop abnormally low.[2,59-61] In this case, water passes into the irritated tissues of the eyes, nasal membranes, intestinal tract, brain—as during allergic headaches—or any affected area, and results in swelling.[1,25] Almost immediate relief often occurs if the blood sodium is replaced by taking ½ teaspoon each of ordinary salt and baking soda in a little water, a procedure that can be repeated when allergic symptoms again become severe. Increasing the blood sodium frequently relieves an asthma attack provided some food containing sugar is taken simultaneously: orange juice; or milk, juice, or tea sweetened with honey. Such attacks occur when the blood sugar is low—an added stress—and the adrenals are too exhausted to form sugar by breaking down protein.

When cortisone or ACTH is given for allergies, however, sodium is held in the body and little or no salt should be eaten.[59-62]

Allergies wrongly blamed. Because allergies can result in a variety of symptoms, they are frequently blamed when they do not exist. For instance, in one study of 50 babies with skin rashes, all supposedly allergic to milk, none showed improvement when milk was denied them.[63]

Such rashes are usually caused by a lack of B vitamins or linoleic acid and clear up when the missing nutrients are supplied. Physicians have pointed out that migraines, or so-called "histamine" headaches, are rarely due to allergies,[35] but occur when the blood sugar is low (p. 277).

I frequently find persons living year after year on severely restricted, inadequate diets because of "allergies" even though their symptoms persist or become progressively worse. When a food is vital to health, it should not be withdrawn from the diet except temporarily and then only if disturbing symptoms disappear as soon as it is withheld.

Allergies resulting from emotional problems. Certain foods are emotionally "loaded" with symbolic meaning in that they unconsciously remind us of early traumatic experiences. For example, individuals allergic to milk have become violently ill when "blind" fed, by stomach tube, distilled water which they were told was milk. Conversely, milk itself caused no reaction as long as they believed it to be water.

During sleep, the unconscious mind recalls past unhappinesses and the accompanying desire to cry or express anger, pushed back during the day; hence allergies of emotional origin usually become worse during the night. Swelling or puffiness around the eyes, a stuffy nose, postnasal drip, and other hay-fever-like symptoms are often particularly noticeable on awakening and indicate a need to cry; and they frequently disappear when the individual permits himself the freedom of tears.

Similarly, asthma attacks that occur at night are usually of emotional origin. Long-forgotten but intense anger, which once caused a primitive desire to claw, can induce allergies in which itching becomes so severe that scratching (clawing) is a necessity. Eczemas, skin rashes, and hives are examples. Such allergies clear up much more rapidly when the primitive emotion is expressed harmlessly (p. 112) than when medication or diet therapy is used. Asthma and migraine headaches are also often caused by early anger and frequently disappear during psychotherapy. Parents of asthmatic children can gain understanding of the emotional origin of this illness by reading the book *One Little Boy* by Dorothy Baruch.

Persons with severe buried hostilities customarily hide them by having misleadingly sweet dispositions. Unfortunately, parents are invariably proud of children with such dispositions and ignore, deny, or fail to suspect that they could have an emotional problem. Unless the emotional origin of allergies is recognized, the allergic symptoms persist year after year while such people often live on severely limited diets, take quantities of medications, and go from doctor to doctor without improvement. Instead, negative feelings should be expressed and, when possible, psychotherapy obtained.

The stress brought on by negative feelings, like any other form of stress, increases the need for all body requirements, and particularly for vitamin C, pantothenic acid, protein, and the antistress factors.

Diet for the allergic person. Allergens vary widely from time to time;[64] many are only transitory.[65] A food that causes an allergy when a person is emotionally upset may be completely digested when he is happy; hence skin tests are unreliable.[66] If the nutrition is improved and digestion made efficient, all foods can be well tolerated and offending ones need not be sought out.

In an effort to build up the adrenals, an antistress program (p. 31) unusually high in all nutrients including salt should be followed and, at first, supplements heavily relied upon to furnish every vitamin and mineral. To saturate the tissues, the antistress formula (p. 31) might be taken every three hours, preferably around the clock, and continued until health is restored, the amounts depending on the severity of the allergy. During a severe attack, even larger quantities of vitamin C and pantothenic acid, dissolved in water and sweetened, can be given every hour. If food allergies exist, lecithin, acidophilus culture, digestive enzymes, and hydrochloric acid (ch. 13) should be used with every meal. When these steps are taken, mild allergies can usually be overcome without any health-building food being eliminated from the diet.

Elimination diets, in which many excellent foods are withdrawn,[1,25,67,68] are usually inadequate in almost every nutrient. Such diets prevent allergens from being detoxified. They exhaust the adrenals even more, cause digestion and liver function to be further impaired, and increase the permeability of the cells to foreign substances. The lack of pantothenic acid alone causes faulty digestion within two to three weeks,[19-21] thus making all food allergies worse and more numerous.

When a valuable offending food is avoided temporarily, adequate substitutes for it must be found. After being on a health-building program for perhaps a month, a few drops or ⅛ teaspoon of this food should be tried with digestive enzymes and 500 milligrams of vitamin C. If no reaction follows, the amount of this food can be gradually increased. After an allergy has been severe, however, an offending food should be reintroduced with great caution and only if it is nutritionally important; and to prevent a large amount of allergen from reaching the blood at one time, small, frequent meals should be eaten. In no case, however, should allergies be looked upon as permanent.

Finding adequate substitutes. The most common allergy in children is to wheat,[68] partly caused by giving babies solid foods before the digestive tract is mature enough to handle them;[65,69] but wheat can be avoided without detriment. Chocolate, another common allergen, should certainly be dispensed with.[25] An allergy to eggs is usually to undercooked egg white, and hard-cooked eggs or yolks alone are well tolerated.[9] The most serious allergy is one to milk.

Goats' milk can often be substituted successfully for cows' milk[66,70] although allergies to it can exist. Allergic people can usually take yogurt or acidophilus milk, and buttermilk is sometimes well tolerated by adults. Thin yogurt prepared from fresh cows' or goats' milk, beaten until the curds are small, can be given to infants instead of a formula. Yogurt has been widely used in Europe in feeding ill infants, and should be relied upon here more than it is. Acidulated milk, made by adding lemon juice to fresh milk, can sometimes be taken successfully. Canned milk is frequently well tolerated,[70-72] and, though somewhat harmed by heat, should be used more liberally by adults allergic to fresh milk. I have yet to find any person, young or old, who can maintain an adequate diet without drinking milk.

Most physicians agree that soy milk lacks much of the value of cows' milk and should be used only as a last resort.[70,73,74] Death caused by a lack of vitamin D_1 has been reported in infants fed soy-milk preparations,[74] and the worst vitamin-B_2 deficiency I have ever seen was in a child given only soy milk. Such milk also lacks calcium, and is so deficient in iodine that goiter has developed in children receiving it.[75] Soy milk is low in the amino acids methionine and cystine,[76] and will not support the growth of valuable intestinal bacteria (p. 144). Commercial infant formulas prepared with soy or peanut flour are deficient in so many nutrients and so extremely high in refined sugar that I consider them to be dangerous. These deficiencies, however, can be overcome.

Soy milk may be prepared by blending with 1 quart of

water, 1 cup of full-fat soy flour or powder to which has been added ⅓ cup of calcium lactate per pound. This milk can be used as a basis for pep-up (p. 329) or other fortified milk. If gas occurs or if it is to be used for an infant's formula, it should be cooked 20 minutes in the top of a double boiler and strained. For a formula, 2 tablespoons of oil, 1 teaspoon of lecithin (to homogenize the oil), ¼ teaspoon of a magnesium salt, a few drops of Lugol's solution, 1 to 4 teaspoons of yeast, 1 tablespoon of acidophilus culture, and ¼ cup of milk sugar, or lactose, should be added to each quart.

Yeast is rich in the amino acids that are low in soy or peanut flour;[77] and when given to young infants by outstanding pediatricians, it has produced better growth than when the many vitamins it contains have been administered separately.[78,79] No more than ¼ teaspoon of fortified yeast (p. 320) per bottle should be given at first; the amount can be gradually increased to 1 to 3 teaspoons per bottle.

Allergies are extremely rare in breast-fed children; and babies nursed for a single month have far fewer allergies than those artificially fed.[70,80,81] When a hereditary tendency to allergies exists, special effort should be made to nurse an infant. Allergic symptoms usually do not occur until the third month,[81] and if the diet is adequate in linoleic acid, magnesium, vitamins C, D, E, and especially pantothenic acid, and more B vitamins are supplied by yeast, allergies need not be produced even in bottle-fed babies. The only sugar in breast milk is lactose which supports billions of intestinal bacteria capable of producing B vitamins. Similarly, all infant formulas should contain some milk sugar (lactose), and a tablespoon of acidophilus culture should be added to each quart to supply valuable bacteria. Other kinds of sugars, none of which can support bacterial growth, should be avoided.[82,83]

Unsuspected allergies. In addition to the millions of people known to have allergies, numerous medical articles have pointed out that thousands more go unsuspected, especially among children.[16,64,84-89] These children are characterized by stuffy noses, dark circles under their eyes, puffiness, fatigue, pallor, unco-operativeness, and antisocial behavior; and they usually show an increase in eosinophils.[16,22,85,86] Many of these children are described as "character problems."[87] When their allergies—or pantothenic-acid deficiencies—have been successfully diagnosed and treated, they have shown dramatic improvement in schoolwork,[16,87] and have changed so drastically in emotional behavior as to be compared with Dr. Jekyll and Mr. Hyde.[88]

Perhaps no other abnormality shows the appalling extent of malnutrition in our country as do the vast number of allergies. Yet probably all of them could be prevented if the nutrition were kept adequate and emotional needs met.

16

Liver Damage Has Become Widespread

Although a healthy liver is vital to well-being and is perhaps a main defense against cancer,[1] the incidence of liver damage in the United States, including often fatal cirrhosis, is said to be increasing rapidly even among children.[2-4] This problem, once confined to chronic alcoholics, is now common among social drinkers, overweight individuals, people harmed by drugs or chemicals, and those whose diets are inadequate.[5,6]

Some physicians consider that the appalling consumption of soft drinks—60 million bottles daily of one brand alone—is a major cause. Any toxic substance can harm the liver. Since all of us consume with our foods DDT and other pesticides, food additives, preservatives, nitrates from chemical fertilizers, and often detergent-contaminated water from reclaimed sewage, probably everyone has liver injury to some extent. To prevent such damage must now be a constant goal of good nutrition.

Liver functions. The liver, located under the diaphragm just above the stomach, is the largest organ in the body; and thousands of chemical reactions take place in it every second during life. When healthy, it inactivates hormones no longer needed, synthesizes many amino acids used in building tissues, and breaks proteins into sugar and fat when required for energy or eaten in excess. The liver also produces lecithin, cholesterol, bile, blood albumin vital to the removal of tissue wastes, prothrombin essential to the clotting of blood, and innumerable enzymes and coenzymes. It converts sugar into body starch, or glycogen, stores it, and reconverts it to sugar when needed; and it stores iron, copper, several trace minerals, vitamins A and, to some extent, D, E, K, and the B vitamins. A healthy liver destroys harmful substances such as hista-

170

mine, and detoxifies drugs, poisons, chemicals, and toxins from bacterial infections.[7,8] Liver damage interferes with all of these functions and many more.

Mild liver damage. Slight liver injury causes vague symptoms such as digestive disturbances, loss of energy, and inability to detoxify harmful substances,[9] but damage is rarely suspected until it becomes severe. For example, a close friend who was neither old nor an alcoholic went into the hospital last Monday afternoon; Wednesday night he died of advanced cirrhosis, apparently an aftermath of lead poisoning contracted while working in a battery factory. Although he had felt fatigued for the past year, a recent physical examination had revealed nothing. A general feeling of illness, some swelling of the "stomach," and a slight cast of jaundice caused him to consult his doctor again two days before his death.

In one study liver-function tests and biopsies showed that each person of a group with no apparent liver damage had degeneration of liver cells, a high infiltration of fat, much scar tissue, and other abnormalities.[6] Such people may have an enlarged liver yet think they have merely put on weight around the waist; and if pain is present, they often consider it to be indigestion. Long before actual liver injury can be detected, enzymes and coenzymes are so reduced in number that the utilization of all foodstuffs is interfered with.[5,10] Body starch (glycogen) can neither be formed readily nor stored, a condition which can cause both chronic fatigue and overweight. An unhealthy liver may produce only half the normal amount of bile,[7,11] causing chronic indigestion to result. It can neither synthesize lecithin normally[12] nor utilize fats efficiently.[10]

Failure of the liver to synthesize enzymes needed to inactivate various hormones allows excessive amounts to accumulate in the body, resulting in a variety of unpleasant symptoms. For instance, inability to inactivate the antidiuretic hormone controlling urine production allows the tissues to become waterlogged.[13,14] Too little insulinase permits the insulin in the blood to be excessive[15] and the blood sugar to remain consistently low (p. 72). Hyperinsulinism, or hypoglycemia, describing this situation, has become a common diagnosis within recent years, though easily prevented or corrected by an adequate diet.

When insufficient enzymes are produced to inactivate the thyroid hormone, a condition known as toxic thyroid (hyperthyroidism) results;[16] the accumulated hormone causes the body cells to race like a hotrod gunned by a teen-ager. This condition, strikingly similar to a magnesium deficiency,[17] causes such severe stress that the diet should be extremely adequate. It can often be overcome if calcium, magnesium, iodine, and vitamins A, E, and all the B vitamins are supplied in particularly generous amounts.[18] Taking 2 to 6 milligrams of iodine daily has proved especially beneficial.[19-21]

When an injured liver permits female hormones to accumulate, men occasionally develop enlarged, swollen breasts.[16,22-25] I have seen a surprising number of such cases, all of them college boys living on the cheapest food available. One shy, bookish law student told me he did not have time to date, but he became so alarmed over the implication that his masculine prowess was below par that three weeks later he had a wife and soon a very pregnant wife. Another was a divinity student who was deeply shocked because his physician had asked him if he were homosexual. The swelling of the breasts subsides a few weeks after the diet is made adequate. Failure to inactivate male hormones has been produced in female rats by diets inadequate in protein and the B vitamins.[22] To my knowledge it has not been studied in women, but liver damage probably accounts for excessive growth of hair on the face and upper lip.

Limited enzyme synthesis allowing the accumulation of hormones has been produced in animals by diets deficient in vitamin B_1,[26] B_2,[15] niacin,[22] pantothenic acid,[15] the amino acid tryptophane,[22] and especially cholin, vitamins C and E, and the sulfur-containing amino acids.[27] Such injury is prevented or corrected when the missing nutrient is added. Vitamin A—generally 50,000 units daily—has been used successfully in treating swollen breasts and in inactivating excessive thyroid in humans.[28]

In any case where foods are inefficiently utilized or hormones appear to be excessive, liver damage should be considered as a possible cause and the diet improved accordingly.

Experimental liver damage. Unfortunately, the American diet is the very one by which liver damage is produced in animals. Massive areas of the liver are replaced by scar tissue when rats are given diets high in refined carbohydrate and saturated fats[6] or slightly deficient in magnesium.[29] The damage is far worse if calcium is also low, phosphorus high,[29] and protein or the sulfur-containing amino acids, cystine and methionine, are undersupplied.[30]

If generous amounts of vitamin E are added to the low-protein diet, however, no scar tissue is formed.[30] Vitamin E also prevents experimental liver damage produced by a variety of industrial chemicals.[31]

When rats are kept on diets deficient in both protein and vitamin E, massive areas of cells die, much liver tissue is completely destroyed, and extensive hemorrhages occur; and the damaged areas become filled with scars incapable of carrying on the work of normal cells.[32-34] The more saturated fats added to such a diet, the more extensive the injuries become.[34] If generous amounts of vitamin E or the sulfur-containing amino acids are added to this doubly deficient diet, however, damage can still be entirely prevented. The addition of yeast alone can keep serious injury from occurring.[34]

A lack of vitamin C causes severe liver degeneration in animals unable to synthesize this vitamin. The livers of these deficient animals become severely inflamed and infiltrated with fat; and numerous hemorrhages occur, resulting in the death of cells no longer supplied with oxygen and food.[35] When drugs, chemicals, and other foreign or toxic substances are injected into such animals, liver damage sets in quickly and becomes severe with startling rapidity. If vitamin C is generously supplied, however, the liver is amazingly protected, even from highly toxic substances.[35] Vitamin A and cholin also protect the liver against toxic drugs and chemicals.[24]

When rats are deficient in cholin, fat starts to accumulate in the liver cells within a few hours, and in a short time causes them to become so inflamed, swollen, and engorged with fat that the flow of blood and lymph is pinched off.[36] Cells gradually become so filled with fat that many actually burst, and the fat combines into pools and seeps into the blood and bile, especially when saturated fats are fed rather than oils.[37] Unless cholin is added to the diet, scars replace most of the liver tissue,[36] a condition comparable to human cirrhosis,[38] fatal to animals and people alike. If cholin is given early enough, however, the liver again becomes healthy. Even without cholin, generous amounts of vitamin E or the sulfur-containing amino acids markedly prolong survival.[36] Of these nutrients, vitamin E is far the most important.[10]

If a diet is adequate in calories and rich in both protein and vitamin E, the liver can be completely protected without cholin.[12] In this case, the amino acid methionine pinch hits for the vitamin. If the diet is so low in calories that protein must be used to produce energy or if the protein requirement is unusually high, as it is during growth, the liver is not protected. When diets are deficient in both protein and cholin, severe cirrhosis results quickly. Many investigators believe that liver damage in animals and humans alike progresses from inflammation and swelling to fatty degeneration, then to cirrhosis, and, unless death intervenes, to cancer.[1,27]

Fortunately, the liver has an amazing capacity to regenerate itself. If the diet is adequate and two-thirds of a rat's liver is cut away, the entire organ grows back within three weeks.[39] Even if experimental cirrhosis is produced before part of the liver is removed, regeneration takes place quickly provided all essential nutrients are supplied.[40] In fact, how rapidly the liver grows back is a method of determining the curative value of various nutrients.[39] Diets high in complete proteins,[30] vitamin C,[35] the B vitamins, particularly cholin,[36] and especially vitamin E[30,31,34,36] hasten its regeneration.

Recovery from liver damage. As with animals, people with damaged livers or even cirrhosis can recover rapidly provided their diets are markedly improved. In one study of 102 persons who had lived largely on refined carbohydrates and were grossly deficient in protein, fatty livers caused mild to severe abdominal pain, enlargement of the organ, and tenderness to the touch.[37] Weekly biopsies and numerous tests showed that after their diets were made high in protein and supplemented with cholin, methionine, and vitamin B_{12}, even the worst cases had recovered within six weeks. Improvement is usually much faster when lecithin is given as a source of cholin rather than the vitamin itself, which at times can be destroyed by certain intestinal bacteria.[41]

In a study of 68 people seriously ill with cirrhosis, a high-protein diet supplemented with a multivitamin capsule and 2 tablespoons of yeast at each meal induced "rapid recoveries" in all, including the most advanced cases.[42] In another group of patients with cirrhosis, the severest scarring was replaced by normal tissue within a few months after the diet was made adequate; and as long as such a diet was adhered to, there was no return to liver damage.[43]

When persons with cirrhosis have been given 10 grams each of cholin and methionine daily but the general diet was not improved, biopsies still showed vast areas of dead cells and extensive scarring months later.[44] If a completely adequate diet is carefully followed, cirrhosis is remarkably reversible,[43,45] but an irreparable stage is reached if such steps are not taken promptly.[38]

Liver damage caused by various industrial poisons—benzene, nitrobenzene, leaded gasoline, and numerous hydrocarbons—has been corrected by diets high in protein and vitamin C; and damage from such chemicals was found to be greatest when these nutrients were undersupplied.[46,47] High-protein diets, used as a preventive measure, have also reduced the toxicity of many poisons.[48] Injury to the liver brought on by inhaling carbon tetrachloride has likewise been corrected by an adequate diet.[40] Damage from toxic drugs usually goes untreated; though the drugs may be discontinued, all nutrients which help regenerate the liver should be simultaneously increased.

I can find no medical reports of patients with liver disease having received vitamin E, though they have abnormally small amounts of this vitamin in their blood.[49,50] Hospital diets given to patients with cirrhosis have been found to supply daily only 17 milligrams of vitamin E;[51] and autopsies on persons who died of cirrhosis reveal depositions of the brown pigment characteristic of severe vitamin-E deficiency.[4] In cirrhosis, the liver becomes so full of scars that circulation is impaired and hemorrhaging is a frequent cause of death.[7] As in other injuries, the massive scarring forms after damage has been done.[38] Yet, if generously supplied, vitamin E would not only help to prevent scarring (ch. 4), but also could decrease the need for oxygen (p. 64) and thus keep many cells from dying when swelling and inflammation impair circulation.

During exposure to toxic substances, whether in spraying the garden, taking medication, or working with industrial poisons, cholin, vitamins C and E, and protein, particularly the sulfur-containing amino acids, should be immediately increased; and during sober periods, alcoholics who are especially subject to cirrhosis, should try to obtain these nutrients.

Special problems in severe liver damage. Often during liver disease, quarts of liquid accumulate in the abdominal cavity, a condition known as ascites. In this case the injured liver is unable to produce enzymes needed to inactivate a urine-controlling (antidiuretic) hormone, and too little urine is formed.[26] When 2 tablespoons of yeast have been given at each meal to patients with ascites, rapid recovery occurred.[42] A few times I have been consulted by people who accumulated liquid so rapidly that for months their abdomens had been tapped frequently and the liquid removed; yet after the diet was made adequate, the condition was corrected within a few days.

When the severe stress of liver damage has been so prolonged that ascites occurs, sodium is rapidly lost in the urine; hence a salt-free diet, which is usually recommended, often induces weakness, muscle cramps, lassitude, and low blood pressure.[3] In most cases, instead of salt being withdrawn, salty foods should be eaten. If too much salt is retained, water is held uniformly in all tissues, and not in a localized area.

During severe liver damage, large amounts of amino acids are lost in the urine at the very time quantities of protein are needed for repair.[52] Yet often a high-protein diet cannot be given because toxic quantities of ammonia accumulate in the blood. This ammonia comes from the breakdown of body proteins, accelerated by the stress of the disease, and from the intestine, where it is liberated by bacteria living on undigested protein.[53,54] Ammonia formed within the body is normally changed to harmless urea by enzymes, provided vitamin B_6 and magnesium are adequate, but it accumulates when either is lacking.[54,55] It can be markedly decreased by an antistress diet, which prevents such unnecessary breakdown of body protein. The formation of ammonia from undigested proteins can be stopped by taking yogurt or acidophilus milk,[53] digestive enzymes, lecithin, hydrochloric acid, and small, frequent meals (ch. 13).

Hepatitis. Inflammation of the liver, or hepatitis, can be caused by viral or bacterial infections or a variety of toxic substances including drugs, chemicals, and pesticides.[7,11] Hepatitis was a major problem during World War II,[56] and in some theaters of operation the cause was thought to be overexposure to the then-new DDT. Virus hepatitis is said to be increasing and frequently results in cirrhosis, especially in children.[2,4,37] A similar increase in toxic hepatitis parallels the use of drugs and of chemicals in both industry and the home.[11]

In hepatitis, which is often accompanied by jaundice, the liver is frequently damaged to the extent that fatty degeneration or even cirrhosis develops.[56] If the illness is acute, excessive ammonia in the blood often becomes a problem.[57] The diet for hepatitis, therefore, must be designed to render harmless any toxic substances or, if it is infectious, to build resistance at maximum speed (ch. 11) so that jaundice and ammonia formation do not occur.

Such patients utilize protein well,[58] but they develop fatty liver if high-fat diets are given without added cholin.[56] When persons with hepatitis received 1,000 to 2,000 milligrams of vitamin C every three to four hours,[60-63] they made "dramatic improvement," sometimes in a single day,[60] and liver biopsies showed rapid recovery.[63] Before vitamin C was given, some of these patients had been ill for weeks without improving.

Jaundice usually does not occur until one to three weeks after the onset of the illness. If, for a few days, large amounts of cholin or lecithin, vitamins C and E, and the antistress formula (p. 31) are taken around the clock with fortified milk (p. 329) containing many eggs or egg yolks and undiluted concentrated fruit juices, jaundice can usually be avoided. Eggnogs and malted milk, each fortified with oil, lecithin, powdered milk, and perhaps soy flour, can be used to relieve monotony. Recovery is generally rapid provided the patient can force himself to eat small, frequent, highly nutritious meals rich in both proteins and calories.[11,59] When calories are undersupplied, proteins must be used to furnish energy, and liver damage can become severe in spite of a high protein intake. If acute jaundice has already developed, the same procedure should be followed, though even more carefully.

When a transfusion, which often causes virus hepatitis, is necessary, large amounts of vitamins B_6, C, and pantothenic acid should be taken before and for several days afterward. Virus hepatitis is so contagious that members of a family, nurses, physicians, and anyone in contact with a patient suffering from this disease would also be wise to increase their vitamin-C intake.

Even after apparently complete recovery from hepatitis, unless the diet is kept highly adequate for many months or years, unusual sensitivity to toxic substances may persist. For instance, a friend who had acute hepatitis recovered sufficiently to become a trophy-winning tennis player, seemingly in excellent health, yet when she took a single birth-control tablet, well tolerated by thousands of other women, she became so seriously ill that she had to be hospitalized for several weeks. In any case where a medication seems to be particularly toxic, liver damage should be suspected and steps taken toward improvement.

The desirability of liver-function tests. Because liver damage is so often unrecognized, it seems to me persons should have one or more liver-function tests taken annually, particularly if they are overweight, have had hepatitis or jaundice, work with industrial chemicals, are enthusiastic drinkers, or have taken large amounts of medication. When liver damage is known to exist, its correction can usually be both swift and easy even for the person who wishes to continue enjoying his highballs. For a time the late W. C. Fields consulted me and somehow managed to mix every food I recommended with alcohol, his specialty being golden fizzes. Alcoholics who eat well even part of the time have been found to have healthy livers.[37]

The need to maintain the health of the liver is far more important than has heretofore been realized. Of all the organs, the liver alone can protect the entire body as well as itself from the thousands of toxic substances to which we are continuously exposed.

17

Problems Involving
the Gall Bladder

The gall bladder, a pear-shaped sack hanging between the lobes of the liver, is a reservoir for bile. A small, Y-shaped canal, or duct, carries bile from both the gall bladder and the liver to the small intestine. When food containing fat leaves the stomach, hormones cause the gall bladder to empty by inducing vigorous contractions in its muscular walls and simultaneously stimulate the liver to produce more bile at an accelerated rate. A diet rich in B vitamins also stimulates the emptying of the gall bladder by increasing energy production.

Although bile contains only water, lecithin, cholesterol, minerals, acids, and pigments, it is vital to health. Its lecithin content breaks fats into microscopic droplets that can be readily surrounded by enzymes, digested, and absorbed; and its bile acids are essential before digested fats, carotene, and vitamins A, D, E, and K can be carried across the intestinal wall into the blood.

Inadequate bile flow. When a diet is low in protein or high in refined carbohydrates, little bile can be produced.[1] If the amount of bile is insufficient or the gall bladder is not made to empty itself and/or the liver is not stimulated to produce bile, fats remain in such large particles that enzymes cannot combine readily with them; hence fat digestion is incomplete and fat absorption markedly reduced.

Part of the undigested fat quickly combines with any calcium and iron in the food to form insoluble soaps; thus these minerals are prevented from reaching the blood, and the hard soaps, causing overly firm stools, bring about constipation. If this condition is prolonged, it can cause severe anemia,[2] porous bones, spontaneous fractures, and the crumbling or collapse of one or more vertebrae.[1,3,4]

179

Poor elimination associated with gall-bladder problems invariably indicates a major loss of vital minerals.

Most solid fats obtained in foods quickly melt at body temperature. If little bile is present, this melted, undigested fat coats all foods, preventing enzymes from combining efficiently with proteins and carbohydrates, thus decreasing their digestion. Simultaneously, the lack of bile acids prevents the absorption of carotene and vitamins A, D, E, and K and whatever fat has been broken down by enzyme action; hence deficiencies of linoleic acid, carotene, and the fat-soluble vitamins are produced. People with insufficient bile flow are usually so deficient in vitamin A that they have difficulty in driving a car at night, sewing, or doing other close work.

Intestinal bacteria multiply enormously on this huge mass of undigested food, releasing quantities of histamine and gas, which cause discomfort, halitosis, and a foul-smelling stool. Much undigested food is usually lost in the stools, and becomes a serious problem when the calorie requirements are high and proteins badly needed for repair.

Although a low-fat diet is customarily recommended to decrease these digestive disturbances,[1,5,6] obviously it cannot rectify this situation or increase the absorption of vitamins.

Dangers of a low-fat diet. The purpose of any diet must be to build health, yet to prevent the gall bladder from emptying by adhering to a low-fat diet can actually be harmful, though such a diet may be temporarily desirable before and after surgery to keep the gall bladder quiet until healing has occurred.

The American Medical Association suggests that a diet for people with gallstones, obstruction of the bile duct, and gall-bladder diseases contain 25 per cent of the calories in the form of fat.[7] It emphatically states that low-fat and fat-free diets should be avoided, pointing out that such diets both undersupply and prevent the absorption of essential fatty acids, carotene, and vitamins A, D, E, and K, thus causing deficiency states that may be far more devastating than gall-bladder problems.

Individuals who have suffered acutely while passing a gallstone or when the gall bladder has been inflamed often become so fearful of food that they frequently live on self-imposed, severely restricted diets free from all fats without realizing that they are making their condition continuously worse.

Experimentally produced gallstones. Autopsies indicate that 10 per cent of our population have gallstones,[3] most of which consist largely of cholesterol,[8] though a few are formed from bile pigments. Cholesterol stones have been produced in rabbits in a single week by substances causing the walls of the gall bladder to become inflamed; in three weeks their gall bladders were completely filled with stones.[9] The inflammation apparently injured the mucous membrane lining the gall bladder, causing cells to slough off upon which cholesterol could deposit.

When hamsters have been given a diet deficient in vitamin E, all developed cholesterol stones, though no stones occurred in animals receiving the vitamin.[10] It has been generally believed that diets high in fat and/or cholesterol produced stones,[11] but animals given large amounts of cholesterol or saturated or unsaturated fats developed no stones as long as vitamin E was adequate.[12] Conversely, hamsters fed no fat or cholesterol whatsoever all formed stones without vitamin E.[10] The stones developed before any signs of a vitamin-E deficiency could be detected[13] and while the amount of cholesterol in the bile and blood was the same as that in animals having no stones.[12]

Moreover, when animals were kept on a vitamin-E-deficient diet until all had stones and the vitamin was then given them, the stones dissolved. Even a diet still deficient in vitamin E but containing yeast and generous amounts of fat (natural lard) caused half the stones to dissolve; the remainder were small and contained little cholesterol.[14] Yeast and soy flour, added to the stone-producing diet, prevented stones from forming; and the addition of natural grains, peanuts, and minerals decreased the number of stones to half.[15]

The reasons why stones form or are prevented from forming by these diets are not yet clear. It is known that vitamin A is quickly destroyed in the absence of vitamin E; that without vitamin A, millions of dying cells from mucous membranes covering the walls of the gall bladder slough off into the bile; and that stones form around a base of organic material. It would therefore appear that dead cells may catch and hold the cholesterol. Foods such as yeast, nuts, and unrefined grains, containing B vitamins and/or oils, increase the production of lecithin (ch. 5); and they as well as lard stimulate the emptying of the gall bladder. Because lecithin breaks cholesterol into tiny particles and keeps it in suspension,[16-18] a high lecithin content of bile would appear to be vitally important in preventing stones.

During pregnancy, when women are notoriously deficient in vitamin E,[19] stones often form;[20] and women who have had many children have far more gallstones than do men or unmarried women.[21] Individuals with gallstones may have normal blood cholesterol,[6] but stones are particularly prevalent among those who are obese or have heart disease, diabetes, or other cholesterol problems.[1] Population groups living on refined foods also have far more stones than those eating only unrefined products.[21]

Can human gallstones be dissolved? I can find only a few reports of gallstones having dissolved spontaneously.[22,23] For example, a young woman developed a large stone during pregnancy which two months later was found to have disappeared.[22] I have worked with a number of persons, however, who have had gallstones, but after they adhered to an adequate diet, no stones showed in later x-rays.

The general medical opinion is that gallstones cannot be dissolved and that sooner or later surgery is required. Many people with stones, however, have no digestive or gall-bladder disturbances;[3] and others apparently have had stones for years without knowing it until a chance x-ray revealed them. There are situations, of course, where surgery is imperative, but if a physician's decision is to postpone surgery, it is worth the effort to try to dissolve such stones.

Investigators have pointed out that the low-fat diets customarily recommended can actually cause stones by preventing the gall bladder from emptying vigorously.[10] The longer bile remains in the gall bladder, the more concentrated it becomes.[5,6] When the gall bladder fails to empty, thick stagnant bile high in cholesterol may slosh about with each body movement for days or weeks. Cholesterol and bile pigments are thus constantly brought into contact with any dead cells present. Under such circumstances it would be strange if stones did not form.

Human gallstones, implanted in a dog's gall bladder, dissolve quickly.[24] This fact indicates that some constituent in bile keeps cholesterol from settling out; therefore the bile of persons who had had stones removed was studied after various nutrients were given them.[8] Cholesterol settled out quickly when saturated fats were eaten. A teaspoon (3.5 grams) of arachidonic acid—the essential fatty acid in peanut oil—or linoleic acid with 20 to 60 milligrams of vitamin B_6 increased the cholesterol-holding capacity of bile as much as 200 per cent. Vitamin B_6 is necessary before linoleic acid can be changed into arachidonic acid,[25] needed to produce lecithin.

The diet to prevent gallstones or to help them dissolve, therefore, must be high in vitamins A and E to keep cells from sloughing from the mucous membranes. It should contain sufficient oil and B vitamins to stimulate the gall bladder to empty vigorously during each meal; and it must supply all nutrients known to increase lecithin production (ch. 5) so that cholesterol can be held in suspension.[16-18] Saturated fats should be kept to a minimum, and hydrogenated fats and excess carbohydrates, which change into saturated fat, should be avoided.

Large gallstones cannot enter the bile duct, and tiny ones pass readily through it; hence only medium-sized stones may become troublesome. Possibly because many nutrients aid relaxation and decrease sensitivity to pain, some individuals for whom I have planned diets have passed gallstones with little difficulty. Physicians have given others medication to ease the pain while a stone is passing. The discomfort lasts only a few hours, and as soon as the stone is forced through the bile duct, it is gone forever. The over-all pain and certainly the expense is considerably less than that incurred by surgery.

Inflammation of the gall bladder and bile duct. Autopsy studies and examinations of inflamed gall bladders removed surgically show that bacteria are rarely involved.[1] Inflammation of the gall bladder can be caused by drugs, chemicals, and bacterial toxins,[5] in which case the liver should be built up to the extent that such substances can be detoxified (ch. 16). Two sisters who incurred this type of gall-bladder inflammation from spraying roses recently reported a rapid recovery after taking 1,000 milligrams of vitamin C and 200 units of vitamin E every three hours with pep-up containing 4 egg yolks per quart.

Usually, inflammation occurs only when cortisone is not being produced in adequate amounts;[26] hence emphasis must be placed on helping the adrenals function with maximum efficiency (ch. 2). I recently planned a diet for a busy attorney who had acute inflammation of the gall bladder. Because he had low blood pressure and had been under severe stress, I suggested that he have ¼ teaspoon of salt in water every morning for a few days. For a week he stayed on the entire antistress program (p. 31). Although his physician had told him he could not go to his office for six weeks or longer, he was permitted to return in ten days.

Jaundice. When pigments from the breakdown of worn-out red corpuscles, excreted in bile as a waste product, cannot reach the intestine, they accumulate in the blood and are deposited in the tissues, thus giving the skin and whites of the eyes the yellow coloring characteristic of jaundice. Any condition that causes a rapid destruction of red blood cells can bring on jaundice (p. 229), but more often the disease results from surgical trauma, severe swelling or spasms of the bile duct, or obstruction caused by a stone, cancer, or cyst that prevents the bile from reaching the intestine.[1,5]

During World War II, when jaundice was a chief cause of illness, army doctors found that recovery could be markedly speeded up by a diet extremely high in protein (250 grams daily) provided the patient could consume such a huge amount.[27] Fats were not limited, and carbohydrates were generously supplied to prevent proteins from being used for calories. Most authorities have recommended 100 to 150 grams of protein daily with a diet moderate in fat and rich in natural starches and sugars.[5,6] During jaundice, the backing up of bile acids into the blood breaks down fat in the walls of the red blood cells, thus causing anemia. For this reason, the diet should be high in all nutrients needed to rebuild blood (ch. 23). If the diet is faulty, severe liver damage or even cirrhosis may occur; therefore adequate nutrition should be continued long after recovery.

When jaundice is brought on by spasms of the tiny muscles of the bile duct, nutrients that aid tissue relaxation should be immediately emphasized: vitamin B_6, magnesium, calcium, and sufficient vitamin D to insure calcium absorption (p. 254). To stimulate cortisone production, the antistress formula should be taken with highly fortified milk around the clock. When these measures cannot be started quickly enough, bile is sometimes forced into the pancreas, where it can cause severe inflammation, acute pain, and hemorrhage.[1,5] If pancreatitis does develop, an antistress diet rich in the above nutrients should be given as soon as the patient is able to retain food.

Diet for gall-bladder abnormalities. At the onset of hepatitis, pancreatitis, an inflammation of the gall bladder, or when a stone first obstructs the bile duct, nausea and vomiting usually become so severe that little food can be eaten. A physician should be called immediately. Every effort should be made, however, to prevent acidosis (p. 123) and to meet the demands of stress (ch. 2).

After the acute stage has passed, small two-hour feedings are gradually replaced by six light meals daily. The bile flow is inadequate during most diseases of the gall bladder, but lecithin can be taken to homogenize fats, thus increasing their absorption.[16-18] Though bile acids, necessary to taxi digested fats and fat-soluble vitamins across the intestinal wall, can be increased 100 per cent by using oils instead of solid fats,[28] they should be supplied temporarily by tablets of dried bile.[3] Generally a teaspoon of lecithin and 1 to 3 tablets of dried bile with enzymes per meal and mid-meal are sufficient to assure efficient digestion and prevent gas formation. Soft stools would indicate that enough bile is being obtained and that insoluble soaps are not being formed (p. 179). Beacuse the blood levels of vitamins A, D, and E are especially low during diseases of the gall bladder,[29] these fat-soluble vitamins should be taken with the lecithin and bile.

Gas distention can be further reduced by taking 1 or 2 cups of yogurt or acidophilus milk daily. If an odor to the stool persists, indicating that protein digestion is still incomplete, lecithin, yogurt or acidophilus. and bile tablets with enzymes should all be increased: and conversely, when no digestive disturbances occur, amounts of these foods may be decreased and the tablets discontinued.

Diets for gall-bladder diseases usually have a long list of "avoids," for which there appears to be no scientific basis (p. 322). Actually, no food need be forgone as long as it builds health; even salads are not taboo. To stimulate bile flow, no less than a teaspoon of oil should be obtained at each meal and mid-meal, always used appetizingly in food. At first milk and milk soups, whole-grain breads and cereals, lean meats and fish, eggs, cottage cheese, fruits, vegetables, custards, and simple milk desserts are customarily allowed.[2,6] When weight permits and recovery is well under way, small servings of pork, steak, gravies, and gently fried foods can usually be eaten without discomfort provided lecithin and bile tablets are taken at each meal.

Because oils are more readily absorbed than solid fats and increase the production of bile acids and lecithin while decreasing the cholesterol content of bile,[28,30-32] they should be used for cooking and seasoning. Eggs are well tolerated, and several whole eggs or yolks should be eaten daily, especially if the liver is damaged. Enough whole milk, cream, and butter may be used to make food appetizing, the quantity gauged by the need for calories and completeness of digestion. All hydrogenated fats should be strictly avoided.

To obtain a high-protein diet needed for repair without getting excessive amounts of saturated fats, one can rely on yeast, soy flour, wheat germ, fresh and powdered skim milk, nuts, non-hydrogenated nut butters, and liver lightly sautéed in oil. Many of these high-protein foods can be incorporated into delicious breads, waffles, muffins, and hotcakes baked on a dry griddle.

The purpose of a diet for diseases of the gall bladder, it seems to me, has all too often been overlooked. It is to build such a degree of health that you can forget you have a bile duct and, if you still have one, even a gall bladder.

18

Gout Is on the Increase

Gout is a painful disease in which one is literally stuck by thousands of needles. These needles, which settle in the soft tissues around joints and cause inflammation, are crystals of uric acid combined with sodium. When substances forming the nuclei, or business centers, of cells break down, uric acid is liberated.

Provided pantothenic acid is present, uric acid is converted into urea and ammonia,[1,2] both of which are quickly excreted in the urine. Individuals with gout may be too deficient in pantothenic acid to change uric acid readily into these harmless substances or they produce uric acid in such excessive amounts that it cannot be eliminated quickly. Some patients with gout excrete 18 times more uric acid than do normal persons.[1] Gout has been accidentally produced by drugs that have injured the kidneys,[3] thus preventing uric acid from being excreted at the normal rate.[4]

Another stress disease. Long before the body's reaction to stress was understood, medical dictionaries listed "poor man's gout" as being caused by "hard work, exposure, ill feeding, and excessive use of alcohol." It is now recognized that attacks of gout occur immediately after some form of stress.[5] The millions of body cells destroyed during the alarm reaction free quantities of uric acid, which may be neutralized by sodium and shunted into the tissues.[3] Young men submitting to the stress of being immersed in cold water for only eight minutes showed a marked rise in blood uric acid, which was "significantly decreased" when the same experiment was repeated after lárge amounts of pantothenic acid had been given daily for six weeks.[2,6] Furthermore, the amount of uric acid remained low for four months after the vitamin was discontinued.

In contrast, during the severe stress of several weeks of fasting, the amount of uric acid in the blood of obese

187

patients became increasingly higher until some developed gout.[7] These patients were given vitamins A, B_1, B_2, D, and niacin amide but only 75 milligrams of vitamin C daily and no pantothenic acid whatsoever.

An inadequate diet alone can impose sufficient stress to cause gout. For instance, persons deficient in vitamin B_1 have developed gout which was relieved when 10 to 20 milligrams of the vitamin were given daily.[8-10] Similarly, gout has been produced in animals by the stress of a vitamin-A-deficient diet. Since gout occurs in families,[8] people subject to this disease may have hereditarily high requirements for pantothenic acid or other nutrients necessary to protect the body from stress.[11] Any form of stress quickly exhausts the supply of pantothenic acid, thus preventing uric acid from being changed to urea;[2] therefore uric acid accumulates, resulting in gout. The fact that stresses come and go appears to be the reason gout is characterized by attacks and periods of quiescence.

The role played by vitamin E. A lack of vitamin E particularly damages the cell nucleus from which uric acid is produced;[12-15] and persons deficient in this vitamin form uric acid in excessive amounts.[16] Without sufficient vitamin E, essential fatty acids forming part of the actual structure of the cell walls, cell contents, and nuclei are so harmed by oxygen that the cell disintegrates;[14,15] simultaneously, cell-destroying enzymes in the tissues increase 15 to 60 times more than normal.[13,17] Though most animals change uric acid into a substance known as allantoin, when kept on a vitamin-E-deficient diet for only a month, they may produce eight times more uric acid (allantoin) than do normal animals.[17,18] Even if the deficiency is only slight, they excrete twice as much uric acid (allantoin) as when adequately fed,[19] though production of uric acid decreases quickly when vitamin E is given.

Centuries ago gout was extremely common among the wealthier class, who, because little other food was available, lived mostly on meats. Without refrigeration, so much of the meat became putrid and the fat rancid that the demand for spices to make such meat edible caused the great urgency to find trade routes to the Orient. Though I do not know why, it amuses me to point out that America was discovered because of spoiled meat. The fact that rancid fat destroys vitamin E with lightning speed[20] undoubtedly induced deficiencies of this vitamin, which in turn caused a tremendous destruction of body cells; and the excessive release of uric acid resulted in a high incidence of gout. After many types of foods became available and refrigeration was introduced, gout became less prevalent, but now that diets are markedly deficient, it is again on the increase.

A lack of vitamin E may still be a causative factor in gout. Oils, mayonnaise, or salad dressings not refrigerated after being opened, fats kept in a dripping can on the back of a range, and nuts not packed in vacuum cans are often sufficiently rancid to destroy this vitamin. Moreover, our diets today contain only a fraction of the vitamin E they did a century ago;[21] and what little there is available is largely destroyed in cooking.[22] Because fresh oils are being used now in greater quantities than formerly, the need for this vitamin has increased tremendously.[20,23]

Danger of protein imbalance. In animals given incomplete proteins or diets lacking any of the essential amino acids, the production of uric acid increases.[24] Similarly, if separate amino acids are fed and too much of some and too little of others allowed, again the blood uric acid soars. The amino acids from the proteins we eat become the building blocks of which body tissues are made, but it now appears that all ten of the amino acids the body cannot synthesize must be available at the same time and in roughly the proportion found in human tissues.

When the most common amino acid, glycine, is radioactively labeled and fed to animals or humans, it can be recovered from the blood and urine as uric acid.[16] Furthermore, persons with gout change labeled glycine into uric acid much more quickly than do normal individuals.[8,16] This change appears to be the means by which the body rids itself of a waste product when many incomplete proteins have been eaten. Any person with gout, therefore, should be particularly careful to obtain complete proteins; and gelatin, which lacks several essential amino acids but supplies excessive amounts of glycine, should be strictly avoided (p. 310).

Role of intestinal bacteria. During periods of quiescence, the body produces much smaller quantities of uric acid. At such times, however, large amounts of uric acid have been injected into gouty persons without bringing on an attack.[25] One reason appears to be that normally much of the uric acid produced passes into the intestine and is utilized by bacteria,[4] but the amount of uric acid disposed of in this manner depends on the bacterial growth. If the bacteria are destroyed by oral antibiotics, the amount of uric acid in the blood immediately increases.

Such a finding indicates that the individuals with gout should insure the growth of intestinal bacteria by the generous use of yogurt and/or acidophilus milk or culture.

Psychosomatic causes. Psychological stresses are far more frequently the cause of gout than is generally recognized. For instance, a friend in excellent health suddenly developed such acute gout in his right foot that he had to be immediately hospitalized. He wrote me, asking for dietary advice. In my answer, after suggesting several antistress measures, I added facetiously, "Sounds to me as if you want to kick the daylights out of someone." It so happened that my guess was correct. The day he had become ill a majority stockholder had threatened to take steps that would ruin the company of which he was president, a situation causing him intense justified anger, which he dared not express. When he understood the cause, his gout quickly cleared up and has never returned. Unfortunately physicians frequently overlook psychosomatic diseases or lack knowledge of them. Later this man's wife remarked, shaking her head, "We had a whole battery of doctors here trying to find what was wrong, and you, 3,000 miles away, put your finger on it."

It has been my experience that attacks of gout brought on by such emotional upsets are common rather than unusual. Men are instinctively the fighters of the race and are often sufficiently angered to fight—sometimes unconsciously—but are in situations where they dare not. I suspect such suppressed anger accounts for the fact that gout is more prevalent in men than in women, and why, since fighting and kicking are done with hands and feet, it more often afflicts the extremities than other parts of the body. When such persons are angered, they should work out on a punching bag or hurriedly arrange to play football before the stress of their emotions has had time to cause the destruction of body proteins.

Diet for gout. Unfortunately, the diet customarily recommended for gout completely ignores the needs of stress (ch. 2). Its emphasis is on restricting purines, the substances in cell nuclei from which uric acid is formed; hence it is made up of foods which contain few cells. Because liver, yeast, wheat germ, and whole-grain breads and cereals are forbidden, such a diet is extremely deficient in B vitamins and almost devoid of vitamin E and pantothenic acid. Furthermore, medical investigators— though not practitioners—now agree that the tiny amount of uric acid in foods is insignificant; and that the uric acid which causes gout is formed in the body from the break-down of tissue proteins and has never been proved to come from foods.[1,26]

Because a low-purine diet for gout was drilled into us so thoroughly during dietetics training, I formerly recommended it, though I have never known any person adhering to it to recover quickly despite the many excellent foods allowed. Perhaps 25 years ago, a woman told me proudly that she had given her husband, who had gout, large amounts of yeast and liver. "That's exactly what you mustn't do!" I exclaimed in alarm. "But he's well for the first time in years," she answered.

Since this incident, I have refused to plan a low-purine diet. Not only do stress and the pain of gout quickly exhaust the adrenals, but also inflammation (caused by the uric-acid crystals) invariably indicates that too little cortisone is being produced. Giving cortisone for this disease "has proved to be of great value."[5] The dietary approach, therefore, must be to help the adrenals produce cortisone by eating large amounts of liver, yeast, wheat germ, yogurt or acidophilus, and green leafy vegetables; and by taking the antistress formula (p. 31) around the clock during the acute stage. Usually such a diet brings marked improvement in two or three days. Persons fearful of deviating from a low-purine diet should at least obtain generous supplements of all vitamins, especially of vitamin E and the B group.

A urine made alkaline by a high intake of fruits, vegetables, and juices, particularly orange juice, helps to keep the uric-acid crystals in solution and to facilitate their excretion. During gout attacks 3 quarts of liquid daily are usually recommended to carry off the uric-acid crystals, but recovery is more rapid if juices and milk are drunk instead of water. Although any food can be eaten provided it builds health, incomplete proteins such as corn, dry beans, lentils, and cereals should be taken only with milk, eggs, cheese, and/or meats, to prevent an amino-acid imbalance.

If the person who has once had gout keeps his diet unusually adequate, further attacks can often be prevented. He should eliminate as much stress from his life as possible, but, like an individual subject to ulcers, he would probably be wise to keep vitamin C and pantothenic acid with him at all times and to take them with protein every two or three hours during periods when he is emotionally upset.

19
Diseases of the Kidneys

To me, few parts of the body seem so amazing as the kidneys. These bean-shaped organs, lying below the waist on either side of the vertebrae, are only about four inches long, two inches wide, and an inch thick. Yet arranged in orderly precision around the outer portion are millions of tiny balls of capillaries, or glomeruli—the Latin plural for ball. Long, slender tubes, or tubules, curve around each miniature ball, then after winding like hairpin loops on a mountain road, converge into ever larger tubules until all combine into a single canal, the ureter, leading to the bladder. Capillaries carrying fresh blood surround each tubule; and the whole is held together by connective tissue. Thus incredible miles of capillaries and tubes form the working mechanism of the kidneys.

An adult has about 12 quarts of blood, yet because of continuous circulation, the kidneys filter approximately 4,000 quarts daily.[1] Elevated blood pressure in the capillary balls forces protein-free plasma into the tiny tubules; and as this plasma trickles down its long path, water and nutrients are reabsorbed into surrounding capillaries much as foods are absorbed from the digestive tract. In this manner, healthy kidneys prevent dehydration, throw off wastes (largely urea from the breakdown of worn-out cells), and keep the body from becoming acid or alkaline.

Infections of the kidneys and bladder. As with other infections, inflammations of the kidneys and urinary bladder, known as pyelitis and cystitis respectively, call for an antistress diet (p. 31) and increased amounts of all nutrients needed to build resistance (ch. 11). Because a highly acid urine, produced by eating meats, eggs, milk, cheese, breads, and cereals, retards bacterial growth, vegetables, fruits, and especially citrus juices should be largely avoided for a week or more.

During cystitis, ulcers sometimes cover the walls of the bladder, and unless vitamin E is kept unusually adequate,

192

massive scarring can form, contract, and drastically reduce its capacity for storing urine.

Problems with voiding. Inability to control the passing
of urine, or "bed-wetting," has been produced in volunteers by a deficiency of magnesium.[2] Conversely, inability
to pass urine occurs when the blood potassium becomes
low following severe stress;[3] and it has been produced in
animals by diets deficient in vitamin B_2 or pantothenic
acid. Supplying the missing nutrients rectifies the situation.

Bright's disease. The term Bright's disease is applied to
many types of kidney damage, including nephritis, an
acute inflammation most often affecting children but usually not involving bacteria. Blood albumin, antibodies
(gamma globulins), and millions of dead cells are lost in
the urine, and the blood serum is often milky with fat and
cholesterol.[4,5] This disease can become progressively
worse and result in death, or it may subside into a chronic
stage where the patient gets better but not often well.

Nephrosis refers to less acute kidney damage generally
affecting older people. Its onset is usually gradual, though
puffiness under the eyes, frequent urination, perhaps
headaches, and excessive blood cholesterol may precede it
for years. Fatty deposits in the arteries and tiny tubules
decrease the blood supply to the kidneys, the amount of
nutrients reabsorbed, and the quantity of urine excreted.
Entire areas may be filled with dead cells and scar tissue,
yet recovery is still possible.[6] Usually when urine formation is severely inhibited, highly toxic urea cannot be
excreted and may cause fatal uremic poisoning.

Numerous other names given to kidney disease refer to
the part of the organ most damaged and are transitional
phases of the same abnormality.[7]

Experimentally produced kidney diseases. Nephritis has
been produced in many species of animals by diets deficient
in the B vitamin cholin.[8,9] The coils of capillaries are
particularly damaged, severe hemorrhages occur, blood
lecithin drops far below normal,[10] deposits of cholesterol
and fats become so excessive that urine formation is
decreased, circulation inhibited, and so much albumin is
lost in the urine that dropsy results.[4,11,12] Vitamin B_{12},
folic acid, or the amino acid methionine alone can correct
the dropsy, but only cholin can stop the hemorrhaging.

When diets high in calories, especially alcohol or refined
sugar, are given, the need for cholin is markedly increased
and kidney damage becomes much more severe.[13] If the
diet is low in both cholin and protein, such acute dropsy

develops that digestion, circulation, and other body functions are interfered with. Although cholin deficiency also harms the liver, kidney disease is produced long before liver damage can be detected.[14-16]

Cholin can be made from methionine, but when growth is rapid, the building of body protein has priority and leaves none of the amino acid to be changed into the vitamin.[10,17] For this reason, the young of any species are particularly susceptible to nephritis.[17] Even when adequate protein is given, young, rapidly growing rats on a cholin-deficient diet develop nephritis within four to seven days, and most of them soon die, their fat-filled kidneys swollen, discolored, and containing large areas of dead tissue.[18] Because the illness stops growth and decreases the need for cholin and methionine, the kidneys of the animals which live gradually improve.[10]

Like the animals, a rapidly growing child not given cholin may be unable to obtain enough from methionine. When methionine is radioactively labeled and injected into humans, it is recovered not as cholin but as lecithin.[17] The cause of the fatty deposits that damage the kidney appears to be identical to that which induces atherosclerosis (ch. 5). In Bright's disease the blood lecithin decreases in proportion to the severity of the illness,[19] cholesterol is extremely high,[20] and milky blood serum caused by fatty substances is particularly characteristic;[5] when lecithin is given these conditions are rectified.[21-25]

If cholin is added to an otherwise adequate diet, experimental nephritis is quickly corrected. Calves receiving no cholin die within seven days of severe hemorrhaging nephritis.[15] Other calves, kept on the same diet but given 1,000 milligrams of cholin as late as the sixth day, make "dramatic improvement" within 24 hours. Giving cholin with inositol or as lecithin, however, is much more effective than cholin alone.[26]

Though the experimentally produced nephritis, "strikingly similar to the disease seen in man,"[27] is corrected as soon as cholin is added to the diet,[27-30] this vitamin is rarely given to humans with kidney diseases. Yet more than half of 102 people with fatty livers, recognized as cholin deficiency, had high blood urea and albumin in the urine, showing mild nephrosis, which quickly disappeared when cholin was given with an adequate diet.[81] In another study of 48 persons, the blood pressure fell to normal and albumin cleared from the urine when cholin was taken.[32]

Other causes. As with atherosclerosis, any deficiency

that prevents lecithin production appears to cause kidney disease. Nephritis has been produced in almost every type of animal, including insects, by diets deficient in essential fatty acids.[33] Cholesterol and fats are deposited in kidney tissues; the coils of capillaries break down, blood and albumin are lost in the urine, dropsy develops, large areas of tissue are destroyed, and the tubules often become calcified.[33-36]

Animals lacking magnesium also develop nephritis and show the same degenerative changes, made worse after the kidney has once been damaged,[37-39] because this mineral is more readily lost in the urine. When the diet is only slightly deficient in magnesium, the kidneys become tremendously swollen, and 25 times more calcium than normal may be deposited in the kidney tissues.[40,41] This condition becomes much more severe if phosphorus is high and calcium low.[40]

When both vitamin B_6 and magnesium are undersupplied, the kidneys are further damaged by sharp crystals of oxalic acid combined with calcium,[42] and as much as three-quarters of the kidney may be replaced by scar tissue.[43,44] Children with oxalic-acid kidney stones (ch. 20) frequently have high blood pressure and kidneys so damaged that they become progressively worse, causing death from kidney failure early in life.[45]

The typical American high-phosphorus, low-calcium diet, given to animals, causes kidney tissues to become calcified, though such calcification is prevented when the amount of dietary calcium is doubled.[46]

Influence of other vitamins. Since the tiny kidney tubules are lined with mucous membrane, if too little vitamin A is given, they soon become plugged with dead cells; less urine can be formed, excessive water held in the body causes the blood pressure to increase, and urea backs up into the blood;[47-49] and vitamin A is rapidly lost from the liver and body tissues[14,16] into the urine at the very time it is most needed.[47,50-52] When patients with nephritis have been given for a few days 50,000 to 75,000 units of vitamin A daily, urea excretion has increased as much as 90 per cent,[53] showing that kidney function had markedly improved.

If vitamin E is deficient, nephritis occurs in which the tubules become so plugged with dead cells that urine cannot pass;[54,55] and dropsy and progressive degeneration become marked.[54] Should this deficiency be prolonged, even the large collecting tubules are completely destroyed,[54] yet adding the vitamin corrects the condition.[56] Vitamin E has largely prevented the calcification of the kidneys caused by excessive vitamin D and other toxic substances.[57]

Dozens of physicians have reported the marked beneficial effects of giving vitamin E to persons with kidney diseases.[58-62] When children with acute nephritis took 300 units of vitamin E daily, their dropsy promptly disappeared and blood and albumin were no longer lost in the urine.[63] Adults with Bright's disease showed similar improvement after taking 300 to 600 milligrams of the vitamin daily.[64] Vitamin E helps cells survive by decreasing their need for oxygen;[65] it prevents scarring, a severe problem in both kidney diseases and kidneys damaged by toxic chemicals;[66] and at times it lowers high blood pressure associated with kidney disease,[67] and increases the flow of urine.[68]

The effect of stress. Bright's disease has been produced in animals by giving salt and the adrenal hormone DOC,[7,69] a situation comparable to that of humans eating well-salted foods while under stress but unable to produce sufficient cortisone. These animals develop high blood pressure, dropsy, enlarged hearts, narrowed, rigid-walled blood vessels, albumin in the urine, and extensive degeneration and scarring of the kidney. If cortisone is given or the body is allowed to produce cortisone normally, no kidney damage occurs.

Nephritis frequently develops after such stresses as severe infections, particularly strep throats, poisoning from lead or bichloride of mercury, and the taking of toxic drugs.[1,6,70] Even healthy soldiers submitted to the stresses of extreme cold, running, long hikes, or diets low in protein or fat showed kidney damage to the extent that albumin and blood were temporarily lost in their urine.[71] Because cortisone, given for nephritis, has been "strikingly beneficial,"[4] every effort must be made to stimulate natural cortisone production the minute the disease is diagnosed.

Dropsy. Excessive water retention, spoken of as dropsy or edema, may be noticeable only as swollen ankles or puffiness around the eyes yet be so extensive that an emaciated person appears overweight. Such a condition usually indicates adrenal exhaustion.[7]

Giving large amounts of pantothenic acid to young men under stress increased the excretion of sodium,[72] which holds water in the body. A diet high in calcium and adequate in vitamin D likewise increases the excretion of salt, thus reducing edema,[73,74] whereas one high in carbohydrate holds both salt and water in the tissues.[75,76] The stress of nephritis may also cause the adrenals to produce excessive amounts of aldosterone, which holds so much salt and water in the body that edema and elevated blood pressure result.[7] Animals given diets deficient in nutrients that limit cortisone production, such as pantothenic acid and vitamins B_2 and B_{12}, develop edema, which is corrected when the missing vitamins are supplied or cortisone is given.[77-79]

Another cause of dropsy is that, when the kidneys are damaged, blood albumin is lost in the urine. Frequently as much protein as is supplied by a quart of milk is excreted daily over a period of years,[80] all of it coming from body tissues unless supplied in foods. Much additional albumin passes into the intestines and is lost in the feces,[81,82] particularly in persons who are anemic,[83,84] a common abnormality during nephrosis, when iron, copper, and numerous blood-building nutrients are so easily lost through the damaged kidneys.[4] Because blood albumin is vitally important in collecting urine, when it drops abnormally low, fluids and wastes remain in the tissues. Edema occurs readily when the diet is too low in protein or supplies so few calories that protein must be used for energy, but the rate of albumin production can be doubled by an adequate diet extremely high in protein.[85]

Because cholesterol deposition of long standing damages the kidneys and heart alike, severe nephrosis is often associated with a tired, slow-pumping heart which can force relatively little blood through the diseased kidneys, thus resulting in still greater fluid, salt, and urea retention and still higher blood pressure.[86] This condition, often treated only by restricting salt and liquid,[87] calls for maximum dietary improvement.

Increasing urine flow. Years ago it was shown that vitamin C markedly increased urine production,[78,88-92] and that only 300 to 500 milligrams daily were as effective as many medicinal diuretics.[90,91] Vitamin C is less effective when the salt intake is high,[89] and if given by injection, is lost so rapidly through the injured kidneys that it has little value.[92] Vitamin E at times also acts as a diuretic;[68] and urine production has been increased by giving large amounts of natural vitamin A daily.[53,93]

A potassium deficiency, which can further harm the kidneys, can be produced by eating too much salt,[94-96] by cortisone therapy, or by diuretics used in treating kidney diseases.[6,97] In animals, this deficiency causes the blood

pressure to soar,[94] the kidneys to swell to twice their
normal size, and the cells of the tubules to become so
engorged with water that they burst.[97] When the kidney
arteries of animals are tied to simulate those plugged with
cholesterol and such animals are given salt, severe nephrosis develops, but similarly treated animals kept on a low-
salt diet have no kidney damage.[94]

Provided nephrotic patients are given tablets supplying
several grams of potassium chloride daily, such kidney
damage is prevented; and the amount of salt and water
held in the body decrease, especially when cortisone is
administered.[1,97] Many physicians believe that tablets of
potassium chloride should be taken whenever salt is restricted;[95,96] and salt substitutes containing potassium chloride should be used liberally as a source of this nutrient (p.
216).

Unfortunately, taking diuretics, given to increase urine
flow, imposes serous nutritional problems. Large amounts
of every nutrient soluble in water appear to be lost in the
urine, and the more liquid taken, the greater become
these losses.[4,92,98-103] The tragedy is that such losses occur
when cholin, pantothenic acid, vitamin C, magnesium, and
many other nutrients are vitally needed. The same problem arises when patients with nephritis without edema are
asked to drink 3 to 5 quarts of fluids daily.[104] In this case,
even dangerous salt (sodium) deficiencies have been produced.[6]

Kidney hemorrhages. Because of stress, medications,
and high urinary losses a vitamin-C deficiency can be
readily produced during any kidney disease; hence the
danger of hemorrhaging is tremendously increased.[1] Even
a mild lack causes blood to appear in the urine.[1,97]

The passing of bloody urine or hemorrhaging have
sometimes been quickly stopped when huge amounts of vitamin C and/or "bioflavonoids" (p. 316) have been given
to persons with severe nephritis.[1,105,106] I once opened the
door to my waiting room to find a pleasant woman who
greeted me with the words: "May I kiss you? You saved
my granddaughter's life." She then told me that after
doctors had believed the child to be dying from nephritis,
giving her vitamin C and an extract made by boiling the
white of lemon rind which I had suggested had stopped
severe hemorrhaging and allowed the child to recover.

Since a cholin or vitamin-E deficiency can also cause
hemorrhages, large amounts of lecithin, cholin, and vitamin E should be given with vitamin C the minute kidney

disease is diagnosed, and all increased immediately if blood appears in the urine. Kidney hemorrhages have sometimes been stopped by giving vitamin E alone.[64,107]

Uremic poisoning. A nitrogen-containing substance known as urea is formed from the breakdown of body cells and from food proteins used as calories.[80] Since concentrated urea is toxic, if the amount of this substance in the blood becomes excessive, uremic poisoning can result.

A low-protein, high-calorie diet or even a protein-free diet is customarily given to patients threatened with uremic poisoning.[80,108,109] The stress of an extremely low protein intake, however, can cause so much body protein to be broken down that more urea is formed than if a high-protein diet is eaten.[110,111] Because the blood urea usually increases if fewer than 40 grams of protein are given daily,[1,80] at least this amount should be obtained. Though extremely low-protein diets have proved to be dangerous,[108] they are still being used.

Urea in the blood rises rapidly during a vitamin-B_6 deficiency.[112] Giving the amino acid alanine or an excessively high-protein diet, either of which increases the need for vitamin B_6, makes uremic poisoning markedly worse.[70,111,113,114] When 200 milligrams of vitamin B_6 were taken daily by deficient volunteers, the urea level quickly fell to normal;[113] and the blood urea, which is particularly excessive during the toxemia of pregnancy, also dropped to normal after vitamin B_6 was given.[115] Such findings indicate that this vitamin should be increased immediately if uremic poisoning threatens.

Low-salt diets. Because sodium is usually held in the body during dropsy, ordinary table salt and foods containing baking soda are customarily restricted. Though low-salt diets are relatively unappetizing, foods may be well seasoned with herbs, condiments, and salt substitutes.[80] If the diet can meet all the needs of stress and generous amounts of potassium are obtained from foods and/or supplements, salt restriction may be only temporary.

Deficiencies of salt, or of sodium and chlorine, have been produced in patients by too severe salt restriction; and weakness, muscle cramps, vomiting, and an elevated blood urea have resulted.[116] Such symptoms should be watched for, especially during hot weather.[117] Because a salt deficiency can be dangerous,[1,4,117] no fewer than 500 milligrams of sodium should be obtained daily,[118] and a low-salt diet should not be adhered to after dropsy has been corrected. Taking generous amounts of potassium—physicians sometimes give 12 grams or more daily—causes salt to be excreted and often makes salt restriction unnecessary.

The present state of chaos. The famous urologist Dr. Thomas Addis described the dietary management of kidney diseases as being in an "extraordinary state of disorganization" and "chaos";[119] and many investigators have pointed out that diets used today for kidney diseases are 40 years behind research findings.[6,109]

On three occasions I have watched beautiful children die of nephritis while being given diets almost totally lacking cholin, pantothenic acid, magnesium, essential fatty acids, vitamins B_6, C, D, and E, and whose protein intake was drastically curtailed even though their blood urea was not high. In each case, their mothers were afraid to improve their diets without a physician's permission. On the other hand, I have worked in clinics with outstanding urologists, one of whom once told me, "I love to get the patients you've seen. They get well so fast." It was not I, but adequate nutrition that speeded their recovery.

All experimentally produced kidney disease is corrected provided the nutrients needed for repair are amply supplied. The problem is that irreparable damage can be quickly done unless the diet is promptly improved. When the disease is allowed to become serious, so many nutrients are continuously lost through the damaged kidneys that dietary help becomes an uphill task.

Diet for kidney diseases. Because each case of Bright's disease varies during the course of the illness, a doctor must determine the amount of protein, salt, and fluid to be allowed daily. As with a diabetic diet, all nutritional improvements must be made within the framework of these allowances. He will emphasize that calories must be kept high at all times to prevent either food proteins or body proteins from being used for energy and the urea formation increased; and that six meals or more must be taken daily.

Despite years of controversy, authorities now agree that protein must be unusually high except when uremic poisoning threatens. It must be sufficient to replace all albumin lost in the urine and feces, and to rebuild tissues, meet the general body needs, and fulfill the demands of stress.[1,4,6,80] Patients able to take 150 to 200 grams of protein daily recover much more rapidly, and kidney biopsies show greater healing than in others obtaining less protein.[4,6,97] Persons in charge of feeding nephrotic patients should use the tables of food composition to count both the grams of protein and the calories obtained daily (pp. 405–435).

If sodium is restricted, ocean fish and proteins from animals which eat salt—meats, eggs, cheese, milk—may be limited. Low-sodium milk and cheeses are available. Torula yeast is particularly low in sodium, and wheat germ, soybeans, soy flour, nuts, and salt-free nut butters are all excellent and contain far less sodium than animal products. If eggs are limited, use 2 yolks instead of 1 whole egg. When protein is drastically restricted, only egg yolks, liver, yeast, yogurt, milk, and cheese should be used, and incomplete vegetable proteins should be avoided.[108] Pep-up (p. 329) can be prepared with low-salt milk or any fruit juice. Oils should be used for cooking and seasoning instead of solid fats. As long as meat is allowed, fresh and/or desiccated liver may be taken several times daily, especially when anemia is severe.

Supplements should be heavily relied upon to furnish all nutrients not obtained from food. The following amounts have been given daily to persons with kidney disease in the studies cited earlier: 3 to 6 tablespoons of lecithin and 1,000 milligrams of cholin, usually as 250 milligrams at each meal and before bed; 30 milligrams of vitamin B_6 or more; and 25,000 units of natural vitamin A, with 300 to 600 units of vitamin E. If little or no milk is allowed, 250 milligrams of calcium should be taken four to six times daily, preferably with magnesium and 10 milligrams of vitamin B_2. I feel that the antistress formula should be taken around the clock; that the blood cholesterol be known and supplements given accordingly (ch. 5); and because digestion is usually below par, that hydrochloric acid, digestive enzymes, and yogurt or acidophilus milk or culture be taken each time food is eaten. The more liquid the patient is asked to drink, the more carefully the diet must be planned and the larger the amounts of supplements used. When diuretics are given, the situation becomes one of hoping that enough nutrients be retained in the body to rebuild kidney tissue.

The success of a nutrition program depends largely on how promptly dietary improvement is initiated. If an adequate diet is given from the moment the diagnosis is made, the usual attitude that kidney diseases are "not amenable to cure"[109,120] appears to be unjustified. If given a chance, our bodies have an amazing ability to heal themselves.

20
Kidney Stones Can Be Dissolved

Any of the thousands suffering from kidney stones should know the story of a man I shall call Joe. "That kidney of mine's one of the seven wonders of the world," Joe told me. "Works perfectly. It was so full of stones the doctor was sure he'd have to remove it. When I asked him about seeing you, he said, 'Sure. Try anything. I can get you to the hospital in five minutes if you have trouble.' At that time x-rays showed five stones the size of pigeon eggs, nine like your big fingernail. The rest of the kidney looked like it had been shot with a BB gun. Every bit of it was full of stones.

"I've no idea how many stones I've passed. Got a whole bottle of them. My back ached day and night for 20 years and never let up. And renal colic! I've walked the floor, known the agonies of the damned. Doesn't ache a bit any more.

"I've only passed five stones since I started the diet. At the end of the first year, x-rays showed only three little stones left, and I've had no trouble since."

When Joe first consulted me in 1952, little was known about kidney stones except that they sometimes developed in animals lacking vitamin A. It was known that calcium is lost in the urine when protein is low or too little calcium is supplied in proportion to phosphorus; and I reasoned that if the acid in a well-known soft drink would dissolve a tooth, a much softer kidney stone should dissolve in acid urine. I therefore planned a diet which would produce an acid urine and was high in calcium, protein, and vitamin A. Because I believe every diet should be adequate, other nutrients important in dissolving stones were accidentally included.

Several persons with whom I have worked have had stones dissolve or become small enough to pass without difficulty, but none had as many stones as Joe.

Kinds of kidney stones. Kidney and urinary-bladder

stones, which range from grit, sand, and gravel to the size of bird eggs, are mostly formed of crystals of calcium combined with phosphorus or oxalic acid. They are often removed surgically, but more stones usually form within weeks unless preventive measures are taken.

A few stones are mostly uric acid or the amino acid cystine. To prevent such stones, large amounts of fruits and vegetables, especially citrus fruits, should be eaten, thus producing an alkaline urine which keeps crystals of these substances in solution. When a sodium-urate stone has been passed, the dietary measures suggested for gout should be followed (ch.18). The loss of cystine in the urine is said to be a hereditary error, which often means an unusually high genetic requirement for certain nutrients; a few cases have been helped by giving large amounts of cholin.[1] To limit the cystine intake, protein may be restricted to 70 grams daily.

The remainder of this chapter deals only with the more common stones formed from calcium phosphate or oxalate.

The remedy may be simple. Oxalate and phosphate stones develop most rapidly when the urine is alkaline. Normally citric acid, synthesized in the body from carbohydrate, causes the urine to be sufficiently acid to keep minerals and oxalic-acid crystals in solution. If magnesium is lacking, however, citric acid cannot be produced, and the quantity in the urine immediately decreases, but it increases again as soon as magnesium is given.[2] Persons unfamiliar with these acids and perhaps confused by them might think of oxalic acid as the villain and citric acid as the rescuing hero.

Kidney stones have now been repeatedly produced in animals deficient in magnesium.[3,4] When groups of rats lacking vitamin B_6 were kept on diets containing 20 to 400 milligrams of magnesium per 100 grams of food, the animals allowed generous amounts of magnesium had seven times more citric acid in their urine than those receiving small amounts.[4] Each increase in magnesium decreased the number of stones. Oxalic acid remained high, however, as long as vitamin B_6 was lacking. A vitamin-B_6 deficiency alone causes both a tremendous increase in the oxalic-acid content of the urine[5] and a decrease in the amount of citric acid.[2] Giving adequate vitamin B_6 with inadequate magnesium causes kidney stones to be largely calcium phosphate, the kind most common in America. Adequate magnesium with inadequate vitamin B_6 results in oxalate stones, the variety particularly prevalent in England but rapidly increasing here.[3,6]

These experimental findings appear to apply equally to humans. Patients who had passed kidney stones (both oxalate and phosphate) over a ten-year period were given 250 milligrams of magnesium oxide daily.[7] While taking magnesium, they passed no stones or grit; and the urinary losses of calcium and phosphorus dropped markedly, though they became excessive again when magnesium was withdrawn six months later. Immediately small stones began passing, but they stopped as soon as magnesium was resumed.

People who have passed oxalic-acid stones have been found to be deficient in vitamin B_6, and some seem unable to absorb it.[8] The absorption is increased by both magnesium and vitamin B_2; and an injection of vitamin B_6 enables such individuals to absorb the vitamin well thereafter by mouth.[8] Persons who have passed calcium-oxalate stones excrete 16 to 30 times more oxalic acid than do normal individuals;[9] and volunteers on diets lacking vitamin B_6 have excreted increasingly larger amounts of this acid as the deficiency became more severe, though the excretion stopped when the vitamin was allowed them.[10] Similarly, pregnant women, notoriously deficient in vitamin B_6, excrete oxalic acid, which has decreased markedly after 10 to 20 milligrams of this vitamin are given daily.[11]

The source of oxalic acid. The amino acid glycine, improperly utilized when vitamin B_6 is undersupplied, changes into oxalic acid, which forms stones and also often causes sharp oxalate crystals to damage the kidneys.[12,13] Radioactively labeled glycine, given to stone-formers, can be recovered as oxalic acid; in healthy persons it can be found only in body protein.[13] When experimental animals are deficient in vitamin B_6, the more glycine given them, the greater is the urinary excretion of oxalic acid;[11] this excretion decreases immediately if the vitamin is given with glycine.[11]

Individuals who have passed calcium-oxalate stones are often given diets excluding dozens of excellent fruits and vegetables because they contain some oxalic acid. Unfortunately, oxalate stones are still formed even when no oxalic acid whatsoever is obtained in the diet.[1] If fruits and vegetables are restricted, more proteins are eaten; therefore, the need for vitamin B_6 and the intake of glycine both increase while the magnesium intake decreases; thus the stage is set for more stones to form. No healthful food should be avoided but to prevent protein imbalance, complete proteins should be eaten with all incomplete ones; and gelatin, which supplies such an excess of glycine that it can increase stone formation,[13] should be given a wide berth.

Other influences. So many stones have been produced in rats and guinea pigs lacking vitamin A that the kidneys have been filled with them,[14,15] yet this finding has not been consistent. Dead cells, sloughing from the mucous membrane of the kidney tubules when vitamin A is undersupplied, have apparently formed a base upon which calcium crystals are deposited.[16] Similarly, kidney stones in man have at times been associated with symptoms of too little vitamin A,[17-19] yet autopsies of persons who have died with stones have often revealed no signs of this deficiency.[1] Obviously, other factors must be associated with a vitamin-A deficiency before stones are produced.

Stone-formers usually have an alkaline urine that contains bacteria and much ammonia.[16] When vitamin A is inadequate, dead cells support the growth of millions of bacteria which quickly break urea into ammonia, causing the urine to become alkaline. Calcium crystals, which cannot dissolve in an alkaline urine, are therefore readily deposited as stones.[1] In all probability, if bacteria reach the kidneys, a lack of any nutrient allowing cells to slough off, whether cholin or vitamin A or E (ch. 19), contributes to stone formation by supplying food for their growth.

A potassium deficiency, brought on by eating refined foods, too much salt, or too few fruits and vegetables, causes the urine to be so extremely alkaline that minerals cannot be held in solution;[20-22] hence they are easily deposited as stones.

Calcium retention. The loss of calcium in the urine is influenced by many conditions. When the kidneys are healthy, 99 per cent of all calcium passing through the tubules is absorbed back into the blood.[23] Vitamin D, however, is essential before the kidney tubules can reabsorb calcium efficiently. If this vitamin is undersupplied, as it frequently is in stone-formers, large amounts of both calcium and phosphorus are excreted in the urine.[24] Excessive synthetic vitamin D, or irradiated ergosterol, such as 5,000 to 25,000 units daily, likewise causes a heavy loss of these minerals.[24-26]

During any type of stress, self-produced cortisone draws minerals from the bones and increases the urinary losses of both calcium and phosphorus;[2] and these losses usually continue to be abnormally high until the stress is relieved. Cortisone medication, thyroid, aspirin, and numerous other drugs also increase the urinary losses of calcium and phosphorus.[2] An antistress diet (p. 31) high in calcium and adequate in magnesium largely prevents these losses and the accompanying demineralization of bones (ch. 26).

The severe stress of immobilization and the illness that makes it necessary cause a marked loss of minerals, which may persist for many months.[27] Even when healthy volunteers were immobilized by casts from the waist to the ankles, excessive amounts of calcium, phosphorus, and many other nutrients were continuously lost in the urine.[28] Persons whose immobilization is prolonged are particularly subject to the calcium-phosphate type of kidney stones and to spontaneous fractures of the vertebrae.[2,27] Instead of being recognized as a typical stress reaction, however, it is usually assumed that bones, like muscles, degenerate when unused, thus causing the high urinary excretion of minerals.

During stress calcium is so readily withdrawn from the bones that the urinary losses are high when no calcium whatsoever is obtained in the diet.[2] Calcium in the urine of paraplegics has not been reduced by a low-calcium diet.[2] On the contrary, when they received 2.5 grams of calcium daily—an amount obtainable from 2½ quarts of milk—the urinary losses of both calcium and phosphorus were markedly reduced. The investigators therefore recommended that supplements of calcium always be given to immobilized people.

Much of the calcium and magnesium is carried and retained in the blood by being combined with albumin. When the diet is low in protein, so little albumin can be produced that these minerals are lost in the urine,[16] a situation conducive to stone formation. Both of these minerals, however, compete for the available albumin. If excessive magnesium is taken, it combines with so much of the albumin that calcium is crowded out, thus causing it to be lost in the urine.[29] Excessive calcium can crowd out magnesium in the same manner.[16] Individuals who take huge amounts of calcium carbonate in antiacid preparations frequently produce such severe magnesium deficiencies in themselves that they develop kidney stones. Similarly, laboratory and farm animals kept on milk diets develop magnesium deficiencies. Studies of persons in Finland and Africa, who eat unrefined foods high in both magnesium and calcium, however, revealed no kidney stones in spite of a calcium intake of 4 to 5 grams daily.

An imbalance of calcium in relation to phosphorus can also cause calcium to be lost. Because the body uses a large percentage of available calcium and phosphorus together to give rigidity to the bones, if excessive amounts of either mineral are obtained, much of the excess cannot be used for lack of a "companion." This situation is like having too few men to marry the available women, though the reverse is just as bad. When too little calcium is obtained and the diet is high in phosphorus—a typical American diet—much of the phosphorus, though perhaps severely needed, is excreted in the form of a calcium-phosphorus salt; thus the urine is high in both calcium and phosphorus.

Conversely, if a diet is low in phosphorus but high in calcium, which usually occurs only in a laboratory, such large amounts of both calcium and phosphorus are lost that stones are formed;[30] yet this diet has actually been recommended for persons with kidney stones.[27] Even when losses of these minerals are high, if they stay in solution, no stones can form.

Danger of inadequate diets. People with kidney stones have had low-calcium, low-phosphorus, and low-protein diets recommended to them, often forbidding milk and milk products, eggs, liver, and whole-grain breads and cereals;[1,31-33] yet such diets are inadequate in almost every respect. Moreover, they are frequently given gels, which cause phosphorus—needed daily by every cell in the body—to be excreted in the feces and thus have the same effect as a low-phosphorus diet. To prevent the urine from becoming too concentrated, stone-formers are frequently asked to drink 4 to 5 quarts of liquid daily, though such a quantity might easily wash out so much magnesium, vitamin B_6, and other nutrients that stone formation could increase. When adequate magnesium and vitamin B_6 keep minerals in solution and reduce their loss, excessive amounts of fluid are not needed.

Several rapid stone-formers have consulted me who had been kept for several years on inadequate diets with gels and a high fluid intake. Two young women, 19 and 26 years old, both of whom looked like walking ghosts, had had repeated surgery for the removal of stones. The younger one died following further surgery shortly after I first saw her; I am convinced that her adrenals were too exhausted to withstand more stress. The second, whose doctor feels that she has made a remarkable recovery, is no longer a stone-former, but her body is old, and irreparable damage appears to have been done.

Probably every person who has passed a stone should take 250 to 500 milligrams of magnesium and 10 to 20 milligrams of vitamin B_6 daily. As I see it, except for these supplements, nothing more is needed either to prevent or to dissolve kidney or bladder stones than a diet that furnishes adequate amounts of every nutrient including calcium (ch. 32).

21
Your Blood Pressure

Before writing this chapter, I asked several persons—all intelligent individuals—to define or describe blood pressure and received the following amazing answers: "That's how hard your heart pumps," "What you feel in your ears," "It means you get a stroke," "A squeeze put on something 'til you explode," and "It's when your pulse is abnormal." By then I decided blood pressure should be explained.

The function of blood pressure. The force exerted by the blood against the walls of the blood vessels is the blood pressure, and it is similar to the pushing of water against the sides of a garden hose. Decreasing the water in a hose or replacing a small hose with a large one and keeping the amount of water the same reduces the force against the walls, simulating low blood pressure. Conversely, if the amount of water in a hose is increased or a standard hose is replaced by a small one, the pressure against the walls is raised, as in hypertension. In atherosclerosis, arteries normally large enough to slip a little finger into may be so plugged with fatty substances that a match can scarcely be inserted; when most of the arteries are thus clogged, the blood is squeezed into a relatively little space, and the blood pressure naturally becomes high.

It is the blood pressure which forces oxygen and food, or plasma carrying sugar, amino cids, fatty acids, vitamins, and minerals, into the tissues through porous microscopic capillary walls; hence normal blood pressure is vital to the nutrition of the cells. When the blood in the capillary beds becomes concentrated from the loss of plasma, the blood protein, albumin, attracts tissue fluids carrying wastes into the vessels, causing the quantity of blood to remain remarkably constant. Thus by virtue of the blood pressure, all tissues are constantly bathed in fresh, nutrient-laden fluid and the breakdown products from worn-out cells are removed.

When larger amounts of oxygen and nutrients are needed, the contraction of tiny muscles in the arterial walls causes the pressure to increase and supplies to be pushed more quickly to the cells. Conversely, if few nutrients are required, these muscles relax, the pressure decreases, and food is conserved. When I was doing graduate work, a medical student showed our physiology class a graph of his wife's blood pressure which he had taken at hourly intervals throughout a day, starting before she awoke. Since few nutrients are needed during sleep, the first reading was low. Each meal, particularly a large dinner, caused a marked rise to supply plasma required to produce quarts of digestive juices; this pressure gradually dropped. It soared during a game of tennis, fell when she read, and reached a peak after a quarrel over a bridge game. Such normal fluctuations occur in all of us from birth to death.

With each heartbeat, a fresh spurt of blood is forced into the arteries, temporarily increasing the pressure against their walls. This pressure, spoken of as systolic, is normally 120 to 130 millimeters when measured by a standard column of mercury. The pressure, naturally lower when taken while the heart is resting, or dilated, is known as diastolic and is normally 80 to 90 millimeters.

Increasing low blood pressure. Faulty nutrition allows the tissues forming the walls of the blood vessels to become overly relaxed and perhaps flabby or stretched; hence less oxygen and nutrients are supplied the tissues. As a result, the person with low blood pressure suffers needlessly from fatigue, usually lacks endurance, is sensitive to cold and heat, requires more sleep than healthy individuals, develops a rapid pulse on exertion, and often has little interest in sex. These symptoms become worse when superimposed on normal decreases in blood pressure. Such people usually feel more tired when they get up in the morning than before they went to bed.

Low blood pressure has been produced in volunteers by diets only mildly deficient in calories,[1] protein,[2] vitamin C,[3] or almost any one of the B vitamins.[4] Of all nutrients, however, a lack of pantothenic acid most quickly causes low blood pressure.[5] Since an undersupply of this vitamin inhibits the production of adrenal hormones, excessive amounts of salt and water are excreted and the amount of blood—the volume—actually decreases. Adrenal exhaustion brought on by prolonged stress, which greatly increases the need for pantothenic acid, is invariably accompanied by low blood pressure. Obtaining sufficient pantothenic acid alone often raises the blood pressure to normal.

An adequate diet which emphasizes complete proteins, the B vitamins, the antistress factors, and particularly the nutrients that stimulate adrenal production (ch. 2) quickly normalizes low blood pressure. For several years I planned diets for all the patients of three obstetricians, hundreds of whom had low blood pressure; usually it was corrected in two or three weeks. Until the blood pressure reaches normal, however, salty foods and/or ½ teaspoon of salt in water should be taken daily. Since vitamin E reduces the need for oxygen,[6] it is especially helpful in relieving the fatigue that results when the tissues are oxygen-starved.

High blood pressure, or hypertension. The blood pressure becomes elevated when larger-than-normal amounts of water (and sodium) are held in the body, a situation that invariably occurs during the alarm reaction to stress. In this case, the quantity of blood plasma, or the blood volume, increases. On the other hand, arteries can become smaller when tension causes the muscular walls to contract or when they are plugged with cholesterol, compressed in beds of fat, or shrunk by scar tissue that may be calcified. Most persistent high blood pressure results from a combination of these factors.

In order to form urine, the blood pressure in the capillary coils of the kidneys is already unusually high (p. 192); therefore when an elevated blood pressure is superimposed on such tiny, strained capillaries, they can easily be damaged. Simultaneously high blood pressure forces the heart to pump against a greater resistance, putting it under constant strain. For these reasons, hypertension is associated with and often a symptom of diseases of both the heart and the kidneys. When prolonged high blood pressure occurs without apparent damage to the heart and/or kidneys, it is spoken of as essential hypertension.

The usual symptoms of high blood pressure are headaches, dizziness, noises or ringing in the ears, and, sooner or later, hemorrhages in the eyes.[7] When the marked elevations of blood pressure that occur normally are superimposed on high blood pressure, capillaries can easily break and result in a heart attack or cerebral hemorrhage (stroke). It has been suggested that the brain is particularly susceptible to hemorrhages because it is imprisoned in the skull and cannot expand when the blood volume increases or heightened pressure drives excessive fluids into its tissues.[8]

Moderately high blood pressure is 150 to 180 systolic over 90 to 100 diastolic. Pressures above 180 systolic and 100 diastolic bring grave danger of blood vessels breaking. A minor break can cause a clot to form and perhaps cut off circulation to millions of cells, whereas a major break may result in paralysis or death.

Effect of kidney damage. One function of the kidneys is to control blood pressure. When oxygen is inadequate, they appear to secrete a hormone-like "pressor factor" which elevates the blood pressure, thus increasing the oxygen supply.[9] Because vitamin E decreases the need for oxygen, it is especially important for persons with high blood pressure.[10] Deficiencies of cholin or of vitamin C or E cause hemorrhages in the kidneys and bring oxygen starvation to cells formerly depending on the interrupted blood supply (ch. 19); thus such deficiencies may stimulate the pressor factor and elevate the blood pressure.

High blood pressure has been produced in animals by removing part of a kidney to simulate human kidney destruction caused by Bright's disease.[9,11] Marked and prolonged elevated blood pressure can even result from mild kidney damage. For example, an insignificant lack of vitamin B_6 can cause hypertension due to damage to the kidney by sharp crystals of oxalic acid.[12,13] This form of kidney injury, quickly corrected after the vitamin is given, is probably responsible for the high blood pressure so common in pregnant women. Hypertension resulting from kidney damage is still further elevated by diets excessive in salt, calories, or hydrogenated fats, and by taking ACTH or cortisone.[11]

In any case of hypertension, the first emphasis must be placed on maintaining the health of the kidneys (ch. 19).

Effect of cholin. Because high blood pressure has been repeatedly produced in animals on diets deficient in cholin,[14,15] 158 patients with dangerous hypertension were studied while being given cholin daily.[16] Of this group, 133 had essential hypertension of unknown origin; and 22 had had hemorrhages in the brain or eyes, three had diabetes, three heart disease, and 19 nephritis. Since each person had been on various medications for a year or longer without improvement, all medication was discontinued before cholin was given.

Such symptoms as headaches, dizziness, ear noises, palpitation, and constipation improved or disappeared completely five to ten days after the vitamin was started. The blood pressure, which began to fall within three weeks, decreased in every case, the average drop being 31 millimeters systolic and 20 diastolic; in more than a third of these patients, the blood pressure dropped to normal, but none fell below normal. Insomnia, trembling, dropsy when present, and visual disturbances were gradually relieved, and improvement was noticed in speech and mobility.

Before cholin was given, the capillary walls were extremely weak in 97 per cent of the cases; a marked increase in strength occurred almost immediately and "vast improvement" took place over a period of five months. Simultaneously, the blood vessels dilated, blood flow was accelerated, and the work of the heart was markedly decreased. In some individuals, the blood flow in the eyes showed steady improvement over a two-year period. When cholin was withdrawn, however, the capillary walls again became weak, and the blood pressure sometimes increased.

Cholin has rarely been given to persons with high blood pressure. Since it is essential for the synthesis of lecithin and the utilization of fat, cholin deficiencies may be responsible for the hypertension that is particularly prevalent among overweight individuals, diabetic patients, and those suffering from nephritis and/or heart disease. Reducing weight, for instance, does not necessarily reduce the blood pressure.[17]

Giving a diet high in complete proteins sometimes decreases hypertension,[2] possibly because cholin can be made from the amino acid methionine; and any nutrient that increases lecithin production may be equally valuable. Animals deficient in magnesium, for example, often develop high blood pressure accompanied by the deposition of calcium in the arterial walls,[18] but whether this deficiency is a major cause of hardening of the arteries is not known.

Sodium and potassium. High blood pressure has been produced in animals merely by keeping them on a potassium-deficient diet or by feeding them excessive amounts of salt which causes so much potassium to be lost in the urine that a deficiency results.[19-24] In either case, so much water is retained that the volume of blood increases and the blood pressure is elevated.

Human potassium deficiencies as a cause of high blood pressure have been little studied. The incidence of hypertension throughout the world, however, is greatest and develops at the earliest age in populations having an excessive salt intake; and high blood pressure is virtually unknown where little salt is used.[25] In Japan, for instance, heart disease is rare, yet brain hemorrhage brought on by high blood pressure is the leading cause of death.[26] In northern Japan, where salt fish is a principal food, the salt intake averages 27 grams daily, and deaths from brain hemorrhages are much higher than in the south, where the daily intake averages 17 grams.[22] In America also the incidence of high blood pressure parallels the salt intake of 1 to 5 teaspoons (4 to 20 grams) daily,[25] especially among overweight persons;[22] and the tissues of American stroke victims have a much higher salt content than those of individuals dying from other causes.

Decreasing the salt (sodium) intake has long been used successfully to lower blood pressure,[27] but because severe salt restriction can be dangerous,[28] this approach may not be the wisest one. Adequate calcium and vitamin D help to increase the loss of salt in the urine,[29,30] and in rats, high blood pressure caused by salt toxicity can be decreased or prevented by giving generous amounts of cholin, pantothenic acid, vitamins B_2 and C, and particularly potassium.[31]

The quantities of sodium and potassium in the blood constantly teeter-totter, and an excess of one causes the other to be lost in the urine. Thus persons eating salt as they wished excreted nine times more potassium than when their salt intake was limited;[32] and human volunteers kept on diets deficient in potassium retained so much salt that they developed high blood pressure.[32-36] Conversely, potassium obtained from leaves and grass caused such high sodium losses that wild animals used to walk hundreds of miles to salt licks.

Healthy kidneys, which conserve sodium far more efficiently than potassium, readily lose potassium in the urine; and when kidneys are damaged, this nutrient is lost even more quickly.[32] If foods rich in potassium are eaten or a potassium salt is taken, a high blood pressure drops to normal provided its only cause is an excessive salt intake. Similarly, when sodium is restricted, potassium is conserved, excessive amounts of water and salt are no longer retained, and the blood pressure, if high, decreases.

Under normal circumstances potassium remains largely in the cells and sodium in the surrounding fluids; thus placed, both play vital roles in controlling the passage of dozens of substances into and out of each cell. When the potassium content of the cells decreases because of a potassium deficiency, sodium passes into the depleted cells and attracts so much fluid that tissues become water-logged.[32] For this reason, high blood pressure is often accompanied by dropsy.

Physicians have given patients with hypertension 5 to 20 grams of potassium chloride (or other potassium salts) daily and have found this approach equally as effective in reducing blood pressure as restricting salt (sodium).[37-42] Furthermore, because many of these patients had both heart disease and high blood pressure, electrocardiograms were taken at 15-minute intervals after potassium was given; the changes toward normal were identical to those occurring when salt (sodium) was restricted.[1,38-42]

Unfortunately, a diet consisting of rice, fruit, and sugar[43] is frequently given to people with high blood pressure despite the fact that it is criminally deficient in cholin, pantothenic acid, all other B vitamins, iodine, vitamin E, complete proteins, and many other nutrients.[11,44] Furthermore, carbohydrates cause salt and water to be retained in the body.[45] Although the stress of this diet has induced ulcers,[47] it does supply 20 times more potassium than sodium; and in persons able to endure it for two to five months, it has reduced blood pressure.

Quantities of potassium are discarded during the refining of foods, and the richest sources, cooked green leafy vegetables, are now rarely eaten. These factors, combined with excessive urinary losses induced by our high salt intake, have now caused potassium deficiencies to be commonplace. Both sodium and potassium should be adequate, yet neither excessive. If salt is used in moderation, refined foods avoided, and fruits and vegetables generously supplied in the diet, a potassium deficiency is improbable unless the kidneys are damaged. Because my husband enjoys salt but looks on salads and many vegetables with a jaundiced eye, I keep ordinary salt mixed with an equal amount of a potassium-chloride salt substitute in all our salt shakers. No one has ever discovered this subterfuge. Such salt substitutes, however, vary from horrible to excellent.

Persons whose blood pressure is already high should use a salt substitute entirely for a while; and, as a temporary measure, take 1 or 2 grams of potassium chloride at each meal unless they are being given digitalis. The diet should also be particularly adequate in every nutrient shown to reduce blood pressure.

The effect of atherosclerosis. Atherosclerosis is a major cause of high blood pressure in the United States;[7,26] and autopsies have shown that the degree of hypertension during life parallels the extent of cholesterol deposition in the kidney arteries.[7] High blood pressure can be produced in animals merely by tying threads around arteries in the kidneys, thus simulating blood vessels in human kidneys plugged with fatty substances.[9,48] The kidney arteries are so tiny that relatively little cholesterol can reduce the oxygen supply and release the "pressor factor" (p. 213);[9] thus the blood pressure can become elevated while the blood cholesterol is still normal. This mechanism, triggered by a lack of oxygen, can be delayed by giving vitamin E, which reduces the oxygen requirement.[6]

Conversely, high blood pressure hastens the deposition of fatty substances and makes atherosclerosis much worse;[49] hence almost twice as many people with high blood pressure die of heart attacks as do individuals whose blood pressure is normal.

Hypertension of emotional origin. Any form of stress, even such a simple thing as low blood sugar, can increase the blood pressure.[37,50] ACTH or cortisone medication, simulating the outpouring of hormones during stress, invariably elevates the blood pressure, and thus prepares the body for "fight or flight."[8,51] Such emotional stresses as anger and fear, which particularly make us want to fight or escape, cause the pressure to rise by the contraction of tiny muscles in the arterial walls; and such hypertension continues as long as the emotions exist provided the adrenals do not become exhausted. If the emotions causing it are expressed, however, the blood pressure subsides.

A woman consulted me whose hypertension had developed soon after she married a well-to-do man who maintained three homes, one in the city and others at a lake and a mountain resort. She told me that he expected her to entertain continuously and, because help was difficult to find, she "spent her life" cleaning a dozen or more bathrooms. Quite justifiably, she smoldered with resentment. I suggested that she take up several hobbies as a means of blowing off steam. Two years later she came to see me bringing a small golf trophy and several pictures she had painted. The bathrooms were not quite so clean as before but her blood pressure was normal.

The prolonged stress of accumulated unexpressed negative emotions (p. 113) is a major cause of essential hypertension. During psychotherapy, such high blood pressure usually drops to normal as soon as "hostilities" are expressed. In any case where essential hypertension is not corrected by adequate nutrition, psychosomatic causes should be looked for.

Strokes. Surely no tragedy is so great as the degeneration of a brilliant mind following a stroke. To prevent such a living death, certain steps can be taken immediately if the blood pressure is found to be high. Only small, frequent meals should be eaten. The cholin and potassium intakes may be increased and sodium reduced. All nutrients needed to meet the demands of stress (ch. 2), to lower blood cholesterol (ch. 5), and to rebuild kidney tissue (ch.19) should be generously supplied. Because even a slight lack of vitamin C or E allows blood vessels to break easily, large amounts of these nutrients may prevent a cerebral hemorrhage.[48,52] As much stress as possible should be removed, and some means found to blow off steam.

High blood pressure can slow up the blood flow to the extent that oxygen consumption is low and the need for vitamin E is increased.[10] Because this vitamin decreases the oxygen requirement, if a hemorrhage does occur, cells that might otherwise be destroyed may survive. Since vitamin E can increase the strength of the heartbeat, it sometimes elevates the blood pressure temporarily if introduced in large amounts; therefore when hypertension is severe, no more than 300 units should be given at first and the amount gradually increased to 600 units daily.[53]

Usually one stroke follows another because the conditions that led to the first remain unchanged. Yet marked improvement has resulted when vitamin E has been given, even long after a stroke has occurred.[54] A completely adequate diet started immediately can sometimes restore health.

The goal. An ideal diet must not only lower elevated blood pressure but also gradually rebuild damage in the blood vessels, kidneys, heart, and brain which usually accompanies hypertension.[16] It is tragic indeed that vast numbers of people are content to alleviate the exhaustion of low blood pressure with pep pills or the symptoms of hypertension with such tranquilizers as rauwolfia, thus allowing the body to continue to degenerate. Far more constructive is the attitude of a woman who once rushed in to see me. "I've got to bring my blood pressure down right now," she exclaimed excitedly. "My son's on the Stanford football team and my doctor won't let me go to a single game unless it comes down." Fortunately, she followed advice carefully, and never missed a game.

Sound nutrition relieves symptoms by improving the health of the body as a whole. Its reward is a renewed zest for living.

22
Disorders of the Nervous System

Nervousness is such a vague term that in scientific circles it barely escapes being classified as a dirty word, though companies making millions from tranquilizers must bless it. Probably every person knows the miserable feeling we think of as nervousness. It has dozens of causes: low blood sugar; a drop in blood calcium; a magnesium deficiency; unconscious anxieties and fears; and a lack of almost any of the ten B vitamins, each of which is essential to the normal function of every nerve in the body.[1]

Symptoms that are all too familiar—tension, insomnia, irritability, quarrelsomeness, butterflies in the stomach, unsteadiness, trembling, and tingling—have been produced in persons denied vitamin B$_6$.[2] Volunteers made deficient in pantothenic acid became easily upset, irritable, quarrelsome, depressed, and suffered from tension, dizziness, and numbness and tingling sensations.[3] Similarly, human subjects lacking niacin, biotin, or any other B vitamin, so readily discarded during refining, have also developed extreme nervousness.[4]

Calcium is essential for the relaxation of nerve tissue, whereas magnesium is particularly involved with the normal function of the brain, spinal cord, and all nerves.[5] Our average daily intake of magnesium appears to be only half the adult requirement.[6] Because alcohol causes a high urinary loss of magnesium (p. 65), nervousness resulting from this deficiency is especially common among social drinkers.[7] Magnesium deficiencies, produced by meals consisting of "enriched" white bread, macaroni, spaghetti, noodles, tapioca, sugar, honey, and hydrogenated fats, caused volunteers to become overly keyed up, high-strung, unable to sleep, and jumpy at the slightest noise.[8]

Such symptoms—call them nervousness or what you will—palliated by tranquilizers only become worse. When endured, they bring unhappiness, loss of patience, and irritability. Corrected by simple nutritional improve-

220

ments, they are often gone in a few days or sometimes even in hours.

Epilepsy. Convulsions apparently identical to epilepsy have been produced in many species of animals and in infants and adults by a lack of vitamin B_6.[1,9] Almost 25 years ago, the late Dr. Tom Spies gave vitamin B_6 to persons subject to epilepsy and achieved excellent results.[10] More recently a well-known proprietary baby formula contained so little vitamin B_6 that more than 300 infants given it developed severe convulsions,[11] an inexcusable tragedy which could have been prevented had the formula been tested on animals before being marketed or had physicians who gave it checked its vitamin-B_6 content. In our community, one exhausted and worried young mother committed suicide because her infant, receiving this formula, had such seizures, though the child is healthy today.

Babies given this formula were irritable, sensitive to noises, showed abnormal electroencephalograms, and had repeated seizures brought on by handling, feeding, or loud sounds. Though these convulsions stopped and the electroencephalograms became normal within minutes after vitamin B_6 was given, some infants needed only 1.2 milligrams daily to prevent further seizures, whereas others required 5 milligrams.[11,12] In one case where the mother had epilepsy unless she took vitamin B_6 regularly, her infant's requirement was particularly high.[13]

If large amounts of vitamin B_6 alone are given, the need for other B vitamins, particularly vitamin B_2 and pantothenic acid, is so increased that harm can be done unless they, too, are supplied.[14,15] Streptomycin, which appears to destroy vitamin B_6 or perhaps increases the need for it, has also caused epileptic-like convulsions in children. Tests for xanthurenic acid (p. 96) have shown, however, that many persons with epilepsy are not deficient in vitamin B_6;[16] and in such cases, the vitamin has no corrective effect.[12,16]

The results of giving persons with epilepsy adequate magnesium have been more consistently favorable. Thirty epileptic children, all previously on anticonvulsant drugs, were given 450 milligrams of magnesium daily by mouth, and the drugs were discontinued.[17] A 13-year-old boy who had had epilepsy for ten years was extremely depressed, showed signs of mental retardation, and his seizures could not be prevented by drugs. After receiving magnesium, his epilepsy disappeared and he became mentally alert. The more serious type of epilepsy, or grand mal, was found to be as easily corrected by magnesium as was the milder form, or petit mal. Of the 30 children, only one child, who may have been deficient in vitamin B6, failed to show marked improvement.

Epilepsy so severe that it could not be controlled by drugs has been brought on by nephritis, which allows magnesium to be lost in the urine; the seizures stopped a single hour after magnesium was given.[18] Muscle biopsies of babies who developed convulsions resulting from magnesium losses through diarrhea showed only half the normal magnesium content. These infants also had intermittent foot and wrist spasms, rigidity of the back and neck, and tremors of the arms and legs, all of which became worse when water, given to overcome dehydration, diluted their magnesium supply. As soon as 500 milligrams of this nutrient were given them, all symptoms promptly disappeared.[5] Because of a high calcium intake, infants are especially subject to a magnesium deficiency (p. 207).

Through the years I have planned nutrition programs for perhaps 50 persons suffering from epilepsy, and know of none who has not stayed free of the illness without anticonvulsive drugs. Dozens of letters have told of similar results. Some of these individuals obtained their vitamin B6 and magnesium entirely from foods, whereas others took supplements of both nutrients. Several have remained free from seizures while following an adequate diet at home, but when hospitalized for one reason or another and not allowed vitamin B6 and magnesium, severe epilepsy has recurred. Poor absorption of vitamin B6 may account for the rare cases where the disease is not alleviated (p. 205).

Babies have been kept on purified diets lacking vitamin B6 until convulsions were produced.[20] Electroencephalograms and muscle biopsies indicate that these convulsions and those produced in adults from a lack of vitamin B6 or of magnesium are identical in every respect to spontaneously occurring epilepsy.[1,5,21] Certainly both nutrients should be adequate in the diet of every individual, particularly one who suffers from convulsions. Such symptoms as extreme sensitivity to noise, irritability, twitching, muscle spasms, apprehension, and perhaps bed-wetting and tremors usually become apparent long before convulsions occur.[22] If both vitamin B6 and magnesium were increased as soon as any of these signs becomes noticeable, epilepsy could probably be prevented.

Tics and tremors. Human volunteers on diets deficient

in magnesium have developed twitching and tremors in many muscles,[23] and individuals lacking vitamin B₆ developed tremors of the hands.[2] Physicians, however, have rarely bothered to report the correction of tremors or tics alone. People whose hands twitched and trembled so severely that their signatures were illegible have been given magnesium, and a few hours later, their names could be easily read; photographs of their writing showed the improvement to be unbelievably striking.[24] In one man a magnesium deficiency induced by vomiting and diarrhea not only caused severe trembling and twitching but also such mental confusion that he was described as "severely psychotic"; yet all symptoms disappeared 15 hours after magnesium was given him.[18] A tiny bit of magnesium changed still another from a trembling, irrational, noisy, combative, and "wildly restless individual" into a "charming and delightful gentleman" free from symptoms in 18 hours.[18] The increase in charm, however, is not guaranteed.

It has been my experience that vitamin B₆ and magnesium alleviates tics and tremors quickly or not at all. A tic under one young woman's left eye had caused her to wink continuously for months, yet an hour after she took 10 milligrams of vitamin B₆ it disappeared. The hands of a beautiful 17-year-old girl trembled so severely that she could not write, type, play the piano, or eat without jostling food from her fork or spoon; after taking only 20 milligrams of vitamin B₆, her trembling stopped completely and never recurred. An elderly man who claimed that the trembling of his hands had been severe for 40 years recovered within 24 hours after he took vitamin B₆. A minister whose lower lip quivered so persistently that he could no longer enunciate his words clearly and feared he would have to give up his work had the identical experience.

The strangest case that has come to my attention was a 12-year-old boy whose eyes turned upward until only the whites showed when he was particularly tired. This characteristic, which had caused him endless embarrassment, had been noticed in the delivery room at the time of his birth, yet to my amazement it cleared up when vitamin B₆ and magnesium were given him. Undoubtedly certain individuals have unusually high requirements for these two nutrients.

Palsy. If tics and tremors can be nipped in the bud, perhaps such serious diseases as St. Vitus's dance (chorea) and palsy (Parkinson's disease, or paralysis agitans) can be prevented. The symptoms of these diseases are remarkably similar. Young girls with acute chorea have experienced rapid and progressive improvement to normal health after 10 to 60 milligrams of vitamin B_6 have been given them daily.[4,25,26] Vitamin B_1, the entire B complex, and magnesium have also produced good results.

People with Parkinson's disease given 10 to 100 milligrams of vitamin B_6 daily have reported feeling stronger, walking with a steadier gait, having better bladder control, a greater sense of well-being, increased mental alertness, and a decrease of muscular cramps, trembling, and rigidity.[25,27-33] When their trembling had been severe for several years, sometimes no improvement could be noted, but individuals who had been ill for a year or less often improved markedly.[29] Some doctors have seen no change after giving vitamin B_6,[34] but unless a completely adequate diet supplemented with all B vitamins and magnesium is followed, no improvement should be expected.

An elderly woman who had been bedridden for more than two years with paralysis agitans once walked into my office unaided two weeks after she had added wheat germ and yeast to her diet. Her gait was unsteady and almost every muscle in her body still trembled, yet she was delighted with her new-found strength. A few others who have had palsy for many years have obtained some improvement, but on the whole, the results I have seen have been disappointing.

It is my conviction that many cases of paralysis agitans are emotional in origin and date back to some terrifying experience early in life. The reaction of shaking because of fear is well known. I was once interviewing a retired pediatrician who had severe Parkinson's disease. He abruptly changed the subject from nutrition to tell me of a time when as a baby he and his terrified mother had been caught in a prairie fire with no apparent means of escape; a change of wind direction had saved their lives. As he spoke, his shaking became markedly worse, and his unconscious terror was so great one felt frozen by it. In another instance, a woman whose tongue trembled so badly she could scarcely eat or talk and who had been confined to a wheelchair for years told me of her early and constant terror of a cruel, domineering father; and she stated frankly that her husband was equally domineering and cruel. When she talked to me alone, all her trembling stopped, but it started with renewed violence almost the minute her husband entered the room. In such cases an understanding psychiatrist could probably help far more than sound nutrition.

Burning or painful feet. Painfully burning feet involving the nerves, which appears to be surprisingly common, occurred in prisoners during World War II and cleared up only when pantothenic acid was given them. It has now been produced in volunteers deficient in pantothenic acid[3] or in vitamin B_6,[35] and disappeared several weeks after an adequate diet was allowed.

When fatty deposits plug the small arteries in the feet, the oxygen supply is so decreased that such pain is made markedly worse. By reducing the need for oxygen, generous amounts of vitamin E bring greatest relief, especially in cases of Buerger's disease and diabetic gangrene, where the arteries to the feet may be completely obliterated.[36] A similar condition, known as Raynaud's phenomenon, sometimes occurs in the hands. Nicotine impairs circulation by causing the blood vessels to contract and makes such conditions worse. The toxic substances from a single cigarette lower blood vitamin C and destroy approximately 25 milligrams of the vitamin;[37,38] hence persons unable to give up smoking should increase their vitamin-C intake.

An adequate diet designed to remove cholesterol deposits (ch. 5) and made particularly high in pantothenic acid, vitamins C, E, and the B vitamins usually corrects these abnormalities of the feet provided it is followed patiently for many weeks.

Neuritis. Vitamin B_1, frequently reported to improve neuritis,[4] is ineffective except when an excessive intake of carbohydrate or alcohol has caused the requirement to be unusually high; even then the aching, stabbing pains are more readily stopped if the diet includes yeast and liver.[39] Large doses of vitamin B_1 alone cause such a high urinary excretion of other B vitamins[40] that deficiencies can be produced,[41] yet each vitamin of the B group is involved in correcting or preventing neuritis.[25,42]

Numbness and tingling of hands and feet, characteristic of neuritis, have been produced in volunteers deficient in vitamin B_6 or pantothenic acid.[3,35,43] Neuritis has been helped when vitamins B_1, B_2, B_6, B_{12}, and pantothenic acid have been given together; and extreme pain, weakness, and numbness have in some cases been relieved in an hour,[25,42,44,45] but yeast and liver have given the most lasting results.[46]

On one occasion, I planned a diet for a man who had

spent years in Santo Tomas prison and whose neuritis was so severe that he was bedridden and constantly writhed with pain. Although huge amounts of many B vitamins had been given to him, the addition of pantothenic acid, yeast, liver, and wheat germ brought such spectacular improvement that his daughter remarked, "Like Lazarus, he rose from the dead."

Various drugs, such as antiacid preparations and streptomycin, cause neuritis by destroying or increasing the need for or excretion of several B vitamins.[47] Such neuritis can be relieved or prevented by giving B vitamins with drugs.[48,49]

Trifacial neuralgia. Trifacial neuralgia, or tic douloureux, has sometimes been treated successfully with the same B vitamins that help other forms of neuritis,[45] but the results have been inconsistent.[50]

In the few cases I have worked with, this localized pain has appeared to be emotional in origin. The blood supplies all organs uniformly, favoring none above others. Occupational neuritis often occurs in the arm of a violinist or the leg of a person who must push a pedal constantly in his work, but individuals do not use their facial nerves excessively. It is common, however, for people to harbor anger or resentment when they would prefer to "tell someone off." If such an emotion is expressed harmlessly (p. 91), the trifacial neuralgia often disappears.

23
Anemia Has Many Causes

The rarity of a ruddy glow which healthy blood casts over the skin is mute testimony of our high incidence of borderline or outright anemia resulting from the consumption of refined foods.

Anemia literally means without blood. Though anemia may result from hemorrhaging, more often the cause is too little red coloring matter, or oxygen-carrying hemoglobin, inside the blood cells. At other times not enough red cells can be produced to carry the oxygen load; or these cells die while still young, stay alive but fail to mature, become misshapen or too large, or disintegrate after reaching the blood stream. Healthy blood cells are produced in the bone marrow provided ample raw materials are supplied.

Red blood cells, which normally live approximately 120 days, are constantly being destroyed and replaced. Each person should have 100 per cent, or about 15 grams, of bright red hemoglobin in a half cup of blood (100 cc) and a blood count of 5 million red cells (per cubic millimeter). Anemia exists when the hemoglobin is less than 80 per cent, or 13 grams, and/or the red-cell count is fewer than 4 million. In all anemia, so little oxygen reaches the tissues that energy cannot be produced normally, and constant tiredness, lack of endurance, pallor, shortness of breath, and perhaps dizziness, headaches, and mental depression result.

Iron-deficiency anemia is so well known that, unless one realizes anemia has many causes, iron is often taken when it may actually be harmful.[1]

Vitamin-B$_6$-deficiency anemia. An anemia in which both the number of red cells and the amount of hemoglobin are decreased has been produced in infants[2] and adults[3] by diets deficient in vitamin B$_6$. This form of anemia, which cannot be corrected by iron, is now found to be common in men, women, and children, and especially in women during pregnancy. Since the cause of such anemia is usually unrecognized, it sometimes persists ten years or longer; and such patients, invariably loaded with iron, often become so ill that transfusions are necessary.[4] When 100 milligrams of vitamin B_6 were given daily to these individuals, the red cells increased markedly and the hemoglobin rose quickly from 8.5 to 13 grams, but the anemia recurred as soon as the vitamin was withdrawn.

The tragedy of loading such persons with iron is that, when vitamin B_6 is undersupplied, iron absorption becomes so excessive that it damages the tissues,[4] causing the formation of scars which readily become calcified.[1] This condition appears to be identical to a fatal iron-storage disease, siderosis or hemosiderosis, which has been rare but is rapidly becoming more common. In experimental siderosis, as much as 18 times more iron than normal is held in the body.[1] The iron is reduced if vitamin B_6 is given, but if withheld, death results.[4] Under normal circumstances iron is absorbed only as needed.

Since vitamin B_6 and magnesium go together like salt and pepper, it is not surprising that anemia has been produced in volunteers (adult men) by a diet lacking magnesium.[5] This anemia was quickly corrected soon after the nutrient was allowed.

Vitamin-E-deficiency anemia. When vitamin E is undersupplied, not only are iron absorption and hemoglobin formation impaired, but also the essential fatty acids forming part of the cell structure are so altered by oxidation that cells break down,[6-14] a destruction that goes on uniformly throughout the body. The speed with which the red blood cells are destroyed when exposed to oxygen, however, has become the test for vitamin-E deficiencies.[15] If vitamin E is undersupplied, so many red cells spill their contents into the blood that the anemia is just as severe as if these cells had never been produced.[16] Furthermore, the life span of the remaining blood cells is markedly reduced.[6,17]

Anemia resulting from a lack of vitamin E has been produced in young men voluntarily deprived of this vitamin[13,14,18] and in almost every species of animal.[19] Biopsies of the bone marrow of anemic babies, adults, and especially pregnant women showed gross abnormalities, but these completely cleared up in five days after 280 milligrams of vitamin E were given daily; and the anemia quickly disappeared.[20] The anemia of sprue,[7] as well as that common in hemophiliacs, has also been corrected by vitamin E.[8] Generous amounts of vitamin C, which decreases the vitamin-E requirement,[21] help to alleviate this anemia, but no amount of iron can correct it. In fact, most forms of iron medication destroy vitamin E (p. 33).

Because premature births are frequently the result of too little vitamin E during pregnancy,[11] such infants are born especially deficient in this vitamin and are particularly susceptible to anemia.[6,9,10,12] When exposed to the high oxygen content of ordinary air, their blood cells break down so rapidly that, unable to excrete the blood pigments quickly enough, they frequently develop jaundice from pigments deposited in the tissues.[6,17] This occurrence is extremely common. It has caused hundreds of babies to become blind (p. 286), and is still a major factor in infant mortality. Yet neither pregnant women nor premature infants are customarily given vitamin E; and the babies are rarely allowed breast milk, which, if from a healthy mother, usually contains 20 times more vitamin E than cows' milk.[9,12,22]

Since vitamin E has a remarkable power of decreasing the body's need for oxygen,[23,24] the symptoms of any anemia, such as fatigue and shortness of breath stemming from oxygen deprivation, are often alleviated when vitamin E is taken. Because "extraordinarily large amounts" of vitamin E are required when oils are used[25] and oil consumption is increasing, more anemia resulting from a lack of vitamin E can be expected.

Folic-acid-deficiency anemia. An undersupply of the B vitamin folic acid causes a "large-cell" anemia common among pregnant women, individuals lacking stomach acid, infants and children following infections, and persons who have a high intake of refined foods, especially alcohol.[26-30] This form of anemia, repeatedly produced in humans, is associated with a sore mouth and tongue and perhaps a grayish-brown skin pigmentation.[30] It cannot be corrected by iron, but within a few hours of adding 1 to 5 milligrams of folic acid to a diet deficient in it, the bone marrow starts producing new blood cells,[31] and the anemia quickly disappears.[27,30,32]

Such anemia, though corrected by folic acid, which is rich in liver, kidneys, chicken giblets, and cooked green leafy vegetables, quickly recurs unless vitamin C is adequate.[33] The vitamin C not only increases iron absorption and the rate of hemoglobin production, but also is necessary before folic acid can be changed into a usable form.[19,31,34] Rats, which synthesize their own vitamin C, nevertheless recover from folic-acid-deficiency anemia much faster when given large amounts of both vitamins C and E.[19]

Sickle-cell anemia occurs in persons who appear to have an unusually high requirement for folic acid.[85,86] Such patients have improved when given 5 milligrams or more of this vitamin daily.

Effect of drugs and insecticides. Anemia can be caused by a variety of drugs that destroy vitamin E[17] and by others that inactivate nutrients needed in building blood cells.[87] When medications must be used, nutrients known to prevent anemia might be temporarily increased. By damaging the bone marrow, several insecticides cause anemia which can be fatal.[88] Since all foreign substances appear to destroy vitamin C (p. 34), anything not occurring naturally in the body undoubtedly contributes to anemia unless the diet is unusually adequate. How much anemia may be caused by food additives and artificial sweeteners, for instance, is not known.

Anemia and stomach acid. An iron-deficiency anemia often occurs when the diet is high in iron but lacking vitamin B_1, B_2, niacin, pantothenic acid, or cholin.[86] If any one of these vitamins is undersupplied, the stomach is unable to secrete sufficient hydrochloric acid to dissolve iron; hence it cannot be absorbed.[86] Because a deficiency of iron itself does not limit acid production, an anemia induced by a lack of stomach acid cannot be corrected by iron but only by obtaining adequate B vitamins and taking hydrochloric acid temporarily.

In children, an anemia associated with a lack of hydrochloric acid and low resistance to infections often occurs because the blood proteins, albumin and globulins (antibodies), pass into the intestines and are lost in the feces.[89,40] The loss of antibodies naturally lowers resistance. Again, giving iron cannot alleviate these abnormalities, both of which result from the lack of stomach acid. A sufficient B-vitamin intake to stimulate normal acid production brings correction.[40]

Iron-deficiency anemia. Iron is so widely distributed that to produce an anemia from a lack of it, one must live largely on refined foods. Hemoglobin, many enzymes, and a substance known as myoglobin, which carries oxygen in muscle cells, cannot be produced without iron. Even a mild deficiency so limits enzyme and myoglobin production that chronic fatigue, headaches, and shortness of breath can occur long before anemia develops.[45] When persons with iron-deficiency anemia eat beets, the red color is said to appear in the urine;[46] hence eating beets may serve as a test to determine whether anemia results from a lack of iron or from other causes.

Iron-deficiency anemia is common in women of reproductive age whose menstrual flow is heavy; among persons of all ages who eat mostlv refined foods; in adolescent girls whose diets are often appalling and whose iron requirements are high because of muscle development, increased blood volume, and menstrual losses; and, because cows' milk contains little iron, among bottle-fed babies and persons who live largely on milk.[47,48] Yeast is such an excellent source of iron that anemia can be easily prevented by taking a few teaspoons daily or adding it to a baby's formula.

Blood examinations of thousands of army recruits have shown that iron-deficiency anemia is common in young men,[49] who have unusually high iron requirements because of the large amount of myoglobin being formed in their rapidly developing muscles. Instead of the normal 15 grams of hemoglobin, some recruits had less than 5, and many less than 10. Their shortness of breath on exertion and chronic fatigue disappeared when iron was given them, and they experienced a marked sense of well-being. Because the body uses iron over and over, before so much refined food was eaten, anemia in men was rare except after a loss of blood.

Years ago a young man with the iron-storage disease, siderosis, requested from me an iron-free diet; he was an identical twin and his brother had already died of the disease. At first I sincerely attempted to comply, only to discover that it was absolutely impossible to plan an adequate diet free from iron. Meats, eggs, whole-grain breads and cereals, fruits, and vegetables all contain iron in considerable quantity; and a general diet of unrefined foods usually supplies twice the amount of iron recommended by the National Research Council. A diet of nothing except milk and refined foods—vitamin and mineral supplements were unavailable then—could not be recommended, and this young man was too frightened to eat anything else. I never heard how long he lived, but the experience convinced me that if refined foods are avoided, iron supplements are not needed.

All nutrients are essential. Almost every nutrient is needed to produce red blood cells, hemoglobin, and enzymes required for their synthesis;[37] and anemia is usually brought on by several subtle deficiencies existing simultaneously. In addition to the nutrients already mentioned, copper is necessary before iron can be absorbed, carried in the blood, or utilized: cobalt is an essential part of vitamin B_{12}; and hemoglobin cannot be produced without pantothenic acid and 19 different amino acids, many furnished only by complete proteins.[41-44]

When blood has been withdrawn from animals, the best food to correct the resulting anemia was liver of every variety.[50] Kidneys, chicken gizzards, and egg yolks ran a close second, and muscle meats and brains ranked slightly above green leafy vegetables. Peaches, apricots, and prunes had half the potency of liver. Unfortunately, yeast and wheat germ were not tested in these studies, but most of the nutrients needed for building blood are rich in these foods.

When liver is eaten, recovery from anemia is much more rapid than if all nutrients are obtained separately; hence some investigators believe an antianemia factor is still to be isolated.[41] A pregnant woman wrote me recently that her physician had recommended ferrous sulfate, which she knew to be toxic (p. 33). Instead she had eaten liver, yeast, and wheat germ daily, and he later remarked that he had never known blood to regenerate so rapidly.

Pernicious anemia. The blood abnormalities characteristic of pernicious anemia can be corrected by folic acid, but a simultaneous deficiency of vitamin B_{12} causes this disease to be accompanied by an irreversible degeneration of the spinal cord.[27] An individual lacking vitamin B_{12} or one with untreated pernicious anemia develops a shuffling gait, loses the sense of position of his feet, and can become completely paralyzed. If the fatigue caused by the anemia is prevented by folic acid, a patient may fail to consult his physician during the early stages of the disease, and permanent crippling can result. For this reason, folic acid is presently sold on prescription. though supplements should supply both vitamin B_{12} and folic acid.

Vitamin B_{12} can only be absorbed with the aid of an enzyme known as the intrinsic factor, normally produced by glands in the stomach.[51] In pernicious anemia, the stomach has become so unhealthy that it can no longer secrete either this enzyme or hydrochloric acid. An injection of 0.1 milligram of vitamin B_{12} each month can prevent the degenerative changes in the spinal cord, but this amount given daily by mouth is ineffective.[52] Some vitamin B_{12} can be absorbed when huge quantities are taken orally, but the cost of such doses is usually prohibitive.[37]

When the stomach is removed because of cancer or ulcers, hence no intrinsic factor is available to assure the absorption of vitamin B_{12}, four or five years can pass before pernicious anemia develops.[53] A person who still has his stomach thus has years in which he can improve his health before pernicious anemia sets in. The same B vitamins that stimulate hydrochloric-acid production (ch. 13) appear to be essential for the secretion of the intrinsic factor; therefore if the diet were adequate during this five-year period, pernicious anemia would be prevented. Because of the assumption that the intrinsic factor can never again be produced after pernicious anemia once develops, persons with this disease rarely make a serious attempt to improve their diets.

Before folic acid and vitamin B_{12} were isolated, Miss Amy Tapping of Plainfield, New Jersey, consulted me because of severe pernicious anemia. At that time her work kept her traveling constantly and, like a sailor with a girl in every port, she had a physician in nearly every major city in the United States. Injections of liver extract were costing her an average of $140 each month. After staying on an adequate diet containing large amounts of liver, yeast, and wheat germ for some time, however, her stomach secretions became normal and all liver shots were discontinued. She has had not the slightest return of anemia and now, almost 30 years later, is still in remarkable good health.

Through the years several persons with pernicious anemia who have consulted me have had equally good results. Physicians examining such individuals, however, have invariably concluded that the original diagnoses were wrong. This conclusion has perhaps been true in some cases, but it is improbable that a dozen or more physicians would all be wrong concerning Miss Tapping's diagnosis. It seems to me, therefore, that a person with pernicious anemia should make every attempt to stimulate normal stomach secretions.

Vitamins B_6 and C increase the absorption of vitamin B_{12}, and adequate protein prevents this vitamin from being lost in the urine, whereas diets low in protein accelerate its loss.[27] Provided iron and vitamin C are obtained with hydrochloric acid, they stimulate the production of the intrinsic factor sufficiently so that persons with mild pernicious anemia can take smaller doses of vitamin B_{12}.[27] Although many persons have died from this disease, it has not yet been proved to be incurable. If individuals with pernicious anemia who take hydrochloric acid with each meal to assure the absorption of nutrients (p. 143) were to adhere to a completely adequate diet containing generous amounts of the antistress factors, pantothenic acid, and all the natural sources of B vitamins, the reverse could probably be shown.

Pernicious anemia among vegetarians. Vitamin B_{12} is almost exclusively associated with animal proteins such as liver (by far the richest source), kidney, muscle meats, milk, eggs, cheese, and fish.[34,54] Vegetarians are particularly subject to pernicious anemia unless they eat generous amounts of milk and eggs. Because a vegetarian diet is rich in folic acid, however, the blood remains normal, and irreparable nerve damage can easily occur before the vitamin-B_{12} deficiency is discovered.

Of all vegetable foods, only yeast, wheat germ, and soybeans contain traces of vitamin B_{12}.[34] People who have followed a vegetarian diet without eggs or milk for five years or longer often develop sore mouths and tongues, menstrual disturbances, and a variety of nervous symptoms including a "needles and pins" feeling in hands and feet, neuritis, pain and stiffness in the spine, and difficulty in walking.[55] All of these symptoms, which are danger signals, dramatically clear up provided vitamin B_{12} is obtained. To prevent permanent damage, persons adhering to a strict vegetarian diet should probably take 50 micrograms, or 1 tablet, of vitamin B_{12} each week while their stomach secretions are still normal. Although vitamin B_{12} is synthesized by intestinal bacteria, human absorption from this source is doubtful.[56] The intrinsic factor is produced only in the stomach whereas the B vitamins are mostly released in the large bowel almost 30 feet away.

The price paid. Except for the occurrence of pernicious anemia in strict vegetarians, all other varieties are part of the price paid for being consumers of refined foods. If natural foods grown on rich soils could be eaten by everyone, most anemia would probably be only of historical interest.

24
Abnormalities of the Muscles

Weak and inefficiently functioning muscles often cause problems about which little is done until they become serious. Yet the strength and normal function of muscles can be judged by excellent carriage and grace of movement, both of which are rare indeed. In America, weak muscles are evident in all age groups, from the wobbly necks of the newborn to the stoop of the aged and far less than aged. And muscle diseases of every variety are said to be increasing rapidly.

Poor muscle tone interferes with the circulation of blood, inhibits normal lymph flow, prevents food from being digested efficiently (p. 143), often causes constipation, and at times makes it impossible to control the passing of urine or even to void. Not infrequently weak muscles allow the internal organs to sag or to loll about on each other like so many soft-boiled eggs, thus interfering with the functions of these organs. Clumsiness, jerkiness, muscle tension, and lack of co-ordination, so frequent in the malnourished child and usually passed over with the statement that "Johnnie is not good at athletics," are symptoms frighteningly similar to those seen in muscular dystrophies and multiple sclerosis.

Muscle weakness. Muscles consist largely of protein but contain some essential fatty acids in their structure; hence these nutrients must be adequate before muscular strength can be maintained. The chemistry of muscles and the nerves controlling them, however, is extremely complex; and because innumerable enzymes, coenzymes, activators, and other compounds are involved in their contraction, relaxation, and repair, every nutrient gets into the act in one way or another. For example, since adequate calcium, magnesium, and vitamins B_6 and D are each necessary for their relaxation, muscular cramps (p. 246) and tics

235

and tremors (p. 222) can usually be relieved when increased amounts of these nutrients are taken.[1,2]

Potassium is essential to the contraction of every muscle in the body. In a single week healthy volunteers given refined foods such as those eaten daily by millions of Americans developed muscle weakness, extreme fatigue, constipation, indifference, and lack of feeling, all of which disappeared almost immediately when 10 grams of potassium chloride were given them.[3,4] Severe potassium deficiencies are frequently brought on by stress, vomiting, diarrhea, kidney damage, the use of diuretics, or cortisone therapy,[5-8] causing sluggishness, flabbiness, and partial paralysis. Muscles of the intestines, thus affected, allow bacteria to form such quantities of gas that colic occurs and/or spasms or twisting of the bowel may result in obstruction.[9] When a potassium deficiency has caused death, autopsies have revealed severe muscle damage and scarring.[10-12]

Some persons have such unusually high potassium requirements that they are subject to periodic paralysis. Studies of these individuals show that blood potassium is decreased by the typical American high-fat, high-carbohydrate diet of well-salted foods, and especially by candy binges, stress, or ACTH and cortisone.[13-16] Even though muscles become weak, lax, soft, or partially paralyzed, recovery occurs within minutes after potassium is taken.[13] A diet high in protein, low in salt, or rich in potassium can prevent this abnormally low blood potassium.[6,16] Such studies help to reveal why American children, who consume so many candy bars, soft drinks, refined foods, and salted popcorn and potato and corn chips, made a poor showing in comparison with European children on recent physical tests.

When weak muscles result in fatigue, gas distention, constipation, and perhaps inability to pass urine without a catheter, the taking of potassium chloride tablets has proved especially advantageous,[8,17,18] Most people, however, can obtain ample potassium from fruits and vegetables, particularly cooked green leafy ones, and by avoiding refined foods.

A lack of vitamin E is a frequent but rarely recognized cause of muscle weakness. In the same way that red blood cells break down when essential fats forming the cell structure are harmed by oxygen in the absence of this vitamin (p. 228), so are muscle cells destroyed throughout the body.[19-23] The muscles are left damaged and scarred, particularly in adults who do not absorb fats readily.[24] The nuclei of muscle cells and the enzymes needed for muscular contractions cannot be formed without vitamin E.[25] Its lack tremendously increases the need for oxygen in muscle tissue,[21,26] inhibits the utilization of several amino acids,[27] and allows phosphorus to be lost in the urine[28] and many B vitamins to be destroyed by rancidity,[29] all of which interfere with the function and repair of muscles.[30,31] Furthermore, enzymes that break down dead muscle cells may increase as much as 6,000 per cent when vitamin E is undersupplied;[19,20,27] and the calcium content of vitamin-E-deficient muscles increases so tremendously that calcium is deposited in them.[32,33]

Muscular weakness in pregnant women caused by a vitamin-E deficiency—frequently induced by iron supplements[34,35]—often makes their deliveries difficult by decreasing enzymes needed for muscle contraction.[36] When 400 milligrams of vitamin E were given daily to 112 persons with muscular weakness, pain, stiffness, wrinkled skin, and lack of elasticity in their muscles, marked improvement was made by elderly and young alike; and those who had suffered from many of these abnormalities for years recovered almost as quickly as did others who had been ill only a short time.[37]

The most spectacular improvement in muscle strength I have seen occurred when 100 to 300 units of vitamin E were given daily to babies slow in holding up their heads, sitting erect, crawling, or walking. Often within a week their muscles became firm, and the child was looking about, sitting up, or crawling or walking normally. Repeatedly mothers of these children have told me their pediatricians have claimed that vitamin E was dangerous.

Johns Hopkins physicians have given massive doses of this vitamin to children with excellent results and could observe no toxic effects.[38,39] Mongoloid and mentally retarded children have received up to 3,000 units daily for years with amazingly beneficial results in some cases;[40] and equally huge amounts have corrected such muscle problems as crossed eyes[41] and been given to volunteers[42] with no sign of toxicity. Many outstanding physicians believe that all bottle-fed infants should be given approximately 30 units of vitamin E daily;[43-45] and that a vitamin-E deficiency can be suspected in any baby unable to sit up well when three months old.[39,46]

Prolonged stress and Addison's disease. Advanced adrenal exhaustion, such as Addison's disease, is characterized by apathy, torturous fatigue, and extreme muscular weakness. Although proteins broken down at the onset of stress come largely from the lymph glands, when stress is prolonged, muscle cells are destroyed as well.[46] Furthermore, exhausted adrenals can no longer produce a hormone that saves nitrogen from the breakdown of worn-out body cells; normally this nitrogen is reused in building amino acids vital to the repair of tissues. Under such circumstances the muscles lose strength rapidly even though the diet may be high in protein.

Exhausted adrenals are also unable to produce sufficient amounts of the salt-retaining hormone aldosterone. So much salt (sodium) is lost in the urine that again potassium leaves the cells,[9] resulting in still-greater muscular weakness, slowed contractions, and partial or complete paralysis of certain muscles. Taking potassium can increase the amount of this nutrient in the cells,[17] but in this case salt (sodium) is particularly needed, and many of the muscle problems can be alleviated merely by eating salty foods. People with adrenal exhaustion usually have low blood pressure, which indicates that salt should be obtained (p. 29).

The adrenals quickly become exhausted during a pantothenic-acid deficiency, causing the same conditions brought on by prolonged stress. When volunteers were deficient in this vitamin for only a short period, the output of adrenal hormones fell quickly and severe urinary losses of nitrogen occurred, showing that muscle tissue was being broken down.[47,48] All experienced muscular weakness. One man developed an abnormal gait, and others had muscular cramps, poor co-ordination, and tremor of their outstretched hands.[48,49]

Because stress plays a role in every type of muscle disturbance, emphasis must always be placed on building up the adrenals regardless of the diagnosis. The antistress program (p. 31) should be carefully followed, especially by persons suffering from Addison's disease; and recovery is more rapid when the antistress formula (p. 31) is taken around the clock. Not one essential nutrient should be overlooked.

Fibrositis and myositis. Inflammation and swelling of the connective tissue of the muscles, especially that covering the muscle sheaths, is spoken of as fibrositis or synovitis, whereas inflammation of the muscle tissue itself is known as myositis. Both are usually brought on by mechanical injury or strain and, being inflammations, always indicate that the body is not producing sufficient cortisone. A completely adequate antistress diet with large amounts of vitamin C and pantothenic acid taken with highly fortified milk around the clock usually brings rapid relief. Because of the damage done, scar tissue may form quickly; hence vitamin E must be emphasized.

These abnormalities are common among women during the menopause, when the need for vitamin E is tremendously increased, especially if estrogen is given;[50] often they result in considerable discomfort and stiffness before the cause is recognized. Marked improvement has occurred when vitamin E was taken daily for myositis;[51-54] and in one study of 300 middle-aged persons with fibrositis, "the vast majority were cured" after vitamin E was given them.[55]

Recently a woman consulted me who, because of fibrositis of many years' standing, spent most of the time in bed. Besides much other medication, she was taking aspirin every three hours to deaden pain. After a single month on an antistress diet, supplemented with 600 units of vitamin E daily, her physician took her off of all medication; and within two months she was leading an unusually active life, doing most of her housework, much entertaining, and, according to her husband, was "an entirely new woman."

Myasthenia gravis. The name myasthenia gravis means grave loss of muscle strength. This disease, another of many said to be increasing rapidly,[56] is marked by exhaustion and progressive paralysis, which may affect any part of the body but most frequently involves the muscles of the face and neck. Double vision, drooping eyelids, frequent choking, and difficulty in breathing, swallowing, and talking, shown by imperfect articulation, stammering, and stuttering, are common symptoms.

Prisoners held in Singapore during World War II developed what appeared to be myasthenia gravis; partial paralysis caused choking, drooping eyelids, blurred and double vision, and difficulty in speaking and swallowing. They recovered completely after being given large amounts of yeast and liver over a long period.[57] A report from the Mayo Clinic tells of a 39-year-old who had had myasthenia gravis for five years yet who made a spontaneous recovery two weeks after a toxic thyroid was removed.[58] In such a case, the nutritional requirements are so tremendously decreased that the effect is the same as adhering to a highly improved diet. Mrs. Donald

Kempton of Horse Shoe, North Carolina, who had this disease for 27 years, before she became interested in nutrition, recently wrote me: "My last physical examination showed no symptoms of myasthenia gravis."

Remarkable recoveries from myasthenia gravis have been reported when patients were given a diet high in protein, vitamin E, all the B vitamins, and, for a short period, 50 milligrams of manganese at each meal.[56] All the classical symptoms and other forms of partial paralysis disappeared within a few weeks. Each of these people had enlarged thymus glands, typical of adrenal exhaustion and/or a severe pantothenic-acid deficiency,[59] but the enlarged glands "virtually melted away" when the diet was improved. The results were said to have been "rapid and astonishing."

Studies with radioactive manganese show that enzymes involved with muscular contraction contain this nutrient,[60] and that the amount in human blood increases when muscles are damaged.[61] The lack of manganese causes abnormalities of the muscles and nerves in experimental animals[62,63] and muscular weakness and poor co-ordination in livestock.[64,65] Although the amount needed by humans has not been established,[19] wheat germ and whole-grain breads, the richest natural sources, may well be emphasized by persons suffering from such muscle weakness.

When given separately, cholin, pantothenic acid, and vitamins B_1, B_2, B_6, C, and E have been reported to have been helpful in treating myasthenia gravis.[56,66] No studies seem to have been made in which diets adequate in all nutrients have been used. Blurred vision and some mild symptoms of myasthenia have been produced in men deficient in vitamin B_6 and pantothenic acid;[67] and monkeys lacking vitamin B_1 have developed symptoms identical to those seen in myasthenia patients.[68]

In myasthenia gravis, some defect occurs in the production of a compound that transmits nerve impulses to the muscles.[69] This substance, made in the nerve endings from cholin and acetic acid and known as acetylcholin, is under normal circumstances constantly broken down and re-formed. In myasthenia gravis it appears to be produced in too meager amounts and/or cannot be re-formed readily. The disease is usually treated with medication that retards the breakdown of acetylcholin, but unless the diet is made adequate, this approach is another example of beating a tired horse.

An entire battery of nutrients is necessary for the production of acetylcholin: vitamin B_1,[70,71] pantothenic acid,[70,72] potassium,[73] and many others. A lack of cholin itself causes a marked underproduction of acetylcholin and results in muscle weakness, damage to the muscle fibers, and extensive scarring; and it is accompanied by the urinary loss of a substance, creatine, which invariably shows that muscles are being destroyed.[69] The daily cholin intake in America is said to be less than one-fifth of the estimated requirement. Although is can be made from the amino acid methionine provided a high-protein diet is eaten, folic acid, vitamin B_{12}, and other B vitamins are necessary before the amino acid can be transformed into the vitamin.

Vitamin E increases the liberation and utilization of acetylcholin, but, if undersupplied, an enzyme essential to the formation of acetylcholin is destroyed by oxygen.[74,75] Again muscle weakness, damage, scarring, and loss of creatine occur, but giving vitamin E rectifies the situation.[76,77]

Because the onset of myasthenia gravis almost invariably follows prolonged stress and is aggravated by drugs known to increase body requirements,[58] an antistress diet unusually rich in every nutrient is indicated. Lecithin, yeast, liver, wheat germ, and eggs are excellent sources of cholin, and each should be taken daily in six small, high-protein meals generously supplemented with vitamin E, the antistress formula (p. 31), magnesium, B-complex tablets high in cholin and inositol, and perhaps manganese. Salty foods should be eaten temporarily, and potassium increased by a generous intake of fruits and vegetables. When swallowing is difficult, all foods can be liquefied in a blender and liquid supplements used (p. 326).

If the diet is completely adequate, such "rapid and astonishing"[56] improvement so frequently follows that there seems little justification for the belief that nothing can be done for myasthenia gravis.

Multiple sclerosis. This disease is characterized by calcified patches on the brain and spinal cord, muscular weakness, inco-ordination, strong jerky movements or spasms of the arm, leg, and eye muscles, and difficulty in bladder control. Autopsy studies show a marked decrease in the lecithin content of the brain and the myelin sheath covering the nerves, both of which are normally high in lecithin;[78] and even this lecithin is abnormal, containing saturated instead of unsaturated fatty acids.[79] Further-more, multiple sclerosis is most common in countries where the diet is particularly high in saturated fats,[80,81] which invariably means that the amount of lecithin in the blood is markedly reduced (ch. 5). Probably because the need for lecithin has been decreased, persons with multiple sclerosis have had fewer bad periods of shorter duration when given low-fat diets.[82] Even greater improvement has been made when 3 or more tablespoons of lecithin have been added to the daily diet.[78]

Probably the lack of any nutrient that prevents lecithin production, whether magnesium, vitamin B_6, cholin, inositol, or essential fatty acids (ch. 5), can make multiple sclerosis worse. Muscle spasms and weakness, involuntary twitching, and inability to control the bladder have been produced in healthy volunteers by a diet deficient in magnesium.[1,83] These symptoms quickly disappeared soon after magnesium was given. Also when patients suffering from multiple sclerosis have been given vitamins E, B_6, and other B vitamins, the illness has been arrested; even advanced cases improved in walking and had better bladder control and fewer arm and leg spasms.[84] The calcification of soft tissues has been prevented with vitamin E.[85,86] It seems to me that all of these nutrients should be emphasized in the diet of any individual suffering from this disease.

Multiple sclerosis in the people I have worked with has invariably been brought on by extremely severe stress during periods when pantothenic acid has been deficient in their diets. In experimental animals, a lack of pantothenic acid causes an actual loss of the myelin sheath covering the nerves,[87] such as occurs in multiple sclerosis. Deficiencies of vitamins B_1, B_2, B_6, E, or pantothenic acid— the need for each of which is tremendously increased by stress—results in nerve degeneration in both humans and animals; and in animals such damage can be corrected by adding the missing vitamin.[88] Furthermore, multiple sclerosis is often treated with cortisone, indicating that every effort should be made to stimulate normal hormone production.

I have seen a number of persons who have recovered completely from multiple sclerosis when dietary improvement was made soon after the disease had been diagnosed. These individuals have stayed on the antistress program (p. 31) and a highly adequate diet such as the one outlined on pages 330–331. In some cases, 600 units of vitamin E taken with each meal—1,800 units daily—have brought spectacular improvement. Recently I was talking to a young woman who told me that for several years she had been an invalid because of this disease but that after following an excellent diet she had no signs of the illness except occasional foot cramps which disappeared when she increased her magnesium intake. In advanced cases, however, irreparable damage may have been done.

Mrs. Violet Kazakoff of Arlington, Virginia, who has applied nutrition conscientiously, wrote me recently: "I have had MS for almost 19 years. In 1956 I became helpless as a baby. I could not walk, could not speak one word, and my hands were too weak to write my name, yet I have recovered and today, although I still have some problems, I go to dances, parties, church, entertain, do much of my housework, and live a very happy life."

Mrs. Kazakoff wisely adds that plenty of rest, a happy mental outlook, and a determination to try to get well are probably as helpful as sound nutrition. I have also seen a few cases in which persons with multiple sclerosis made marked progress when under psychotherapy, which undoubtedly relieved much emotional stress.

Muscular dystrophies. All varieties of animals kept on vitamin-E-deficient diets develop muscular dystrophy provided they can live long enough.[12,89,90] Human muscular dystrophy and atrophy appear to be identical to this experimentally produced illness. In both the laboratory and the human disease the oxygen requirement is tremendously increased; many enzymes and coenzymes needed for normal muscle function are markedly reduced; and muscles throughout the body become injured and weakened as the essential fatty acids forming structural parts of muscle cells are destroyed.[26,91-94] Numerous nutrients leak out of the damaged cells, and eventually the muscles are largely replaced by scar tissue.[89,95] The muscles split longitudinally, which, incidentally, makes one wonder if vitamin-E deficiency plays a causative role in hernia, especially in babies known to be woefully deficient in this vitamin (pp. 228–229).

For months or years before muscular dystrophy can be diagnosed, amino acids and a substance known as creatine are lost in the urine, both showing that muscles are breaking down.[27,96,97] If vitamin E is given at this time, before the disease has progressed too far, the destruction of muscle tissue stops completely, as shown by cessation of creatine excretion.[25,39,98] In animals—and probably humans—the disease is produced much more rapidly if the diet is deficient in protein and/or vitamins A or B_6 as well as vitamin E,[90],[94] but even then the dystrophy can still be corrected by vitamin E alone.[99]

When a severe vitamin-E deficiency has been prolonged, muscular dystrophies in humans are irreversible. Massive amounts of vitamin E and many other nutrients have been repeatedly tried without effect. The facts that this disease is "hereditary"—several children in the same family may suffer from it—and that alterations in chromosomes can be detected have made many physicians believe nothing can be done to prevent it. The hereditary factor may only be an unusually high genetic requirement for vitamin E,[100] which is needed to form the nucleus, including the chromosomes, of every cell.

The point at which muscular dystrophy or atrophy becomes irreversible cannot be accurately determined. In the early stages, either has sometimes been corrected by fresh wheat-germ oil, vitamin E, or vitamin E given with other nutrients.[101],[102] Some patients have recovered after early diagnosis merely by adding to their diets wheat germ and homemade bread of freshly ground wheat.[103] Cases of muscular dystrophy have also been described which, when the diet was made adequate, do not get worse for years; and others have improved without complete recovery.[103] Furthermore, the muscular strength of persons who had had the disease for many years has been markedly improved when a variety of vitamins and minerals was given.[104]

Because five-year-old Michael Donnelly had already had muscular dystrophy more than half of his life when his mother got in touch with me, little improvement could be expected. After an antistress program containing 600 units of vitamin E daily had resulted in a considerable increase in strength, Mike remarked, "Miss Davis knows how to make little boys stronger but she doesn't know what they like to eat."

Children with muscular dystrophy have a history of sitting up, crawling, and walking late, of being slow at running, and of having difficulty in climbing stairs and especially in getting up after falling.[66] Frequently a child is ridiculed for being lazy and/or clumsy for years before a physician is consulted. Because huge masses of scar tissue are usually mistaken for large muscles, mothers of such children are often pathetically proud of their "fine development." Eventually the scar tissue contracts and thus causes extremely painful sway-back and/or short-ened Achilles' tendons, which result in as much disability as the weakened muscles themselves. The Achilles' tendon is frequently lengthened surgically years before the actual disease can be diagnosed, yet no vitamin E is given as a preventive measure.

Any person with a muscle problem should have a urine test immediately, and if any creatine is being excreted, his entire diet should be markedly improved and include gen-erous amounts of vitamin E. Muscular dystrophies might be stamped out if vitamin E were given to all pregnant women and to bottle-fed babies[44,45,105] and if refined foods lacking the vitamin were avoided.

The causes are many. Like most diseases, abnormalities of the muscles stem from multiple deficiencies rather than a few. Unless the diet is adequate in every nutrient, recovery can be neither expected nor maintained.

25
Problems That Concern Women

Faulty nutrition can at times cause women to envy men and mothers to wish they had sons only. Nervous tension, flightiness, irritability, emotional upsets, and much of the erratic behavior of girls at puberty make it difficult for them to live with themselves or anyone else. The output of hormones from the still-immature ovaries, needed for the efficient utilization of calcium, is so small that for about 18 months prior to the onset of menstruation the blood calcium usually remains below normal;[1] and even a slight calcium deficiency allows it to drop still lower. Thus starts a problem that frequently recurs intermittently throughout the reproductive years, becomes worse at menopause, and results in a stooped, brittle-boned old lady nursing an aching back.[2]

Such abnormalities can be prevented at any time in life by increasing the calcium intake and by obtaining adequate vitamin D and the various nutrients needed by the pituitary, sex, and adrenal glands to produce their hormones.

Premenstrual tension and menstrual cramps. When I was an undergraduate at the University of California, each girl in our department gave blood daily for a study being made by Dr. Ruth Okey of the blood calcium levels in relation to the menstrual cycle. Often we took calcium before and during menstruation, and brought in from other departments girls complaining of menstrual cramps. Dr. Okey's work showed that starting approximately ten days prior to menstruation, when the ovaries are the least active, the blood calcium drops steadily and progressively. Such a calcium decrease results in premenstrual tension, nervousness, headaches, insomnia, and mental depression. As one woman put it, "That's the time I spank the kids, yell at my husband, live on tranquilizers, drink too much, and can't stand myself."

Because the decreased blood calcium acts as a stress,

the production of cortisone and aldosterone are stimulated and salt and water are retained in the body, often causing the breasts, hands, face, and feet to swell, weight to increase 5 to 10 pounds, headaches to occur, and resistance to allergies and infections to decrease markedly.[8] Crimes of violence committed by women take place mostly during this period.[3]

The first day of menstruation the blood calcium takes a still-greater nose dive, causing muscular cramps in the emptying uterus and sometimes elsewhere in the body. Should the blood calcium drop dangerously low, convulsions result. Yet if adequate calcium is obtained and efficiently absorbed, both premenstrual tension and menstrual cramps can be prevented.

When cramps occur, 1 or 2 calcium tablets every hour generally bring quick relief. Some calcium supplementation is usually desirable during the second and third days. As menstruation proceeds, however, the blood calcium gradually increases. If the diet is fair, the calcium level in the blood remains normal for the two weeks following menstruation, after which daily calcium supplementation should be started. Since more calcium is retained when magnesium and vitamin D are adequate,[4-6] my 15-year-old daughter takes daily prior to and during menstruation 5,000 units of vitamin D and tablets supplying 250 and 125 milligrams of calcium and magnesium respectively at each meal; and she claims never to have experienced the slightest menstrual discomfort.

If the blood calcium has been allowed to drop so low that it has induced stress, causing puffiness and a weight increase, generous amounts of protein, vitamin C, and pantothenic acid are needed in addition to vitamin D, calcium, and magnesium.

Vitamin D increases calcium absorption, retention, and utilization (p. 254); and because of the demands of growth, the vitamin-D and calcium requirements are both unusually high throughout adolescence. Teen-age girls given 1,250 milligrams of calcium daily and 650 units of vitamin D excreted far more calcium than they retained; when the vitamin D was temporarily increased to 3,900 units daily, ten times more calcium was retained.[1] If continued, this quantity of synthetic vitamin D could be toxic.

The ovarian hormone, estrogen, and the pituitary hormone that stimulates the ovaries play vitally important roles throughout the reproductive period. They can be

synthesized, however, only when protein, linoleic acid, the
B vitamins, and particularly vitamin E are generously
supplied (p. 272). Estrogen increases the intestinal absorption of calcium, causes it to be held longer in the
body, and allows it to be used over and over;[7] hence it
helps to prevent menstrual discomfort when calcium is
undersupplied. If the diet is adequate, these hormones are
produced in normal amounts and menstrual difficulties are
avoided.

Other menstrual problems. Cessation of menstrual flow
or irregular or scanty menstruation are signs of general
malnutrition. Girls and women in prison and concentration camps during World War II invariably developed
these abnormalities. Such problems are accompanied by a
marked decrease in the production of sex hormones and
often by a shriveling of the breasts and ovaries.[8]

Occasionally a single nutrient brings marked improvement. For example, either a vitamin-B_{12} or folic-acid
deficiency causes irregular and decreased flow or cessation
of flow, but normal menstruation occurs as soon as the
missing vitamin is supplied.[9-11] Sometimes the addition
of vitamin E alone corrects the menstrual rhythm and
causes small breasts to develop without a corresponding
gain in weight. When the diet is made completely adequate, especially in the nutrients that aid the pituitary and
sex glands (ch. 28), menstruation usually becomes normal
in a few weeks.

Because excessive menstruation can be a symptom of
uterine cancer, a physician should be consulted immediately should this abnormality arise. A menstrual flow that
continues to be heavy after three or four days has often
been corrected within a single month by taking 600 units
of vitamin E daily.[12] An excessive flow may indicate
that the thyroid is underactive, in which case protein and
especially vitamin E should be increased,[38] and probably
no less than 5 milligrams of iodine should be obtained
daily.[13] Liver damage, which can prevent the inactiva-
tion of hormones regulating menstruation, may be responsible and, if so, should be corrected (ch. 16).

I can find no research on the relation of nutrition to
endometriosis. This abnormality is one in which a network
of blood vessels similar to those lining the uterine walls
prior to menstruation grows uncontrolled outside the
uterus. I suspect that liver damage which prevents the sex
hormones from being inactivated (pp. 171–172) may be
responsible, and that the best diet possible is indicated.

Vaginal discharge, inflammation, and itching. One of
the most common causes of a vaginal discharge, usually
accompanied by inflammation, itching, and perhaps pain
during intercourse, is a parasitic infestation of the vagina
known as trichomoniasis.[14] In animals, this infestation
develops when the diet is deficient in protein, vitamin A,
or any one of several B vitamins.[15] The doctors making
the following reports have not mentioned trichomoniasis,
although it was probably present in each case.

Itching around the genitalia has "responded dramatically" when women have been given as little as 6 milligrams
of vitamin B_2 daily.[16] A rash or dermatitis in the
vagina, accompanied by swelling, itching, and even bleeding, has cleared up when vitamin B_2 or B_6 or both have
been taken.[17,18] Inflammation and itching of the vagina
have also been helped by vitamin E;[12,19] and leukorrhea
and inflammation have disappeared after vitamin A was
given.[13,20] Women who eat no meat and are therefore
deficient in vitamin B_{12} develop irregular menstruation
and a "foul-smelling vaginal discharge" which is corrected
by adequate vitamin B_{12}.[10] I have frequently recommended vitamin B_6 for severe vaginal inflammation, and
a number of women have reported experiencing marked
and almost immediate relief, especially after applying a
salve containing this vitamin.

When nearly 300 obstetrical patients were given 50,000
units of vitamin A daily, inflammation of the vagina and
infections of the ovaries, uterus, and Fallopian tubes were
only 20 per cent of those experienced by an equal number
of women receiving no supplementary vitamin.[21] In case
of such an infection, medical care should be sought and
not only vitamin A but also protein and vitamins B_6, C,
E, and pantothenic acid should be kept particularly high
(ch. 11).

Menopause difficulties. At the end of the reproductive
period, the ovaries gradually become inactive. This process
is the reverse of changes that occurred at puberty, and a
healthy woman on an adequate diet is as unaware of any
disturbances as she was at adolescence. Furthermore, normal adrenal glands produce a number of sex hormones
which take over when menstruation ceases.[3]

Problems at menopause are often much more severe
than at puberty, largely because the diet has been deficient
in many nutrients—protein, calcium, magnesium, vitamins
D, E, and pantothenic acid—for years prior to its onset.
For instance, persons who spend much of their time in-

doors may have no vitamin D whatsoever in their blood.[6] Moreover, women who have a particularly difficult time during this period are usually those whose adrenals are exhausted.

Because calcium is less well absorbed and the urinary losses are greater when the output of estrogen decreases,[7,22] such calcium-deficiency symptoms as nervousness, irritability, insomnia, headaches, and depression are common. These problems can be easily overcome if the intakes of calcium, magnesium, and vitamin D are all generously increased and are well absorbed. Any woman having difficulty at this time should probably supplement her daily diet with the antistress formula (p. 31), 1,000 units of natural vitamin D, and 500 milligrams of magnesium; and obtain daily 2 grams of calcium, which can be supplied by 1 quart of milk fortified with ½ cup of non-instant powdered milk. Approximately 500 milligrams of calcium, preferably with magnesium, should be taken at any meal and before bed when fortified milk is not drunk.

During the menopause the need for vitamin E soars 10 to 50 times over that previously required.[23] Hot flashes and night sweats often disappear when 50 to 500 units of vitamin E are taken daily, but they quickly recur should the vitamin be stopped.[24,25] If estrogen is given, the need for vitamin E increases still further.[23] Because this hormone has been used to induce cancer in rats and mice,[26,27] I personally would prefer to improve my diet rather than resort to hormone therapy. One doctor, stating that 75 milligrams of vitamin E daily had alleviated hot flashes in his patients, pointed out that estrogen, given to any woman who had had cancer, might "activate dormant cells to malignant phases."[31]

Although the effect of cold creams apparently has not been specifically studied, it is known that estrogen, the adrenal hormones, and vitamins A, D, E, and K dissolve in mineral oil,[28-30] from which most cold creams are made; and that mineral oil absorbs through the skin when creams containing it are used. These hormones and vitamins are then lost in the feces. Mineral oil in all forms should probably be avoided, particularly during the menopause. Creams having a base of avocado oil, bone marrow, or other vegetable or animal fat may be used instead.

When menopause symptoms are severe, the condition should be looked upon as another form of stress, and all nutrients needed to stimulate the production of adrenal hormones particularly emphasized (ch. 2). Emotional stresses, such as rebellion at growing older and fear that one will become unattractive or that one's sex life will cease, often play a role in menopausal disturbances; and they increase the need for all nutrients as readily as any other form of stress. There is, however, another point of view. I once interviewed a woman who told me she loved her menopause; that she had been pale all her life, but since she had had hot flushes, she had received many compliments on her complexion.

Varicose veins. Although men have varicose veins, they are far more common among women. Anything that stops or interferes with the normal return of blood through the major veins in the legs, such as a tumor, cut, scarring, or clot, can cause other veins to become overloaded. A clot may form anywhere in the body yet lodge like a roadblock in the large leg vein. As in any detour, the blood is shunted along other roads; thus the smaller veins near the surface are forced to carry so much blood that they become unsightly.

The lack of any nutrient that allows blood to clot too rapidly (ch. 6) may play a role in the production of varicose veins. Blood clots that block circulation have been produced in animals by a diet lacking vitamin E.[32-34] If the vitamin is then given, such clots stop forming, the veins become dilated, and auxiliary blood vessels quickly develop around the clots which soon dissolve.[33,35,36] Similarly, giving vitamin E to humans has apparently prevented clots and embolisms but clot formation recurs if vitamin E is discontinued (p. 264). Varicose veins most frequently appear during pregnancy, when the requirement for this vitamin is unusually high and is both woefully deficient and often destroyed by iron supplements. Vitamins C, E, and several of the B vitamins are said to help dissolve clots.

Some investigators believe the major cause of varicose veins to be faulty elimination, in which an overloaded bowel presses against the veins in the lower abdomen year after year, gradually breaking down the valves in the veins and allowing a reverse flow of blood.[37] Among people on diets of unrefined foods, such as the Zulus in Africa, varicose veins and hemorrhoids (another form of varicose veins) are virtually unknown. In fact only three cases among 115,319 patients were found to have varicose veins compared with 10 per cent of the hospital population in England. To correct the situation, a "1,000-year-old diet" of fruits, vegetables, meats, eggs, cheese, sour milks, nuts, and whole-grain breads and cereals free from all refined foods is recommended. A millennium ago, few methods of refining were known, sugar was rare, and honey such a luxury that it was eaten by the common people only at wedding feasts.

Still another cause of varicose veins is a swollen, enlarged, or fatty liver which slows down the return of blood to the heart. In this case, a diet to correct liver damage (ch. 16) should be adhered to. There is no doubt that varicose veins can be prevented by an adequate diet and that prevention is much easier than correction. When removed surgically without the cause being corrected and preventive measures taken, they usually reappear in a relatively short time.

Various emotional upsets, particularly suppressed anger, can make varicose veins worse. Deep within all of us is a primitive desire to kick when something goes wrong; even if such a desire remains unconscious, large amounts of blood are still sent to the legs. When varicose veins exist, the return of this extra blood to the heart causes the already overloaded veins to swell still more. I have yet to know a woman whose varicose veins did not become severely troublesome if, for instance, she was furious because her husband was divorcing her. When such anger can be harmlessly expressed by kicking a pillow placed securely in a corner, further overloading of the veins can be prevented. One about-to-be-divorced woman told me recently, "It feels so good to kick that I don't care any more whether it helps my veins or not, but it has."

Rewards of minor improvements. A few minor nutritional improvements can help most women enjoy one part of each month as much as another and the middle years as much as the earlier ones. When such improvements are made, women can more fully appreciate their greatest asset: femininity.

26

Bone Problems Need
Early Recognition

A friend in her early forties was waiting for a traffic signal to change when a truck smashed into her car. Because of severe back pain resulting from the accident, she had x-rays taken. On examining them, her physician remarked, "You'd be laughed out of court if you showed anyone these x-rays. You've had osteoporosis for years." She had suffered from less severe backache which she had assumed to be muscular since her college days, when a too-limited budget and lack of knowledge caused her to live on candy bars and canned soup.

In the United States an estimated 4 million persons over 65 years of age suffer from severe backaches caused by abnormal bones, and their vertebrae frequently fracture merely from the weight of the body itself.[1-3] Yet the problem, which can be brought on by stress and/or inadequate diet at any age, is by no means confined to the elderly. This widespread abnormality occurs in undernourished children and adults of all economic brackets, is common in young women after induced menopause and older ones following natural menopause, and in almost every person over the age of 60.[4,5] I am convinced that it starts with the inadequate formulas given to babies, and that millions more backaches are in the making. The tragedy is that people are unaware that such a problem exists. It has long been assumed that porous bones are an inevitable part of growing older, but bones of well-fed animals become progressively stronger with age.

Such backaches can be relieved or prevented provided every nutrient needed to build and repair bones is obtained, efficiently absorbed, and not lost in the urine.

Bones change constantly. Like any other cells in the body, the cells forming the base of bone, or matrix, a

253

cartilage-like structure containing much tough connective tissue, continuously die and must be replaced. Bone repair or development is halted by an inadequacy of protein or of any nutrient required to utilize protein;[6] and/or by too little vitamin C, essential to connective-tissue formation.[4,7] When such deficiencies exist, so many cells die that areas become decalcified; the bones are left weak and brittle, and the minerals are freed into the blood.[8,9] Repair starts immediately, however, if all nutrients are supplied.

Even though some calcium is lost daily in urine and feces, when the diet has been adequate, an excess is stored in the long bones, which, like a bank account, can be used as needed for bone repair and by the soft tissues. Conversely, when sufficient calcium is not supplied by food and none is stored, bones cannot be repaired but are robbed to supply calcium to the soft tissues; thus the amount of calcium in the blood is maintained at approximately the same level throughout life.

Phosphorus is equally as essential as calcium, but the intake in America is excessive, whereas the calcium intake in all age groups is below that recommended by the National Research Council.[10,11] The excessive phosphorus causes a continuous urinary loss of calcium. Furthermore, much calcium is lost in the urine when magnesium is undersupplied; and the magnesium deposited in bones is given up reluctantly even during a severe deficiency.[12-16] These facts indicate that magnesium, which is usually deficient,[17] is important in correcting bone abnormalities.

Vitamin D increases calcium absorption through the intestinal wall and reabsorption from the kidney tubules; and it controls enzymes necessary to deposit minerals in bones and teeth.[18,19] Because this vitamin can be produced on the skin by summer sunshine provided the oils have not been washed off,[20] populations living in the tropics and subtropics have far better bones though a lower calcium intake than those in temperate zones.[21,22] For example, student nurses working indoors in Michigan were found to have no vitamin D whatsoever in their blood even during the summer.[19]

The fact that calcium, magnesium, and vitamin D are undersupplied in the American diet could account for the widespread bone abnormalities, yet poor absorption may be equally at fault (p. 179).

Osteoporosis. Although the word osteoporosis literally

means porous or honeycombed bones, prolonged deficiencies of calcium and vitamin D cause the skeleton to become demineralized and in time shrunken instead of porous.[23-25] The former belief that this disease resulted from the body's failure to synthesize the protein base of bones has proved to be false.[7,26] High-protein diets do not correct osteoporosis.[27] The identical disease develops when adult rats are given low-calcium diets, and made far worse if vitamin D is also undersupplied.[28,29]

Many studies have shown that persons with this disease have had calcium intakes far below the recommended daily allowances and have often lacked protein and/or enzymes needed to utilize calcium and phosphorus, whereas individuals obtaining ample minerals have normal bones.[1,4,6] Usually the calcium intake has been below 500 milligrams daily—the amount obtained from 2 glasses of milk—yet the need for calcium actually increases with age, probably because absorption becomes less efficient.[10] Persons obtaining 1,250 milligrams of calcium daily had much denser bones than ones getting 750 milligrams.[30] Most individuals with osteoporosis have milk and cheese available and can afford calcium supplements, but have rarely been aware of their benefits.[5,6,23] Vitamin D, which has been shown to be as important for adults and especially elderly men and women as it is for children[31,32] is often totally lacking. Some patients have excreted excessive amounts of calcium, most have obtained far too much phosphorus, and many have been deficient in vitamin C, but invariably all have obtained too little calcium.[4,7,18,19,23,25,26]

Because of calcium losses during pregnancies and menstruation, this disease is far more prevalent in women than in men.[3,5] In elderly people it is accompanied by an actual loss of height and by bending, causing a humpback deformity that crowds lungs and digestive organs;[33] yet the amount of calcium in the blood does not drop below normal nor do the bones change chemically.[4-6,34] Thus this disease is particularly difficult to diagnose, and may be detected by x-rays only after 60 per cent of the minerals have been withdrawn from the bones and over 1 pound of calcium lost,[4,35,36] an amount equivalent to that supplied by 500 quarts of milk.

Persons customarily consider a broken hip bone to be the result of a fall, whereas the collapse of the bone is usually the cause of a fall which first calls attention to osteoporosis. Before a diagnosis is possible, backache and spasms of the back muscles, aching of the long bones and thighs, rarefication of the pelvic bones, loss in twisting and bending strength, and spontaneous fractures often occur.[1,2,37] Not infrequently the neck of the femur at the hip gives way or the lower vertebrae crumble merely from the weight of the body.[10,11]

When the diet is made adequate, particularly in protein, calcium, magnesium, and vitamins C and D, and is supplemented by 1 or 2 grams of calcium daily, backaches and other symptoms gradually disappear and new fractures rarely occur.[4,33] Calcium is actually absorbed by people with osteoporosis more rapidly than by normal individuals, and it continues to be stored for several years provided the diet and supplements are taken conscientiously.[33] Many years must pass, however, before a detectable difference can be seen in x-rays.[1,27]

It must be clearly understood that the male and female hormones, androgen and estrogen, currently used in treating osteoporosis, cannot take the place of calcium and other nutrients. When given to young animals, estrogen increases bone growth, but it inhibits bone repair in "middle-aged" or older animals.[38-40] Patients who have reported feeling better after receiving estrogen showed the same or greater improvement when placebos—usually tablets of milk sugar—were given them instead;[5,41] and their blood calcium, if low, increased no more than when calcium alone was taken. Doctors making a detailed study of 200 osteoporotic patients on androgen therapy concluded that amounts small enough to prevent masculinization of women were ineffective,[42] though the hormone may increase the formation of vitamin D in the skin.[43] Those receiving vitamin D alone, however, absorbed more calcium than individuals given androgen.[19] The most adequate diet possible, therefore, should be followed whether these hormones are taken or not.

Of the hundreds of studies made, no person has ever been found to have osteoporosis who had received adequate calcium which was well absorbed and retained.

Osteomalacia. This disease—its name literally means bad bones—results primarily from a severe vitamin-D deficiency. Arabian and Indian women who keep themselves heavily veiled frequently develop such painful backs that they can scarcely rise; and they suffer multiple spontaneous fractures and have extremely rarefied bones, all of which clears up dramatically when vitamin D is given them.[21,25,44] In America osteomalacia is usually associated with kidney damage, which prevents calcium from being retained.[45] It also occurs in people who get little sunshine and/or stay on such low-fat diets that bile flow is inadequate, hence vitamin D is not absorbed. In addition to aching bones and fractures, they suffer from nervousness, twitching, and muscular cramps and spasms.

When bile is prevented from reaching the intestines of adult rats, osteomalacia is produced in every case even though the diet supplies calcium and vitamin D. Persons with osteomalacia recover rapidly when the bile flow is stimulated (ch. 17) and the diet supplies oils, lecithin, calcium, and vitamin D. Enzyme tablets with bile and hydrochloric acid tablets or liquid (p. 142), however, should be used temporarily to increase absorption.

Broken bones. For years I have been appalled at the number of people who have come to me on crutches or in wheelchairs because broken bones have failed to knit. Frequently their diets have been inadequate in almost every respect. When healing is slow, special attention should be given not only to the diet itself but also to all factors that increase absorption and to psychological problems which sometimes make immobilization desirable.

Because of the combined stresses of the broken bone and immobilization of part or all of the body, much body protein is broken down and the urinary losses of nutrients are high. The diet required for repair, therefore, should be particularly rich in protein, all antistress factors (p. 28), vitamin C, and pantothenic acid, as well as calcium, magnesium, vitamin D, oil, and lecithin. One would not expect a normal protein intake to be a limiting factor, yet in one study of 55 persons whose bones refused to knit, giving 160 grams of protein daily as the only dietary improvement brought complete and rapid healing.[6] Digestive enzymes with bile and hydrochloric acid taken with each meal usually accelerate repair; and if the surrounding tissues have been damaged, a high vitamin-E intake prevents scarring and stiffness.

Inflammations of the bone. Osteitis, osteomyelitis, and osteitis deformans are types of inflammation of the bone marked by swelling, tenderness, pain, and perhaps infection. In osteitis deformans, brought on by severe stress, the bones of adults demineralize so rapidly that they actually bend; and the stress inhibits the formation of new proteins needed for the bone base. Studies with radioactive calcium, however, show that when the diet is extremely adequate, recalcification is also unusually rapid.[46]

As always when inflammation is the major problem, the adrenals must first be helped to produce more cortisone. In addition to foods needed for repairing bones, the anti-stress formula (p. 31) should be taken every two or three hours around the clock with highly fortified milk until the inflammation subsides; and liver and a cooked green leafy vegetable should be eaten daily. If the bone is infected, still larger amounts of vitamin C may be needed.

When all nutrients are generously supplied and absorption and retention are increased, recovery is often rapid. Not long ago a man who had been an invalid for more than two years because of osteitis deformans was brought in a wheelchair to see me. He had made no progress on a fairly adequate diet, but recovered quickly after enzymes, hydrochloric acid, lecithin, magnesium, and large amounts of vitamin C and pantothenic acid were taken daily.

Paget's disease is a form of osteitis deformans that, though said to be congenital, can also be helped by an adequate diet. For example, Mr. Husted Meyer, of Leland, Michigan, suffered from this disease so severely that his painful spine bent and became inflexible, his skull narrowed, other bones enlarged, and he could walk no more than 100 yards. Through carefully applied nutrition, he has regained flexibility, stands straighter, walks easily, and leads an active, normal life. X-rays show that the disease has been arrested.

When healing fails. I have before me the case history of a Seattle woman whose hip broke when she was 52. During the past four and a half years she has been under the care of doctor after doctor, has had repeated surgery, and has been unable to walk during this entire period. Although she writes, "the pain is terrific" and "the steel pin and head have slipped down into the marrow of the bone," her menus show not one drop of milk.

In most cases where healing is slow, the calcium intake is far too low. Moreover, there must be adequate hydrochloric acid, fat, vitamin D, and bile to assure efficient calcium absorption (p. 179). The absorption and retention of this mineral are still further increased by vitamin A, many of the B vitamins, citric acid (p. 204), magnesium, and several amino acids from digested proteins.[10,17]

Several studies show that milk sugar, or lactose tremendously increases the absorption of calcium.[47-50] Although intestinal bacteria break milk sugar into lactic acid which helps to dissolve calcium, an increased calcium absorption occurs in the presence of milk sugar even when all bacteria have been destroyed by antibiotics. Animals given calcium with milk sugar deposit some calcium in the femur, or leg bone, in 30 minutes and lay down "highly significant amounts" within two hours.[51] If other sugars are allowed, calcium absorption is so markedly decreased that little of the mineral reaches the bones. This fact undoubtedly explains why babies given formulas containing large amounts of dextromaltose or glucose frequently have faulty bone formation which is shown by abnormal bulging foreheads. The excessive intake of sweets during childhood and adolescence causes facial bones to be underdeveloped and the jaws to remain so small that the teeth are crowded together. Similarly, eating sweets can prevent calcium from being absorbed by an adult.

Normally the hydrochloric acid in the stomach dissolves the calcium supplied by foods and holds it in solution until it can be absorbed through the intestinal walls. Sugar and other sweets, however, stimulate the production of alkaline digestive juices so rapidly that calcium becomes insoluble before it can reach the blood. Thus, after the stomach has been removed because of cancer or ulcers, eating sweets or other concentrated carbohydrates can cause a patient to go into shock; so many quarts of alkaline digestive juices are quickly formed from blood plasma that the blood volume is suddenly decreased, and the effect is much the same as if a severe hemorrhage had occurred.[52,53] Persons with this condition, known as the dumping syndrome because food is dumped directly into the small intestine, get along well on an adequate diet high in protein and fat, but if hydrochloric acid is not taken at each meal, osteoporosis develops quickly. If calcium is to be well absorbed, such individuals and anyone with bone abnormalities should avoid all foods containing refined sugar and obtain calcium from fresh milk and/or yogurt, preferably fortified with powdered milk.

Although no amount of vitamin D can compensate for the lack of calcium, this mineral is lost in the urine at any age unless vitamin D is adequate; and the losses continue even when no calcium is supplied in the diet.[31,45,54,55] If sufficient calcium has been obtained and well absorbed, large amounts can still be quickly lost in the urine should vitamin B_6 and/or magnesium be undersupplied (ch. 20).

Stress, such as the immobilization of a single limb or

the entire body, or the taking of cortisone not compensated for by adequate nutrition, causes calcium to be withdrawn from the bones, the blood calcium to be high, large amounts of this mineral to be lost in the urine, and protein synthesis to be retarded.[9,46,56-58] When the daily diet has supplied 2.5 grams of calcium, healing has been promoted, yet the amount of calcium lost in the urine has not increased.[5,34]

If stress or cortisone therapy is prolonged, demineralization of bones may "develop dramatically" and spontaneous fractures occur.[5,45,46] Recently I received a letter from a man who because of arthritis had been given cortisone; and during the past year alone he had suffered seven spontaneously broken vertebrae. The loss of minerals stops as soon as stress is removed, cortisone is discontinued,[5] and/or the diet meets the needs of stress. In such cases, following the antistress program (p. 31) becomes as important as a high intake of calcium and vitamin D.

What effect strontium-90 has on healing of bone abnormalities is not yet known, but fallout from bombs already tested is expected to continue for the next several years.[59] This mineral is chemically so similar to calcium that it is readily deposited in the bones and teeth whenever calcium is inadequate. Analysis of thousands of deciduous teeth collected in the St. Louis area show that the deposition of strontium has been steadily increasing during the past decade. The body prefers calcium to strontium, however, and if the calcium intake is high, strontium is neither absorbed nor laid down in the bones.[60] Although milk contains some strontium-90, its high calcium content makes this food the best safeguard against harmful deposition.[2,61] Patients with osteoporosis have been found to absorb strontium particularly rapidly,[27] but the radioactive element is gradually replaced by calcium provided the diet is adequate.

Disc problems. The effect of nutrition on discs, or cartilage pillows which, if healthy, are like rubber cushions between the vertebrae, appears to have been little studied. When patients with disc lesions were given an adequate diet supplemented with 500 to 1,000 milligrams of vitamin C daily, their back pains disappeared and extensive surgery was avoided.[62] A diet particularly high in protein, especially in eggs to supply methionine, and in vitamin E is probably as essential as vitamin C before a damaged disc can be repaired.

The diet for bone abnormalities. Persons suffering from osteoporosis or fractured, broken, inflamed, or infected bones should probably have no less than 2.5 grams (2,500 milligrams) of calcium and 500 milligrams of magnesium daily. One 8-ounce glass of milk, buttermilk, or commercial yogurt supplies 250 milligrams of calcium. Calcium lactate and gluconate, which contain no phosphorus, are available in both powder and tablets, alone or with magnesium oxide. The amount of calcium needed could be supplied by a combination of fresh whole or skim milk, buttermilk, yogurt, acidophilus milk, or fresh milk fortified with powdered milk, and calcium tablets or powder. The calcium in yogurt and acidophilus milk is already dissolved; hence it is more readily absorbed than that in fresh milk; and many persons, particularly elderly ones, tolerate cultured milks better than fresh.

The vitamin D given for osteoporosis has usually varied from 1,000 to 5,000 units daily. Even as few as 400 to 700 units daily has increased the blood vitamin D more than exposure to summer sun, yet some patients with osteoporosis had no vitamin D in the blood when this amount was given daily.[19] Such a small quantity allows little or none to be stored, whereas a larger amount is beneficial long after it is taken.[31,55] When 5,000 units of vitamin D have been given daily, the amount of this vitamin in the blood was comparable to that found in elderly women living in the subtropics;[19] hence this quantity appears to be sufficient. If this vitamin D is entirely natural, or supplied only from fish-liver oil, such a quantity is probably never toxic to an adult, but 5,000 units of synthetic vitamin D, or irradiated ergosterol, could be toxic if continued over a considerable period. Read labels carefully and be sure to use only natural vitamin D.

Unless the demands of stress are met and the diet is adequate in every other respect (ch. 32), little improvement should be expected. Usually enzyme and hydrochloric-acid tablets and lecithin should be taken temporarily, especially by older individuals.

To prevent misery and the expense of hospital and medical bills, every senior citizen should be urged to drink more milk and to supplement his diet with calcium tablets and/or powder and vitamin D. In fact, it appears that any person who wishes to enjoy the twilight years without an aching back should give particular attention to his calcium and vitamin D intake from the age of 40 on.

27

Surgery, Accidents, and Burns

It is almost unbelievable how rapidly people with a strong will to live can recover after extensive surgery or horrible accidents or burns. Such patients can be made more comfortable and the work of doctors and nurses easier, however, when the nutrition is kept as adequate as circumstances allow. A malnourished person, for instance, is usually particularly sensitive to pain, whereas adequate calcium, magnesium, vitamins B_1 and E, and other nutrients appear to decrease such sensitivity.[1,2]

Stress with a vengeance. Following severe injury, the outpouring of pituitary and adrenal hormones causes the breakdown of tremendous amounts of body protein which may continue a month or longer, and it inhibits the formation of new proteins needed in large quantities for healing.[3,4] Usually the patient can eat little or nothing; hence still more body protein is broken down to serve as calories. If vitamin B_6 is undersupplied, so much urea may be formed (p. 199) that it decreases healing even further.[5-7] Overweight persons delight in pounds lost at such times, but the destruction of body protein frequently results in ugly wrinkles.

By the second or third day following major surgery or a severe accident or burn, the adrenals are usually exhausted because pantothenic acid and vitamin B_2, which cannot be stored and without which cortisone cannot be produced, have been used up.[8-10] Salt is lost from the body, and potassium leaves the cells (pp. 143–144), resulting in partial or complete paralysis of the intestines, urinary bladder, and uretha.[11-16] The paralysis is made worse by a deficiency of potassium or of vitamin B_1, which is quickly produced if intravenous feedings of sugar are given.[17,18]

Though the paralysis can be prevented or relieved by supplying the missing nutrients, from the patient's point of view it usually brings the major suffering following surgery. Bacteria living on stagnant food in the immobile intestines form tremendous quantities of gas, which can cause excruciating pain when it presses against a raw abdominal incision. The use of a catheter, necessitated by an inability to pass urine, is often agonizing, especially for men.

Inability to urinate has been produced in animals under stress by diets mildly deficient in vitamins B_2, C, or pantothenic acid;[19] and if any of these deficiencies is severe or if too little food is eaten, animals are unable to pass urine even when loaded with water by stomach tube. If sufficient food is eaten and/or the missing vitamins are supplied so that cortisone can be produced or if cortisone itself is given, normal urination occurs promptly.

Exhausted adrenals are a contributory cause of death in cases where severe injury proves fatal. Yet such exhaustion can often be prevented by nothing more than an injection of pantothenic acid.

Vitamin C and injury. The healing of wounds depends on the formation of connective tissue, which, although made of protein, cannot be synthesized without vitamin C.[3] Hundreds of studies have shown that the speed of healing and the tensile strength of the connective tissue are directly proportional to the amount of vitamin C obtained; and that if large amounts are taken, "dramatic results" can be produced,[4] whereas a lack of vitamin C allows incisions to break open.[20]

This vitamin also accelerates the formation of new blood vessels at the site of injury and around clots which may block veins.[20] It activates many enzymes used in healing, speeds the formation of new proteins, and helps to prevent hemorrhages to the extent that without it a minor injury can result in a major loss of blood.[21-23] Its detoxifying action at a time when medications must be given and various harmful substances are formed from destroyed cells[24-26] is particularly important. A single dose of any one of a number of drugs caused the blood of animals to take eight times longer to clot than before the drug was given, and the prolonged clotting time continued for two weeks, yet this effect was entirely prevented when vitamin C was allowed with the drug.[27]

The combined stresses of injury, pain, x-rays, medications, injections, tube feedings, catheterizations, and immobilization can induce a vitamin-C deficiency at lightning speed even when seemingly large amounts are obtained.[28] For example, 300 milligrams of vitamin C daily have proved to be far too little to be effective.[25] A physician recently told me that his patients showed "amazing improvement" when given 500 milligrams every two hours for the first several days after any form of injury.

Vitamin E offers much. When the diet is adequate and vitamin E is amply supplied, wounds can heal without scarring; surgical incisions leave only a thin, soft line free of hard keloid tissue; adhesions can be prevented; and the itching, drawing pain caused by the contraction of scar tissue—excruciating when large areas of flesh have been excised, as after the removal of a cancerous breast—does not occur (ch. 4). By decreasing the need for oxygen, vitamin E allows fewer cells to be harmed when blood vessels have been cut, mangled, or burned;[29] and it increases the number and speed of formation of new blood vessels into a damaged area.[20,30]

A major problem after surgery, injury, or childbirth is that blood clots often form where an incision is made or injections or intravenous feedings are given. Such a clot, carried in the circulating blood and known as an embolism—a clot with the wanderlust—can lodge in any tight quarters. If it blocks a deep vein of the leg, it causes varicose veins and/or phlebitis, or inflammation of the blood vessels. Both varicose veins and phlebitis have been produced experimentally by surgery on animals deficient in vitamin E.[30,31] Dogs and rats not given this vitamin prior to surgery form many more clots than do well-fed animals. These clots block the circulation, causing the nearby veins to become overloaded with blood (varicose veins) and the walls of the blood vessels to become inflamed, swollen, and crowded with dead cells which are replaced by inelastic scar tissue. This effect cannot be produced by diets lacking any other nutrient.[30,31]

I can find no studies in which vitamin E has been taken before operations, but when 100 surgical patients were given 200 milligrams of this vitamin daily after surgery, they had far fewer clots and less severe phlebitis than the same number not receiving the vitamin.[32] In other studies, three times more clots formed when the vitamin was not given and the reaction to the clots was much more severe than in patients allowed vitamin E.[33-35] The inflammation and swelling of phlebitis also disappeared in patients receiving 300 units of vitamin E daily.[33]

All nutrients aid in healing. New cells cannot be made without essential fatty acids;[36] and as with vitamin C, the strength of connective tissue formed at the site of a wound is in proportion to the amount of protein obtained.[8] New proteins needed for healing, however, can be synthesized only when enzymes containing vitamins B_2, B_6, folic acid, copper, magnesium, and several other nutrients are present.[18,20,22,37-41] Vitamin A also plays a role in forming connective tissue.[42] Wounds heal slowly if at all when vitamin B_2 is undersupplied;[39,40] thus unless all nutrients are available, rapid recovery cannot occur.

Even the lack of a single nutrient can prevent healing. For example, when folic-acid deficiencies have been produced in patients, ulcers, bedsores, and tiny wounds caused by taking biopsies have refused to heal.[43] Conversely, wounds, incisions, and bedsores that for months had failed to heal and skin grafts that had consistently broken down have all healed rapidly after an adequate diet unusually high in protein was given.[20,44,45]

Blood clotting. When blood clots normally, hemorrhages are largely prevented and work and anxiety of the surgeon are decreased. Blood clotting involves numerous intricate chemical processes requiring many nutrients, the most important being calcium and vitamins C, E, and K.[21,27,46] Because vitamin K is produced by intestinal bacteria, it is rarely lacking except when the bacteria have been destroyed by oral antibiotics or when bile fails to reach the intestine, conditions easily rectified by taking yogurt or acidophilus milk, bile tablets, and lecithin.[47]

Calcium and vitamins C and E, however, are frequently undersupplied. Vitamin E "constantly and quickly" shortens the clotting time of bleeders[48] and, provided it is taken continuously, has even prevented hemorrhaging in hemophiliacs studied over a period of many years.[48,49]

Shock. When shock cannot be treated quickly, irreversible damage often occurs, which may result in death. The reaction to experimental shock can be made worse by deficiencies of a variety of nutrients, whereas adequately fed animals withstand shock well.[50] Similarly, persons who are malnourished, especially those who have been on low-protein diets, are particularly susceptible to shock.[45] As another form of stress, it causes the amount of vitamin C and most of the B vitamins in the blood to fall drastically;[51] and much harm can be prevented if an injection of these vitamins can be given immediately or be taken before surgery.

In cases where shock has been brought on by acute hemorrhage, damage done by the decreased oxygen supply

to the tissues can be considerably alleviated by giving
3,000 milligrams of vitamin C and 300 units or more of
vitamin E as quickly as possible.[52,53]

Preparation for surgery. When an adequate high-
protein diet has been given patients both before and after
surgery, the destruction of body protein has been almost
completely prevented in spite of extreme stress;[54] and
such a diet often makes the expense and discomfort of
intravenous and/or tube feedings unnecessary.[55] A
month or more of preparation before surgery is important
for all persons, especially those who are already ill.[58]
Malnourished and ill individuals are poor surgical risks,
have adverse reactions to anesthetics, are susceptible to
shock and infections, and heal slowly.[55,56] Animals deficient in protein for only five days prior to surgery require
twice as long to heal as their well-fed litter mates even
though given adequate protein afterward.[3] Because the
blood protein may remain normal, a patient's protein
intake can be far too low without the physician recognizing it.[45]

During the preparatory period, protein grams should be
counted (p. 405), and six small meals supplying at least 25
grams each taken daily.[45] The protein can be supplied
by fresh whole or skim milk fortified with powdered milk,
yeast, soy flour, and eggs (p. 89); and as much meat,
fish, cheese, eggs, yogurt, custard, or cereals cooked in
milk as can be tolerated. Digestive enzymes with bile and
hydrochloric acid should be used to insure greater absorption and yogurt or acidophilus milk or culture taken to
destroy gas-forming intestinal bacteria. Supplements
should be relied upon to furnish nutrients not readily
obtained from foods, and vitamins B_2, C, pantothenic
acid, and the antistress factors kept particularly high.[17]
Because persons mildly deficient in vitamin B_6 are subject to nausea and vomiting (p. 141), taking 10 milligrams
or more daily often pays rich dividends.

Not only does a period of preparation speed up healing
and thus decrease suffering and expense, but at times it
makes surgery unnecessary. My files contain dozens of
such reports: a woman whose bursitis cleared up while she
was preparing for an operation on her shoulder; several
people whose hemorrhoids disappeared; numerous youngsters whose tonsils and adenoids have not had to be
removed; other individuals whose kidney stones, gallstones, or prostates stopped causing trouble; and even one

woman whose inflamed uterus cleared up. Whatever the outcome, the reward more than pays for the effort.

The evening before surgery. The main cause of vomiting after surgery is that the blood sugar is allowed to drop too low. Usually little or no food is eaten the night before and none the day of surgery; hence fat alone is burned for energy and acetone acidosis develops (pp. 97–98). Although retching after abdominal surgery can be sheer torture, vomiting and the need for glucose injections can be largely prevented if during the late evening of the day before surgery the patient will eat a pound of some fat-free candy such as jelly beans, gumdrops, or marshmallows. This large amount of sugar allows the liver and muscles to store a maximum quantity of glycogen, or body starch, which can be gradually converted into sugar during the following morning. A San Francisco surgeon who is a personal friend has used this technique successfully for so many years that he has been given the nickname of "Dr. Jelly Bean." Some physicians recommend that heavily sweetened lemonade be taken throughout the day prior to surgery, but if many hours intervene, much of the sugar is changed into fat.

As a final nightcap on the eve before surgery, 1,000 milligrams of vitamin C, 500 milligrams of pantothenic acid, and 20 milligrams of vitamin B_2 and B_6 might be taken as a gift to the adrenals and to increase antibodies; and 1,000 units of natural vitamin D, 300 units of vitamin E, and 500 milligrams of calcium lactate be given to the blood to insure rapid clotting.

Diet after surgery or injury. To increase the blood sugar and replace salt lost because of severe stress, physicians usually specify that the first meal after surgery or injury be well-salted broth and heavily sweetened tea.[11] If taken, these foods help to prevent vomiting and the intestinal gas and inability to urinate which occur when potassium leaves the cells following a loss of salt (sodium) (p. 262).

All vitamins that dissolve in water, especially those needed by the adrenals, should be increased immediately after any injury and kept unusually high during the entire convalescence;[17,26,39] and "heavy vitamin supplementation" has been found to add tremendously to the comfort of the patient.[18,57] For the first few days, the antistress formula (p. 31) might be taken every two hours, and supplements of minerals and all other vitamins obtained with each meal. To save the time of busy physicians and nurses, these supplements can be brought from home and given by some visiting member of the family.

When food cannot be held on the stomach, physicians give intravenous feedings, which usually supply sugar, salt, digested proteins, and perhaps vitamin B_1. These nutrients are valuable but cannot meet the needs of stress. All vitamins and essential fatty acids, however, absorb well through the skin.[58] If vomiting persists, oils, vitamins A, D, E, and massive quantities of powdered vitamin C and the B vitamins (stirred into salve or cold cream) can be applied directly to the skin several times daily. Often an injection of vitamin B_6 or surface applications of 50 milligrams or more of this vitamin can alleviate vomiting (p. 141).

As soon as the patient is able to eat, the diet should be extremely high in protein. At least 1,000 additional calories must be obtained daily, otherwise this valuable protein will be used for calories and new body proteins cannot be formed or healing set in. If the protein intake can be kept high, repair appears to have priority over the energy needs,[59] and the destruction of body protein can be largely prevented.[54]

One physician, giving patients who have had severe burns, accidents, or major surgery a can of puréed meat per hour or continuously by nasal-stomach tube—16 cans daily supplying a total of 500 grams of protein—reports "dramatic results"; healing sets in immediately and the patients feel stronger, are more cheerful, and have little gas distention.[45] He has found that only 135 grams of protein daily assure rapid healing after hernia repair or the removal of an appendix or gall bladder.[45]

Newly formed tissue is particularly high in the sulfur-containing amino acids, cystine and methionine. Because milk and egg yolks are rich sources of these amino acids, healing has been tremendously accelerated when 6 small eggnogs containing 2 yolks each have been taken daily.[60] Highly fortified pep-up (p. 329) containing whole milk, oil, and 6 or more eggs or egg yolks would undoubtedly accelerate healing even more. Milk, buttermilk, yogurt, eggnogs, and juices should be taken in preference to tea or coffee. When much blood has been lost, liver damage frequently occurs,[8,61] and the diet must be designed to rebuild both blood (ch. 23) and liver tissue (ch. 16).

The disuse of muscles and bones during immobilization has been thought to be the cause of the continuous high urinary losses of calcium, phosphorus, potassium, sulfur, nitrogen, and other nutrients.[61] It now appears that these losses are brought on by the stress of immobilization rather than disuse and can be largely alleviated by an antistress diet (p. 31). To prevent kidney stones, however, vitamins B_6 and D, magnesium, and no less than 2.5 grams (2,500 milligrams) of calcium should be obtained daily;[62] and to compensate for the losses during stress, the diet should be kept highly adequate long after convalescence appears to be complete.

The shock of any injury usually causes a temporary lack of enzymes and hydrochloric acid, and supplements of both can tremendously aid absorption and accelerate healing.[8] Recovery is also much faster when small, frequent meals are served; and the more ill the person, the greater is the necessity for frequent feedings.[63]

Accidents. All the nutrients essential for healing after surgery are equally necessary following accidents. The diet should meet the demands of stress, prevent unsightly scars, knit broken bones (p. 257), keep kidney stones from forming (ch. 20), and build blood to replace that lost (ch. 23).

In cases where a poison has been swallowed, pantothenic acid, vitamin B_2, and huge amounts of vitamin C, needed for detoxifying purposes, should be given around the clock. Generous amounts of vitamin E and a high-protein diet containing 6 or more egg yolks daily can also help the liver detoxify the poison and prevent liver damage (ch. 16). If food cannot be held on the stomach, oil and vitamins should be applied to the skin (p. 268).

When prolonged unconsciousness follows an accident, patients can receive an adequate diet by tube feeding.[55] At a physician's request, I prepared tube feedings for a severely malnourished 12-year-old boy who was unconscious following a car accident. They consisted of fresh and powdered milk, yeast, desiccated liver, wheat germ, egg yolks, vegetable oils, lecithin, frozen undiluted orange juice, 1 tablespoon of cod-liver oil, a solution of vitamin C and pantothenic acid, and the contents of several vitamin-E capsules. Although the child remained unconscious for more than two weeks, during this period his face and body filled out, his color improved, and the texture of his skin and hair changed remarkably. He later made a rapid recovery. Because of shortage of help, physicians are often glad to have such highly nutritious feedings prepared at home and brought to the hospital.

Burns. The excruciating pain of burns appears to result from a lack of oxygen, the supply of which is cut off the minute blood vessels are seared; at the same time, the consumption of oxygen is tremendously increased.[64] When vitamin-E capsules are pierced with a needle and their contents immediately squeezed over the burned area, the pain is dulled and often disappears. More vitamin E should be applied several times daily. If the patient can stand to have the burned surface touched, vitamin-E ointment may be used.[65] PABA ointment (p. 129) also relieves the pain quickly after mild burns, but its effectiveness on severe burns is not known. My conviction is that at least 200 units of vitamin E and 300 milligrams of PABA should be taken after each meal, starting immediately. The PABA may be discontinued when pain is gone, but the vitamin E should be taken until long after healing is complete.

Because huge amounts of toxic breakdown products from damaged tissues are released into the blood, far larger quantities of vitamin C are needed after burns than following other injuries.[66] When a half teaspoon or more of a solution of vitamin C, pantothenic acid, other B vitamins (p. 326), and calcium gluconate, which dissolves readily in water, is given every hour to a severely burned patient for a few days, pain is far less intense and recovery more rapid.[67]

The loss of nutrients in the tissue fluids oozing from the surface of large burns can cause death or quickly produce advanced malnutrition even in a previously well-nourished person.[44,45] Hundreds of studies have emphasized that 400 grams or more of protein are needed daily to replace the tremendous losses, though huge amounts of all nutrients that dissolve in water—vitamin C, the B vitamins, salt, iodine, potassium, and magnesium—are equally needed.[22,26,45] Simultaneously the extreme stress of a severe burn increases all body requirements.[10,26]

On a few occasions I have, with the permission of physicians, worked with mothers of children so severely burned that they were not expected to live. Each time these wonderful women have sat by the bed day and night giving the child almost continuous sips of highly fortified whole milk similar to pep-up (p. 329) and a teaspoon of dissolved antistress formula (p. 31) every hour the patient was awake. Vitamins A and D were supplied once daily in drops, and vitamin-E capsules emptied directly into the mouth as well as over the burned areas. Fortunately, these children have made remarkably rapid recoveries and none have required the expected skin grafts.

It is not easy. Because of nausea, lack of appetite, and extremely high nutritional requirements, obtaining an adequate diet after surgery, a burn, or an accident is not easy. Persons who know the principles of emergency feeding and apply them the best they can, however, are usually rewarded by rapid healing and at times by spectacular and unexpected recovery.

28

And What of Sex?

One of the tragedies of illness is that it usually prevents a normal sex life. Because sex is a means of expressing love and is perhaps the deepest form of human communication, a marriage without it is sterile and often an outright endurance contest. Although major sexual problems, such as impotency and frigidity, and a horde of minor ones are emotional in origin, intercourse is often not enjoyed simply because a partner is tired, has a headache, has not slept well the night before, or feels tense or depressed and wants nothing more than to be left alone.

Any person who is irritable, critical, nagging, or lacks the energy to take a bath is scarcely setting the stage for an evening of ecstasy. During my 37 years of consulting work, dozens of men and hundreds of women have talked to me about their sex problems; and some of the commonest complaints I have heard are that feet smell bad and that the mate has halitosis. Such seemingly insignificant things can prevent a woman from having a fulfilling orgasm and a man a sustained erection.

Much of the joy of sex depends on buoyant good health, which most people can achieve—if they really want it—to a far greater degree than they think possible.

Research is meager. Partly because of reticence, little research has been done concerning the effect of nutrition on sexual performance. It is known, however, that protein, essential fatty acids, vitamin E, and several of the B vitamins are essential before the sex hormones can be produced.[1-3] A lack of protein causes a loss of sex interest and a decrease in sperm count.[4] Unless vitamin E is adequate, the testicles of all varieties of laboratory and farm animals degenerate;[5] and there is a decrease in both the sex hormones and the pituitary hormone gonadotropin, which stimulate the sex glands.[6] Vitamin E also protects the sex hormones from destruction by oxygen.[7,8]

People in famine areas and in concentration camps have invariably reported loss of sex interest; and during World War II men in prison camps found discussions of recipes more fascinating than of sex.[9] Malnourished individuals of reproductive age may have an almost total absence of sex hormones and of the pituitary hormone that stimulates the sex glands,[2,10-12] though recovery occurs when the diet is made adequate.[10,11] Men deficient in vitamin B_6 have become impotent;[13] and during stress, the sex urge and sperm production diminish.[14] The motility and fertility of sperm are in proportion to the amount of vitamin E in a man's semen.[15]

Autopsy studies of poorly nourished people of sexually active age have shown shriveled ovaries and testicles, a decrease in the cells that produce sperm or ova, vast areas of dead tissue, and much scarring; and the ovaries and testicles alike have been loaded with brown pigment characteristic of a vitamin-E deficiency.[2,11] The changes were similar to those seen in advanced senility and in animals deficient in any one of several nutrients, particularly vitamin E.[1,2,11]

Too few calories. During World War II, scientists at the University of Minnesota undertook semistarvation experiments to learn how to rehabilitate persons released from prison camps.[10] When conscientious objectors were kept on diets supplying only 1,600 calories daily, they noticed a marked decrease in sexual desire,[16] became melancholy, morbid, anxious, depressed, subject to hysteria, and were said to be "indistinguishable from many severely neurotic patients."[7] They suffered fatigue, weakness, decreased ability to work, and cold hands and feet, found it impossible to concentrate, and became social introverts.[16,18] When their diet was restricted in both calories and B vitamins, all symptoms became markedly intensified. The investigators concluded that "a superior dietary throughout life may spell the difference between alert, successful living and marginal effectiveness."[17]

Literally thousands of persons, especially women, eat less than 1,600 calories daily, presumably to be sufficiently attractive to be more loved. Yet fatigue, depression, hysteria, and lack of sex interest scarcely make them rollicking bed partners. Men who eat little because alcohol fills their calorie needs usually suffer from general malnutrition associated with a loss of sex interest and inability to maintain erections, both of which are corrected when an adequate diet is adhered to.[19-21]

If the B vitamins are undersupplied. In dozens of experiments men and women volunteers have remained on diets lacking one or another of the B vitamins, and the symptoms produced would invariably make a fulfilling sex life impossible. Individuals undersupplied with vitamin B_1 quickly became fatigued, depressed, forgetful, irritable, quarrelsome, apathetic, confused, restless, anxious, and unco-operative; they neglected their work and appearance, became intolerant of details and noise, and suffered from insomnia, nervousness, paranoid tendencies, and hypochondriasis, all of which were relieved soon after the vitamin was given.[22-26] When volunteers in a mental hospital stayed on a diet deficient in this vitamin, their emotional problems, even though psychological in origin, became greatly intensified.[27]

A lack of the B vitamin niacin amide results in such confusion, disorientation, clouding of consciousness, and hallucinations that it can cause total mental breakdown.[28] One doctor tells of a niacin-deficient woman who thought her neighbors were planning to kill her and who could see and feel vicious animals attacking her; yet 48 hours after the vitamin was given, she was completely rational.[29] Mild deficiencies, associated with irritability, suspicions, imaginary unfairness, and mental depression, usually described as "the blues," are common and can prevent family life from being happy.

Induced pantothenic-acid deficiencies have caused persons to become irritable, depressed, quarrelsome, hot-tempered, easily upset over trivialities, and to want to be left alone;[30-32] they were obviously uninterested in sex. Similarly, volunteers lacking vitamin B_6 not only become highly nervous, tense, irritable, depressed, and mentally confused, but develop halitosis and hemorrhoids and pass quantities of malodorous gas,[33,34] all of which would decrease both sex appeal and sex interest. Fatigue, confusion, irritability, and mental depression have also occurred when deficiencies of folic acid[35] or biotin[36] have been produced. The lack of B vitamins is so commonplace as to affect almost every American family not interested in nutrition. It can wreck a once-good marriage and leave parents not only unable to be loving, kind, and patient toward each other but also quick with harsh words, which cause permanent emotional scarring of their children. In contrast, energetic good health allows richness, joy, harmony, and sexual fulfillment.

Other deficiencies. An undersupply of several other nutrients can also affect sexual expression. Persons mildly deficient in magnesium become highly nervous, irritable, quarrelsome, and may change from friendly, outgoing, co-operative individuals to surly, belligerent, apathetic ones.[37] Yet magnesium deficiencies are widespread indeed.[38] Even the horrible mental torture of delirium tremens, which sometimes occurs in non-drinkers following acute infections, injuries, or surgery, has been corrected merely by giving water, salt, and a small amount of magnesium.[28]

A protein deficiency or an imbalance of amino acids can cause mental depression, apathy, peevishness, and a desire to be left undisturbed;[39,40] and a lack of calcium results in nervous tension and irritability. Such faulty nutrition is largely responsible for the present widespread use of tranquilizers, though a person who is drugged is scarcely a wholehearted sex partner.

Regardless of the cause, the exhausted or depressed individual finds it extremely difficult to eat highly nutritious foods, and his poor food habits result in ever greater emotional upsets and still less satisfactory sex life.[41] A vicious circle is set up which not infrequently leads to a "nervous breakdown."

A woman remarked some time after I had planned a diet for her son, "You saved my husband and me from a divorce." They had both been so tired, irritable, and disinterested in sex, she told me, that they had not had intercourse for two years until they had eaten foods suggested for the child. She felt that the increased milk intake and the addition of wheat germ and yeast had been largely responsible for their recapturing a gratifying sex life.

Fatigue can be prevented. There are many reasons for fatigue, yet any one can interfere with satisfactory sexual expression. Anemia (ch. 23), liver damage (ch. 16), a lack of B vitamins,[30,33,42] nervous tension brought on by deficiencies of calcium or magnesium,[19] the strain of holding in negative emotions (p. 111), and adrenal depletion[43] are all common causes. Millions of people endure daily fatigue due to low blood sugar, which often results from nothing more serious than having missed breakfast.[44]

A few months ago a pale and lethargic young woman

told me she hated preparing breakfasts, and therefore ate none. I suggested that she drink an eggnog, pointing out that if she missed the meal she would be so tired when her husband wanted to make love to her . . . "Oh, shut up," she interrupted, laughing. "You sound too familiar." When I saw her again, her relaxed look of contentment indicated sexual fulfillment long before she remarked, "It really works."

The symptoms of low blood sugar run the gamut of lassitude, fatigue, apathy, tension, nervousness, aimlessness, weakness, trembling, sweating, headaches, and a loathing of daily monotony; if little has been eaten the night before, these symptoms are usually present on waking and often remain throughout the day.[45] Taking potassium chloride (p. 75), which brings almost immediate relief,[47-49] is preferable to pep pills, but it is not needed if small meals low in carbohydrate are eaten frequently and the diet meets the needs of stress. Foods rich in the B vitamins and protein, such as yeast, liver, and wheat germ, often give a marked pickup within a single day. A persistent low blood sugar, however, is typical of adrenal exhaustion,[46] and calls for an increase in salt instead of potassium.

Numerous laboratory tests and physical examinations of 929 people too emotionally ill to work revealed nothing abnormal except slightly low blood sugar; yet they were depressed, apathetic, exhausted, loathed the routine of daily tasks, and had lost their zest for living.[45] Although this study did not include data concerning the sex life of these patients, when they were given an adequate, high-protein diet with mid-meals of milk and toast, and sweets, alcohol, and soft drinks were avoided, improvement was "prompt, striking, and lasting"; and psychotherapy was shortened for those undergoing analysis.

Fortunately, a high energy level can usually be maintained throughout the day by curtailing the evening meal slightly and eating an adequate diet containing some protein and oil at breakfast, lunch, and each mid-meal; thus the absorption of sugar is slowed up, the overstimulation of insulin prevented,[44,50,51] and greater well-being is produced,[52] all making for a more active sex life.

Insomnia. Another common cause of fatigue that interferes with sexual expression is the inability to sleep well. Severe insomnia has been induced in volunteers made deficient in vitamin B_6[33] and insomnia together with sleepiness throughout the day occurred in subjects deficient in pantothenic acid.[31] The intense nervousness resulting from a lack of magnesium is associated with inability to sleep, whereas the addition of magnesium to the diet induces restfulness.[19]

An inadequate calcium intake or poor calcium absorption (ch. 13) can also cause wakefulness. A person suffering from insomnia should probably have 2 grams of calcium daily, an amount that can be supplied by a quart of milk fortified with ½ cup of non-instant powdered milk. A warm milk drink taken with 10, 100, 250, and 500 milligrams respectively of vitamin B_6, pantothenic acid, magnesium oxide, and calcium lactate a half hour before retiring frequently eradicates the problem. The calcium and magnesium also help to prevent or relieve leg cramps and muscular spasms of the toes or feet which frequently wake individuals.[52]

Headaches. Certainly a person with a headache is in no mood for sex. Yet persistent headaches have been quickly produced in volunteers deficient in either vitamin B_6 or pantothenic acid; usually relief came soon after the missing vitamin was given, but in one case they persisted for six weeks after the experiment terminated.[30,33] Iron deficiency with or without anemia causes headaches, which clear up when iron is adequate.[42] The headaches preceding or accompanying menstruation are usually relieved by calcium and vitamin D. Both vitamins B_1 and B_{12} have also helped headaches, including migraines.[53]

Low blood sugar is another frequent cause. For example, 35 migraine sufferers, each studied by electroencephalograms for five hours during severe headaches, all had low blood sugar; and the lower the blood sugar dropped, the more severe the headaches became.[54] Their headaches were present on awakening, when the blood sugar is particularly low, and invariably occurred after little had been eaten the night before. A high-protein diet devoid of sweets and a snack taken before retiring brought permanent relief. Such a finding indicates that taking potassium chloride tablets (p. 276) may be far more helpful than aspirin.

Headaches associated with both low blood sugar and low blood pressure are particularly common after prolonged stress. In this case the adrenals are so exhausted that salt (sodium) is lost from the body (p. 29). Taking ½ teaspoon each of salt and soda in a little water to replace the urinary loss can often bring quick relief, but frequent meals and the antistress program (p. 31) should be carefully followed to prevent further difficulty. Headaches of psychosomatic origin appear to be of this variety.

The unrelenting stress of suppressed, unconscious anger is a frequent cause of headaches. Totally without realizing it, the sufferer turns upon himself a primitive, unconscious desire to bash in someone's head, thus hurting his own head instead. If anger can be expressed harmlessly, such headaches usually disappear (p. 91). A friend who had suffered from migraines for years was told by her physician to take up tennis as a means of blowing off steam; she not only got rid of her headaches but also became a champion.

Low basal metabolism. A hormone thyroxin, produced by the thyroid glands in the neck, controls the speed at which body activities occur. A person who synthesizes too little of this hormone suffers from lack of sex interest, fatigue, lethargy, cold, especially cold hands and feet, and usually has slow pulse, low blood pressure, and gains weight on few calories. Iodine and other nutrients are needed before sufficient amounts of thyroxin can be produced.

Severe iodine deficiencies resulting in goiter have decreased tremendously since iodized salt became available[55,56] but studies of iodine absorption in connection with fallout damage have shown that the iodine intake is still far too low.[57] Mild deficiencies are associated with toxic goiter, a high incidence of thyroid cancer,[58,59] an elevated blood cholesterol, and death from heart disease.[60,61] When only 8.5 milligrams of potassium iodide have been given daily to children for only a few days, iodine was so "avidly absorbed" by the thyroid that its effect lasted six months.[62]

In every variety of experimental animal, an iodine deficiency causes severe hemorrhaging in the thyroid gland, and though quickly stopped when iodine is given, masses of scar tissue form because of damage done.[63] Scar tissue cannot produce the needed hormone nor does it disappear when iodine alone is taken. Substances in peanuts, untoasted soy flour, and vegetables of the cabbage family can combine with iodine and prevent its absorption.[58,64-66] All of these foods increase the iodine requirement.

If vitamin E is deficient, the absorption of iodine by the thyroid decreases to 5 per cent of normal.[8] Because the glands, attempting to compensate for the deficiency, may become overactive, or toxic, anyone with hyperthyroidism should take generous amounts of vitamin E over a prolonged period. Giving adults 500 milligrams of vitamin E daily has caused their thyroid glands to absorb twice as much iodine and the protein-bound iodine in their blood has increased to normal.[8] Individuals with toxic thyroids have also been helped by taking 4 to 6 milligrams of iodine daily.[67,68]

A high-protein diet speeds the activity of sluggish thyroid glands by supplying the amino acid tyrosine, from which the thyroid hormone is made.[69] Tyrosine, however, cannot be used without vitamins B_6 and C,[4] nor can the hormone be made without cholin.[70] Thyroxin itself is inactivated by oxygen if vitamin C is undersupplied or destroyed.[4,71]

All persons should use iodized salt consistently; and research indicates that everyone would benefit by additional iodine as well,[57] especially persons who are ill, inclined to be overweight, or have a high blood cholesterol (ch. 5). An individual with an underactive thyroid should obtain daily perhaps 300 units of vitamin E, 4 milligrams of iodine (a teaspoon of kelp), a high-protein diet, and liberal amounts of vitamin C and B vitamins. If goiter exists, all of these nutrients should be increased immediately and continued until enlargement has subsided. Six milligrams of iodine daily, given for thyroid abnormalities, have produced excellent results,[67] but large amounts are said to be "without merit"[67,72] and can be highly toxic.[73-75] Organic iodine, such as supplied by kelp, is better retained[76] and less readily lost in the urine[77] than potassium iodide.

At times such severe damage has occurred that thyroid medication must be used, but it should not be taken except under a physician's close supervision; even slight excess augments the need for all nutrients and the excretion of most vitamins and minerals.[78] When given to animals, thyroid increases the number and early onset of spontaneous cancers;[59,78] every effort therefore should still be made to restore the health of the thyroid glands.

Sex during the later years. Because sex is a form of expressing love, it can continue as long as life itself, provided physical and emotional health permit. The late Dr. Flanders Dunbar, a noted authority on sex, collected data from 20 per cent of all individuals 100 years old and older in the United States.[79] When asked at what age each had lost interest in sex, these delightfully honest oldsters answered to a person, "Never." Many of the men still retained their potency, and several had remarried after passing the century mark.

Men among the healthiest groups ever to have been studied, the Bulgarians of several decades ago and the Hunzas of today, are reported to have sired children after reaching the ages of 90 and 100 years, indicating that health makes for a prolonged and active sex life.[80] It may be highly significant that the changes in the ovaries and testicles characteristic of senility are the same as those produced in experimental animals by diets deficient in various nutrients, especially vitamin E.[1,2,11]

Although most couples substitute quality for quantity as they grow older, the idea that intercourse should cease after the reproductive period is a heritage from our Puritanical forefathers, who believed sex to be wrong. To feel that intercourse should be discontinued as one grows older is synonymous with believing that one should stop expressing love.

Sexual problems have many causes. The angers, fears, and unfulfilled emotional needs of early childhood have such a marked effect on sexual expression that, when possible, persons with persistent sexual problems should seek psychiatric help. Even a slight understanding of self often brings vast improvement in intimate relationships. For example, if anger must be held back, love also is held back; but if love is expressed, the anger so devastating to marriages must likewise find an outlet. If married couples could look at anger, which is invariably charged with accumulated angers from the past, as vomitus that should be gotten rid of and an indication that love exists, many emotional upheavals could be avoided.

Within every human being is vast warmth, tenderness, love, and a desire to give fully in meeting the emotional needs of the mate. Whether these fine qualities remain uppermost or negative emotions play havoc with sexual expression depends on attitudes, understanding, and the health of both partners.

29
Eye Problems and Diseases

Foods have such a profound effect upon the health of the eyes that in countries where diets have been particularly inadequate—India, Egypt, China—every manner of eye disease, including blindness, has been rampant.

Vitamin A and vision. Visual problems associated with a mild lack of vitamin A include quick tiring of the eyes, sensitivity to bright lights and glare, dimness of vision at night (a common cause of car accidents), less acute day vision, and susceptibility to such infections as sties, conjunctivitis, iritis, and corneal ulcers.[1] Persons taking fewer than 5,000 units of vitamin A daily have an abnormal thickening of the conjunctiva and sometimes degeneration of the optic nerve.[1,2] In America, severe vitamin-A deficiencies are common among persons whose bile flow is inadequate (ch. 17).

An eye abnormality known as Bitot's spots appears to be caused by a combined lack of vitamin A and protein; when 50,000 units of the vitamin have been given daily with milk protein, improvement has been "surprisingly quick."[3]

Retinitis pigmentosa, characterized by a slow but eventually total degeneration of the retina, causes blindness in thousands of Americans annually, and is preceded by years of night blindness and other signs of vitamin-A deficiency.[4] The vitamin A in the blood of persons with this disease is far below normal;[5] they appear not to absorb the vitamin well. When vitamin A has been given by injection "the improvement was prompt and startling."[6] In such cases, water-dispersed vitamin A, oil, bile tablets, lecithin, and generous amounts of vitamin E should be obtained daily.

A lack of vitamin B_2. The eye symptoms occurring when vitamin B_2 is undersupplied vary as the deficiency changes from mild to severe. Sensitivity to bright light, faulty vision in dim illumination, and eyes that water readily are noticeable first. When strained, the eyes may become bloodshot and/or painful on exposure to glare. Bits of mucus often accumulate at the base of the lashes, especially while asleep.[1] If the deficiency becomes acute, the skin at the outer corners of the eyes may split and the eyes burn and become fiery red.

When as few as 5 milligrams of vitamin B_2 have been given daily, a wide variety of eye symptoms have been alleviated: watering, burning, and itching eyes and sandy eyelids; intolerance to light; abnormally dilated pupils; blurred and dim vision; inability to see under poor illumination, or twilight blindness; increased winking of eyelids (also characteristic of vitamin B_6 and/or magnesium deficiencies); inability to focus sharply; and eyestrain, particularly after doing close work.[1,6–10]

Less common symptoms have also been corrected by vitamin B_2: disturbances in recognizing colors, objects, and people; inability to see more than part of an image or a portion of a printed page; conjunctivitis, iritis, and rubiosis iritis, meaning red iris; the seeing of flickering and disappearing images and/or halos around bright lights or objects; and dark spots in front of eyes, or corneal opacities, said to be caused by dead cells, accumulations of white blood cells, and/or bits of scar tissue.

Corneal ulcers have been cleared up when vitamin B_2 has been given, but if allowed to go untreated, can result in scar tissue that causes permanent damage.[1] Such ulcers, bloodshot eyes, dark spots before the eyes, and other symptoms, however, have also developed in persons lacking vitamins B_6, C, and pantothenic acid.[12,13] In animals, corneal ulcers occur when the diet is deficient in protein or any one of the essential amino acids.[14,15] Since such diverse deficiencies can cause visual difficulties, the diet for a person with eye problems should be particularly adequate in all respects.

Cataracts. Experimental cataracts have been produced in every type of animal studied, including fish and geese, by diets low in vitamin B_2; and these cataracts disappear when the vitamin is added to the diet.[1] Cataracts in horses, a common cause of equine blindness, have been corrected by giving vitamin B_2. Excessive amounts of milk sugar or galactose from the digestion of milk sugar, which increases the need for vitamin B_2, also cause cataracts in animals.[16–18] Infants who cannot utilize galactose normally become blind from cataracts unless milk sugar is quickly withdrawn from their diets.[19]

Animals deficient in pantothenic acid develop cataracts which disappear when the vitamin is given.[12] The fact that experimental cataracts can also be produced by an undersupply of any one of the essential amino acids[14] may indicate that cataracts, especially those common among diabetics, can be brought on because the amino acid tryptophane cannot be utilized normally (p. 94) without vitamin B_6.[20] Clouding of the cornea, cataracts, and abnormalities of the retina also occur when diets lack vitamin E; and vitamin E has even corrected experimental cataracts caused from a lack of vitamin B_2 or amino acids.[1]

Cataracts have been produced in animals by giving a variety of drugs or chemicals;[21] and the use of dinitrophinol as a weight-reducing agent has resulted in many cases of human cataract, which cleared up if massive doses of vitamin C were given to detoxify the drug.[22] The formation of human cataracts is hastened when the circulation to the eyes is decreased by the deposition of cholesterol and/or of calcium.[23]

This disease is often brought on by stress; and the fact that cortisone cannot be produced without vitamin B_2 and pantothenic acid may explain why cataracts have occurred when either of these vitamins are lacking.[1,12] Although each year some 200,000 Americans have eye surgery because of cataracts, individuals with this abnormality have invariably been found to be under severe stress and their diets far from adequate. If the stress is removed and they can be helped to relax and are given an adequate antistress diet, the cataracts often disappear.[24]

My files contain dozens of unsolicited letters from persons who have recovered from cataracts after their diets were made adequate, often while they were preparing for surgery. One woman of 86 had cataracts on both eyes, yet her daughter reported that after following a good diet for a few months, her mother was again spending most of her time reading her favorite literature—detective stories. People sometimes take only a vitamin-B_2 supplement and then wonder why their eyes fail to improve. An antistress diet high in protein, vitamins B_2, C, E, pantothenic acid, and all nutrients is essential before good results can be expected. If a cataract has developed, a most adequate diet must be followed to prevent cataracts from forming in the other eye as well.

Nearsightedness. That nutrition plays a role in the prevention of nearsightedness—another manifestation of stress—was forcefully brought out during the depression years, when the incidence in schoolchildren jumped from 25 per cent in 1925 to 72 per cent in 1935.[4] This abnormality is associated with an undersupply or faulty absorption of calcium (ch. 25), which allows tension and sometimes spasms of the tiny muscles holding the lenses.[4] Nearsightedness and crossed eyes have both been corrected by large amounts of vitamin E.[25,26] Children under such stresses as rapid growth, inadequate diet, and allergies are particularly susceptible to nearsightedness.[4] When the adrenals are exhausted, fluids pass from the blood into the tissues;[27] and because the eyes of the young are still slightly elastic, the increased pressure forces the eyeball to elongate slightly and causes images to fall in front of the retina rather than on it. Although eyestrain is often thought to be a primary cause, a large percentage of the children in Egypt and India who do not read or write suffer from nearsightedness.[28]

Symptoms such as eyestrain, squinting, dizziness, fatigue, headaches, pain in the eyes, and perhaps low blood pressure generally accompany the onset of nearsightedness. At this stage, if salty foods are eaten for a week or two and the diet is immediately made adequate in all nutrients, particularly in vitamins B_2, C, D, E, pantothenic acid, calcium, protein, and essential fatty acids, the condition is said to be correctable.[4] Without dietary improvement, permanent correction is possible only with glasses.

Glaucoma. This disease, a major cause of blindness in the United States, results from prolonged stress and is a typical reaction of adrenal exhaustion.[27] When the adrenals cannot produce aldosterone, so much salt is lost from the body that fluids pass into the tissues at a focal point of stress. Because the eyeball is no longer elastic, the intraocular pressure increases. This fluid not only pushes the optic nerve back toward the brain, often damaging it, but also forces the lens forward, distorting vision and perhaps closing off the tiny drainage canal in the lower part of the eye.[28] Scar tissue and adhesions can also prevent this canal from draining.

The symptoms of glaucoma vary from person to person and can come on quickly without warning: pain in the eyes; cloudy vision; failing vision noticeable while doing close work; a need for greater illumination; narrowing of the visual field, as if looking down a hollow tube; seeing halos around lights and bright objects; and the fatigue and low blood pressure typical of adrenal exhaustion.[28] Sudden severe stress can bring on temporary or even permanent blindness. Yet most of these symptoms have been corrected by vitamin B_2,[6-10] essential before cortisone can be produced.

In recent years, glaucoma has fortunately cleared up in every individual with whom I have worked soon after salty foods were eaten, an adequate diet adhered to, and the antistress formula (p. 31) taken six times daily. It cannot be overemphasized, however, that every nutrient be adequate. One elderly man had severe glaucoma in both eyes, and although he adhered carefully to an antistress diet, his intraocular pressure did not decrease. Because of a heart condition, his physician had asked him to forgo salt. After his heart had improved and he was allowed to use salt, his glaucoma quickly disappeared. His eyes have now remained normal for well over a year.

The symptoms of glaucoma can return swiftly if an adequate diet is not continued. The intraocular pressure of one middle-aged woman dropped to normal for the first time in ten years after she adhered to an antistress program. Her doctor, however, permitted her only a pint of fluid daily. Though she cheated by eating copious amounts of watermelon, she had already lost her sight in one eye, and understandably became afraid to take an adequate diet supplying more than a quart of liquid; hence her symptoms soon returned. Happily, they disappeared again when she adhered to the diet more carefully.

A person with glaucoma must be constantly alert to recognize stress and to adjust his diet accordingly. Even a single cup of coffee can increase intraocular tension; many cups can bring on a violent glaucoma attack.[28] Any added stress can have a similar effect unless the nutrients that meet the demands of stress are immediately increased. The unrelenting stress of suppressed negative emotions (p. 111) causes much glaucoma to be a psychosomatic illness.

When surgery is undertaken to drain excess intraocular fluid, the additional stress and increased danger of hemorrhage, infection, and scar-tissue formation make a highly adequate diet imperative. For persons who have already had eye surgery, emphasis must be placed on the removal of scars before improvement can be expected (ch. 4). Even after glaucoma has already caused blindness, unless the diet is adequate, hemorrhages and corneal ulcers can occur, and pain may become so intense and persistent that the sightless eyes must still be removed.[28]

Detached retina. The cause of detached retina is not known. When vitamin E is deficient or when iron salts, which destroy this vitamin,[29,30] are given to pregnant women, however, infants are often born prematurely[30,31] and their retinas frequently become detached if they are exposed to an oxygen concentration greater than ordinary air.[32-35] A few years ago, putting such babies in oxygen tents caused thousands to become permanently blind. This abnormality could be prevented by giving 150 milligrams of vitamin E daily starting immediately after birth[31] or by breast milk, which supplies this vitamin.[36,37] If vitamin E is inadequate, the essential fatty acids in the cells forming the walls of the capillaries in the retina—only one cell thick—are so harmed by oxygen that these cells disintegrate (p. 229).

Studies of newborn kittens exposed to air with a high oxygen content show that the tiny blood vessels in the retina break down first and scars form afterward; as the scar tissue contracts, it pulls the retina away from the underlying part of the eye, forcing it to become detached.[33] Since vitamin-E deficiencies are not uncommon,[38,39] this same process may cause detached retina in humans.

Other eye abnormalities. A number of additional eye abnormalities can be influenced by nutrition. Blurred vision, produced in volunteers deficient in vitamins B_6 and pantothenic acid, was quickly corrected when the vitamins were given.[40] Paralysis of muscles both inside and behind the eyes has been corrected by B vitamins, particularly vitamin B_1;[41] and weaknesses in these muscles, crossed eyes, blurred vision, and double vision have been alleviated by taking vitamin E[25] or liver and yeast.[42] Vitamin C has been used successfully in stopping hemorrhages of the eyes;[43] and retinal hemorrhages have cleared up after yeast and vitamins B_2, C, E, and niacin amide were given.[44] Retinitis occurs when the diet is low in protein[45] and has been corrected by a high-protein diet.[46]

Infections of the eyes call for the same dietary improvements as any other infection (ch. 11). I have worked with a few persons who had such severe eye infections that their physicians had recommended removal of their eyes to prevent the brain from becoming involved. In each case recovery occurred a few days after large amounts of vitamin C were taken around the clock with an adequate high-protein diet.

Protruding eyes are characteristic of people and animals alike deficient in vitamin E.[1,47,48] They are a commonly recognized symptom of toxic thyroid, which may in part be caused by a vitamin-E deficiency (p. 278).

When eye surgery is unavoidable, the preparation should be the same as that for any major operation (ch. 27). All nutrients that speed healing, give protection from stress, and prevent hemorrhages and scarring should be particularly emphasized.

Emotional factors. There are times when persons can no longer bear to look at situations life has forced upon them. Totally without their awareness, the unconscious mind often arranges to "solve" such a problem by the same method a child uses when he closes his eyes to prevent seeing something intolerable. In such cases, any abnormality that can cause blindness may "purposely" be produced. Dr. Arnold Hutschnecker tells, for example, of the wife of a mining engineer who hated the wilds into which her husband took her; she repeatedly developed cataracts on both eyes, which disappeared each time she returned to her beloved New York.[49]

A woman once phoned me to say she had followed a good diet but her cataracts had not improved. After some discussion of nutrition, I explained to her how emotional problems could be a causative factor. She quickly repeated, each time becoming increasingly emphatic, "I know you're *right!* I *know* you're right!" There was a pause, a loud sigh of relief, then a voice filled with determination: "Well, I can conquer that situation! Now I won't have to go blind." With that she hung up.

I never learned her name, but I have often wondered what happened to her cataracts.

30
When the Cause Is Unknown

The sole purpose of nutrition is to build and maintain health. It is not concerned with the treatment of disease. Unfortunately, most people become interested in building health—hence in nutrition—only after they are ill.

My medical dictionary uses 19 columns to describe different diseases and another 13 columns for syndromes, or combinations of symptoms characteristic of other diseases. In literally hundreds of these conditions, the cause is still unknown; yet in every case the same nutrients are required to repair the body.

The cause need not be known. If all nutrients are supplied in generous amounts and no defects have been inherited or irreparable damage already done, the body will in time repair itself without the cause of an abnormality being known.

Mr. Thomas McIlvain, a real-estate broker in Cincinnati, Ohio, is a case in point. Many diagnoses had been made during his severe illness, which cost him $16,000 for medical and hospital bills and $4,000 for drugs. His case had been studied by 24 physicians, including four at the Mayo Clinic and six at Massachusetts General Hospital; and, according to Mrs. McIlvain, dozens more came to look, read charts, and hazard a "guess." She stated that "the only thing the doctors agreed upon was that Tom was dying." After following a complete nutrition program, however, he progressed steadily from bed to wheelchair to crutches to office and during the three years since his illness, he has been working full time, "his health in many ways better than it has ever been." Yet the cause of his illness is still undetermined.

The only advantage of knowing that a lack of certain nutrients may cause an abnormality is that taking these specific nutrients in larger-than-normal amounts often speeds recovery. Any nutrient relieves the symptoms its lack causes. For example, a sore tongue which occurs when the B vitamin niacin amide is undersupplied is said to heal in three or four hours if an enzyme containing this vitamin is given.[1] When large amounts of the vitamin itself are taken, approximately 24 hours are required for healing. If liver is given as the source of the vitamin, three days are needed. Taking yeast, which contains somewhat less niacin, heals the tongue in five or six days, though liver and yeast supply many other nutrients simultaneously.

If the diet were completely adequate, the painful tongue would heal without our slightest knowledge of niacin amide. When all building materials are supplied to the cells and damage is not irreparable, nature will do the healing, and she cares not one whit if we understand how she does it.

What does "incurable" mean? Dozens of diseases formerly considered to be incurable are now readily corrected. The word "incurable," therefore, cannot invariably be defined as incapable of remedy. The method of correction may at present merely be unknown. Because sound nutrition has rarely been tried, its role in rebuilding health in cases of "incurable" illnesses is still a mystery.

I have planned diets for two children with "incurable" Schüller-Christian disease about which I know nothing. Each child's physician referred to his recovery as "one of the few spontaneous cures ever recorded." Similarly, several children with "incurable" heart malformations, kept on excellent diets containing 100 units of vitamin E daily since babyhood, are now 8 to 14 years old and are, with their doctors' permission, active in athletics; none require heart surgery, which had earlier been considered necessary. A few doctors have been correcting congenital heart conditions for years with vitamin E.[2] In my files are dozens of letters referring to the results of good nutrition applied by people with "incurable" illnesses that contain the phrase, "The doctor says it's a miracle." The miracle lies only in the body's fantastic ability to repair itself. Since damage may be irreparable or factors other than nutritional may have caused an illness, good results from an improved diet cannot always be expected.

Until further research can throw light on little-understood diseases, the chance that health may be rebuilt makes adequate nutrition imperative. I have found it particularly exciting to plan nutrition programs for persons suffering from "incurable" diseases. One could expect nothing. The results are frequently most rewarding.

General rules to follow. When the causes of an illness are unknown, the first step is to plan a diet so completely adequate that no nutrient is overlooked. Since all disease is stress, generous amounts of the antistress factors should be included, together with extra nutrients to prevent scarring and to detoxify medications. When the illness in question is similar to a well-known disease, nutrients that help the latter may well be emphasized.

For example, partial or complete deafness, which affects millions of people in the United States,[3] is usually accepted without the slightest attempt to improve the nutrition. Yet deafness caused by neuritis or inflammation of the nerves of the ear has been corrected by giving the B vitamins;[4] and partial deafness has disappeared after yeast and liver were taken.[5] The calcification that causes otosclerosis is not unlike arthritis or that which can be prevented by vitamin E.[6] Deafness caused by cholesterol deposits in the arteries of the ears is said to clear up when the blood cholesterol is kept consistently low. Persons who are hard of hearing have particularly low blood iodine, and a lack of iodine during pregnancy can cause deafness in the infant.[7] Numerous medications that increase body requirements often cause impaired hearing and ringing, roaring, and hissing sounds in the ears;[8] and other forms of severe stress have a similar effect.

Subjects deficient in vitamin B_6 and pantothenic acid developed dizziness and painful throbbing in the ears,[9] symptoms characteristic of labyrinthitis and an abnormality known as Ménière's syndrome. Many cases of Ménière's disease have cleared up after generous amounts of B vitamins were taken; and the vomiting that accompanies it usually ceases when vitamin B_6 is made adequate.[10,11] Like glaucoma, these conditions occur when the adrenals are exhausted, and so much salt is lost in the urine that excessive fluid passes into the tissues at some focal point which, in this case, is the ear. Salty foods[12] and the antistress formula (p. 31) usually allow these abnormalities to clear up rapidly. Of 186 cases of Ménière's disease, most were corrected when the nutrition was adequate and all refined carbohydrates avoided, though some were given small amounts of cortisone.[13]

If the diet were markedly improved as soon as one became aware of impaired hearing, much deafness could be avoided. Not infrequently, however, deafness is psychosomatic in origin. Men with nagging wives and wives with noisy husbands sometimes readily admit that deafness has its advantages. My own children can be remarkably deaf when I ask them to do something they do not wish to do.

Emphysema. This disease is rapidly increasing in our smog-laden cities, yet little is known about its cause. The connective tissue in the air sacs of the lungs becomes filled with millions of tiny air bubbles, like miniature balloons. These air bubbles take up most of the available space, making difficult breathing and a continuous fight for air persistent symptoms of the illness. In time much scar tissue is formed.

Because vitamin E tremendously decreases the need for oxygen,[14-17] generous amounts often bring relief; and the emphysema associated with cystic fibrosis improves after vitamin E is given.[18] Connective tissue, however, cannot be strong without adequate vitamins A and C, protein, and folic acid (p. 265); and a lack of these nutrients may weaken it sufficiently for air to penetrate it.

A friend was recently extremely ill with emphysema. Her voice was so weak she could scarcely speak, and though under an oxygen tent, she fought for every breath. She adhered to an adequate diet, however, and a month later showed no signs of illness, and has had no recurrence. Although I have sometimes been annoyed by physicians declaring that a diagnosis has been wrong when an "incurable" disease has cleared up, her progress was so startling that I caught myself thinking, "The diagnosis must have been wrong."

In most cases of emphysema, the nutrition remains so faulty that scar tissue becomes a major problem; hence rapid results cannot be obtained. If the diet is not improved, however, the illness can be expected to become steadily worse.

Lupus erythematosus. This skin disease, which primarily affects the connective tissue[19] and is characterized by anemia, stiffness of the joints, and numerous symptoms of adrenal exhaustion,[20] is customarily treated with aspirin and cortisone. The amount of vitamin E in the blood is unusually low, and scarring often becomes severe.[20]

Massive amounts of almost every vitamin have been given in an attempt to clear up this disease,[21] but I can find no report in the medical literature where an adequate diet supplying all nutrients has been tried. Patients receiving 1,000 to 2,000 milligrams of vitamin E and 10 to 15 grams of pantothenic acid (10,000 to 15,000 milligrams) daily have responded "most favorably" even though many had suffered from the disease for 10 to 30 years.[20] Their illness recurred, however, when the vitamins were discontinued.[22,23] To me such an approach seems rather like trying to make a cake by adding more and more baking powder and sugar but omitting the other ingredients.

The worst case of lupus erythematosus I have seen was a young girl whose entire body was covered with sores, scales, and crusts which had the appearance of thick layers of grated cheese. This youngster, however, had such an amazing appetite for yeast, liver, yogurt, wheat germ, and other nutritious foods that one suspected she had an instinctive craving for them. Pantothenic acid was scarcely known at that time, hence she received none except in natural food, and she was given only 30 units of vitamin E daily; yet within a month healthy new skin covered her entire body. After first seeing this child, my housekeeper used to shake her head and remark, "I wouldn't have believed such a thing were possible." A month later she was repeating the same remark even more emphatically.

Similar results occurred after a college student developed such acute lupus that she was not expected to live. Physicians gave her cortisone, massive doses of aspirin, and, because of severe anemia, male sex hormones to stop her menstruation. The cortisone caused her to gain 40 pounds; her face became covered with long black hair as a result of the male hormones; and the aspirin so completely destroyed vitamin C that she had internal hemorrhages and bled from the gums, lips, and rectum. At this point her physician suggested that she obtain an adequate diet, which was essentially that outlined on pages 330–331, with most nutrients supplied in unusually large amounts. For instance, her antistress formula (p. 31), taken around the clock, included 900 milligrams of pantothenic acid every 24 hours; and she took 900 units of vitamin E daily. Improvement was so marked that within ten days the doctor reduced both cortisone and aspirin and soon discontinued them. This girl regained her health completely and has remained well during the three years since that time.

Scleroderma and similar abnormalities. Diseases such as scleroderma, myositis, dermomyositis, and bursitis have in common the calcification of the soft tissues. They have now been produced experimentally by Dr. Hans Selye and his co-workers (p. 115). In patients with scleroderma, for example, the calcium content of the skin, muscles, heart, lungs, kidneys, and pancreas becomes excessive. Calcium is laid down only in an injured area in the experimental counterpart, but damaged tissues are not calcified unless this mineral has first been withdrawn from the bones.[24] During stress, however, bones are robbed of calcium; and tissues are damaged by the rapid destruction of protein.[25] Scleroderma frequently accompanies Addison's disease, or extreme adrenal exhaustion, and so often develops after an acute infection, a serious accident, or grave emotional trauma that it has been classified as another stress disease.[24]

The tissues of a person with scleroderma may become calcified following such slight and diverse injuries as sunburns, vaccinations, bumping into furniture, pressure of garters or brassières, or exposure to heat, cold, or chemicals.[24] Even after tissues have been damaged, however, experimental scleroderma can be prevented by large amounts of vitamin E.[6,26] Furthermore, calcium in the soft tissues increases 500 per cent or more when vitamin E is inadequate.[27,28] A person with this disease should undoubtedly obtain generous amounts of vitamin E, though the quantity needed is unknown.

To build up the adrenals at all possible speed, the antistress program (p. 31) should be followed for months; and vitamin D and magnesium particularly must not be overlooked. Unless the calcium intake is consistently adequate—perhaps 2 grams daily—further calcium will be withdrawn from the bones; in my opinion, the worst error one could make is to obtain less than a quart of fortified milk daily. Individuals suffering from scleroderma with whom I have worked and who adhered to a diet similar to that on pages 330–331 have slowly regained their health.

Cystic fibrosis of the pancreas. Another of the "incurable" diseases, cystic fibrosis, which is becoming increasing-in more common,[29-32] appears to result from combined deficiencies of vitamins B_6, E, and pantothenic acid. At the onset, abnormal amounts of salt are retained,[33] typical of the alarm reaction to stress.[25] Cortisone or ACTH therapy, which simulates this stress reaction, frequently causes the pancreas to be damaged.[34]

When cystic fibrosis is first diagnosed, the pancreas produces digestive enzymes normally.[32,35] This organ, however, gradually becomes a mass of scar tissue; yet scars always follow injury and never precede it. Furthermore, scar tissue cannot synthesize enzymes. Digestion and absorption, therefore, gradually become so incomplete that deficiencies of all nutrients quickly occur.[32] Eventually most of the food eaten remains undigested, causing persistent diarrhea with bulky, foul-smelling, greasy stools;[33,36] and persons with this disease soon become susceptible to severe respiratory infections.[32]

Faulty digestion, diarrhea with foul-smelling stools, and extreme susceptibility to respiratory infections have been produced in volunteers lacking vitamins B_6 and pantothenic acid.[1,9,37] Furthermore, damage to the pancreas has been repeatedly produced in animals by diets only slightly deficient in vitamin B_6.[38-42] Such injury is made worse by saturated fats,[42] an excess of calcium or vitamin B_1,[43] a deficiency of magnesium[41,44] or a high-protein, high-calorie diet[41,42] such as is given for cystic fibrosis.[45] If the damage is not too severe, however, healing occurs soon after vitamin B_6[40,41,44,46] or the amino acid methionine[42] is given.

Cystic fibrosis is said to occur with kwashiorkor,[47,48] a disease of malnutrition common in South Africa and Central America. Children with this disease have made spectacular recoveries when given ground whole grains mixed with yeast,[62] but I can find no reports of patients with cystic fibrosis having been given vitamin B_6, pantothenic acid, or any good natural sources of the B vitamins. Antibiotics, which destroy intestinal bacteria, are usually administered continuously; hence the B vitamins normally supplied by these bacteria are not even available.

Autopsy studies of children who have died of cystic fibrosis show multiple signs of vitamin-E deficiencies,[49,50] yet an investigation revealed that not one child had ever received this vitamin.[51] Physicians at Johns Hopkins University School of Medicine, however, have given children with this disease 300 to 1,500 milligrams of vitamin E daily with no observable toxic effects.[50,52] Improvement was quickly noticed, though some youngsters had had the disease for ten years or longer. Both the damage to the pancreas and the resulting scars, however, must be corrected by a diet supplying all nutrients.

When digestive enzymes—powder or tablets—and granular lecithin are given with every meal, the digestion and absorption of an extremely ill person can be markedly improved;[53-58] and both should be immediately increased if digestion is still faulty. With these digestive aids, yeast, liver, wheat germ, perhaps a B-vitamin syrup and/or tablets, and yogurt or acidophilus milk or culture can be taken daily. All of these foods should be started the minute a diagnosis of cystic fibrosis is made.

To protect the adrenals and build resistance, the anti-stress formula (p. 31) could be given every three hours; and the quantity of vitamin C increased at the first sign of an infection. Certainly vitamin E should be generously supplied. Oils are usually well absorbed by persons with this disease,[59] hence they can be used for cooking. Water-soluble nutrients, such as magnesium, vitamin C, and the B vitamins, absorb without difficulty. Because vitamins A, D, and E are well absorbed through the skin, vitamin D can be rubbed directly on the body once daily and vitamins A and E several times daily if the disease is so advanced that little food can be digested. In one way or another, every nutrient can be furnished.

Since life may depend on the B vitamins supplied by intestinal bacteria, sugars which inhibit the growth of these bacteria (p. 145) should be avoided. And if my own child had cystic fibrosis, I would not allow antibiotics to be used until symptoms of an infection appeared. Giving antibiotics when no infection exists seems to me like taking an aspirin now for next month's headache. Building resistance to infections is far more constructive.

It is a heartbreaking experience to watch beautiful children die of this disease while receiving only woefully inadequate nutrition. Invariably young parents are afraid to improve a diet recommended by their physician, whereas I personally would be terrified not to improve the diets I have known to be given.

High hereditary requirements. Certain families and individuals have unusually high requirements for one nutrient or another. Often this requirement is 10 to 20 times greater than that considered to be "normal."[60] Such an extraordinary need apparently accounts for many illnesses thought of as hereditary and therefore "incurable." Examples are persons subject to epilepsy (p. 221), periodic paralysis (p. 236), and perhaps diabetes.

A diet adequate for most people is by no means adequate for such an individual. Until sufficient nutrients are obtained to meet the needs of a person with unusually high hereditary or "genetotrophic" requirements,[61] his illness cannot be considered incurable.

The cause may be psychological. Probably every individual has in early childhood experienced emotional traumas which, under adverse circumstances, can bring about any one of a number of illnesses, many of which have been considered "incurable." Although arthritis is a well-known example, there may be hundreds of others among the less-understood diseases. Usually such persons go from one doctor to another for years and spend thousands of dollars in medical bills without the cause of the problem being found.

When excellent medical attention and a highly adequate diet have not alleviated an illness, emotional causes should be suspected and psychiatric help sought.

After irreparable damage. Often irreparable damage has already been done, and the best of nutrition cannot bring improvement. Within the last few years, for example, some 30 new diseases, called "congenital errors of metabolism" have been identified in which children are born without certain essential enzymes. Even genes and chromosomes, however, require nutrients for their formation. The cause of these new diseases is undoubtedly the appallingly inadequate diets eaten by women during their pregnancies,[63] yet the tragedies have already occurred.

Though permanent repair cannot be achieved, faulty nutrition often adds to the misery of the afflicted and of those caring for him. Usually the symptoms of nutritional deficiencies are thought of as part of the particular illness and are not recognized as unnecessary burdens. A personal friend who worked in a school for children with cerebral palsy improved the school lunches and persuaded parents to give better diets and nutritional supplements to their youngsters. The staff soon noticed less irritability and crying, greater alertness, better bladder control, and fewer colds and general illnesses; and the muscles of some children improved so much after vitamin E was given them that they could hold pencils and write for the first time. In the same way, improved nutrition often makes life easier for both the patient and his family even though little else can be expected.

There comes a time. When I have been asked to plan diets for elderly persons suffering from fatal illnesses, my reply has been, "Adequate nutrition may prolong suffering and do more harm than good." And I have often wanted to add, "Permit them to die in love and peace and with the comfort medical science can give."

Provided we do not die prematurely, there will eventually come a time when each of us no longer cares to live. Because I am personally convinced that we are as dead now as we are ever going to be, and that so-called "death" is similar to a butterfly emerging from the chrysalis, I feel that attempting to apply nutrition during a terminal illness is inappropriate. When I get ready to die, I do not want anyone poking food or vitamin pills down me or making me into a plumbing fixture via stomach tubes or intravenous feedings. I suspect many people feel the same.

History repeats itself. Probably no one could read the history of medicine without being amazed at the number of "incurable" diseases existing in the past which are now readily corrected. Therein lies hope.

31
Nutrition and Cancer

Only a pittance of the millions spent on cancer research has been used for nutritional investigation. The effect of different diets, however, has been studied by giving them to strains of mice that develop spontaneous malignancies; and to animals into which growing cancer tissue has been transplanted or active cancer cells have been injected. Malignant tumors have also been induced in variously fed animals by x-rays or by such materials as thyroid, mineral oil, estrogen, stilbestrol, arsenic, coal-tar or azo dyes, and dozens of other substances.[1-3]

Effect of vitamin A. Massive amounts of vitamin A have stopped the growth of spontaneous cancers in mice,[4] and of transplanted cancers.[5] When 300,000 units of vitamin A and 1,000 milligrams of vitamin C were given daily for three to six months to 218 cases of inoperable cancer, the malignancies regressed in size or remained stationary,[6] but symptoms of vitamin-A toxicity appeared.

The B vitamins and protein. In some experiments, animals given azo dyes when deficient in vitamin B_2 quickly died of cancer, whereas adequate vitamin B_2 completely prevented cancer development. In other studies in which dye-fed rats deficient in vitamin B_2 developed cancer of the lymph glands or liver, giving the vitamin after the cancers were growing "remarkedly delayed" further development; again animals on an adequate diet remained cancer-free.[7,8]

Susceptibility to cancer increases tremendously when diets are deficient in protein or essential amino acids.[9,10] Thus dye-induced cancers have been more numerous and developed earlier when protein was deficient, but these growths were prevented by either additional vitamin B_2 or adequate protein.[11] Moreover, cancer-susceptible mice given diets rich in protein and vitamin B_2 no longer developed spontaneous malignancies.[12] Their requirement for these nutrients is merely higher than those of cancer-resistant animals, a finding that may prove equally true of cancer-susceptible humans.

Several other B vitamins exert a protective influence against many types of malignancies produced by various other means.[13-16] For example, cancers develop quickly when vitamin B_6 is deficient, but excessive amounts cause vitamin B_2 to be excreted, thus increasing cancer growth.[17] Similarly, excessive vitamin B_2, by inducing a deficiency of vitamin B_6, has caused tumors to grow more rapidly.[18] Partly for this reason, I believe that all B-vitamin supplements should contain the same amounts of vitamins B_2 and B_6.

A mild deficiency of cholin lowers the resistance of animals to spontaneous cancer of the liver, especially if protein is also undersupplied.[8,19] Such cancers can be prevented by doubling the amount of milk protein in the diet.[20] If animals with liver cancer are given cholin and a diet containing 20 per cent protein, they recover so completely that no malignancy is found on autopsy.[21] Cancers in rats given low-protein, low-cholin diets are said to show the identical pathological changes seen in human liver cancer.[21] A number of investigators believe that damaged liver and cirrhosis are forerunners of cancer of the liver in humans.[22,23]

A vitamin-like substance, betain, rich in beet tops and roots, can pinch hit for cholin. It also increases the survival time of rats with malignancies. When 22 persons with inoperable cancers ate large amounts of beets daily for several months, 21 showed improvement and their cancers decreased in size.[24] Concentrated beet juice was equally valuable, but when discontinued for financial reasons, cancer growth resumed in three to four months.[24] I know one man with leukemia who has had no recurrence of the disease for over two years; he accredits his seemingly excellent present health to the fact that he has been drinking beet juice and taking desiccated liver daily.

Autopsies reveal that 90 per cent of persons dying of kwashiorkor have cancer.[25] This disease, prevalent in Central America and South Africa, results from diets extremely low in protein and the B vitamins; and it clears up rapidly when milk, rich in both protein and vitamin B_2, is taken. I have yet to know of a single adult to develop cancer who has habitually drunk a quart of milk daily.

Relation of vitamin C. Little is known of the influence

of vitamin C on cancer development; the research has been done largely on animals which synthesize this vitamin. Cancers induced in rats by giving various drugs, chemicals, or dyes, however, have caused the urinary loss of vitamin C to increase 50 to 75 times above normal within six days;[26] and several species of animals with induced cancer have shown symptoms of severe vitamin-C deficiencies.[27,28]

There is growing evidence that many cancers are caused by viruses. Since vitamin C appears to nullify the damage done by viruses (ch. 11), this nutrient may prove to be particularly important. Any cancer is such severe stress that it tremendously increases the need for vitamin C; and most cancer patients, especially children with leukemia, show bruising, bleeding gums, and often outright hemorrhaging characteristic of a vitamin-C deficiency. When 4,000 to 6,000 milligrams (100 milligrams per kilogram of body weight) were given daily to patients with inoperable malignancies, cancer growth was inhibited and in some cases it regressed.[29]

Vitamin E and cancer. Research indicates that vitamin E may be especially valuable in cancer prevention. Malignancies induced in animals receiving varying amounts of vitamin E were fewest, smallest, and slowest in developing when the most vitamin was allowed.[30,31] Certain cancer cells grow rapidly in blood plasma, but their growth has stopped when vitamin E was added; and generous amounts of this vitamin have sometimes caused transplanted cancers to shrivel and die.[30,32] Giving vitamin E has decreased cancers induced in mice.[33] Cancers produced by giving estrogen, which increases the vitamin-E requirement,[34] were also fewer when this vitamin was most generous;[35] and the number of breast cancers in mice has been markedly reduced by vitamin E.[36] When iron salts that destroy vitamin E have been added to the diet of animals, induced cancers developed rapidly, whereas animals not given iron in this form remained cancer-free.[32] Cancers have also been produced by feeding mineral oil in which vitamin E dissolves and is excreted.[37]

Since oils increase the need for vitamin E,[38] cancer-producing substances injected into mice fed corn oil or lard caused twice as many cancers to develop in the oil-fed animals; adequate amounts of vitamin E "remarkedly protected" similarly treated mice.[39] When cod liver oil, peanut oil, coconut butter, or a hydrogenated fat similar to margarine was given to rats fed cancer-producing dyes, the largest number of cancers occurred in animals given the margarine; as long as vitamin E was adequate, no cancers developed even when excessive oils were fed.[40]

Cancers produced in animals by exposing them to x-rays or forms of radiation simulating fallout can be completely prevented by giving vitamin E;[41] and the number is reduced by generous amounts of vitamin C.[42] Unless vitamin E is adequate, x-rays cause toxic substances to be quickly formed from the oxidation of fats, but if sufficient vitamin C is available, the offending materials are detoxified.[41,42] Some 90 per cent of the people whose adolescent acne has been treated by x-rays develop skin cancers later, probably preventable if the intake of vitamins C and E had been increased during the treatments.

Other nutrients. Spontaneous cancers, mostly of the thyroid, have developed in hamsters kept on an iodine-deficient diet, whereas animals receiving adequate iodine remained cancer-free.[43] When rats have been given thyroid or radioactive iodine, the number of spontaneous cancers markedly increased.[44] Cancer of the thyroid is unusually high in countries where the iodine intake is low. In America it decreased after the introduction of iodized salt.[45]

Although over a billion dollars has now been spent on cancer research, the effect of various mineral deficiencies on cancer susceptibility appears to have been studied little. Increasing the copper intake "significantly retarded development" of cancers in animals, and decreased the liver damage and cirrhosis caused by cancer-inducing materials.[46]

In experimental cancers, animals have eventually lacked the ability to form antibodies, and infections rather than the malignancy appear to have been the actual cause of death.[112] The bacteria involved were not "outside invaders," but common putrefactive organisms of the intestinal tract. To me, this finding indicates that emphasis must be placed on maintaining intestinal health by the generous use of yogurt or acidophilus milk or culture to supply valuable bacteria and by avoiding refined foods which inhibit the growth of these valuable bacteria (p. 145); and on making every effort to build resistance to infections (ch. 11.)

Interferon, a substance that has been isolated from normal cells, appears to give protection from cancer-producing viruses and the nucleic acid made by such viruses. Although little is yet known about interferon, adequate nutrition possibly increases its presence in the cells.

Effect of overheated fat. Overheated fats and especially burned fats induce cancers in animals so readily that many investigators believe broiled and barbecued meats may be dangerous.[47-52] Repeated heating appears to be particularly harmful. When a cancer-producing substance was fed or painted on the skin of rats given fresh, unheated corn oil or corn oil that had been used commercially for frying potato chips, 50 per cent of the animals receiving used fat developed cancer; the rats on fresh oil remained cancer-free.[48]

Liver damage. Any form of liver damage causes increased susceptibility to experimental cancers.[23,53-55] Malignancies associated with such injury have been produced in animals on diets inadequate in vitamins B_1, B_2, E, cholin, protein, or the amino acid methionine; and by a wide variety of drugs, chemicals, and insecticides.[23,56] Generous amounts of methionine (p. 194) have "completely prevented" experimentally induced cancers and the accompanying liver damage, whereas small amounts of methionine or cholin were less effective.[57] Cancers have been produced in animals merely by injuring the liver.[19,58] In fact, it is largely by damaging the liver that azo dyes and many other substances readily induce cancers in animals.[56]

Investigators have pointed out that we are continuously exposed to a large number of substances many of which are known to injure the liver[23] and which, collectively at least, are potentially cancer-producing: smoke, smog, pesticides, chemicals of many varieties, drugs, nitrates, preservatives, and food additives (dyes, sweeteners, softeners, synthetic flavorings, etc.), and hundreds of others. Almost any one alone may be innocuous, but accumulatively and in combination they are probably far more deadly than is yet realized. Certain food additives and insecticides are known to be dangerous only when combined with others.[59,60]

There can be little doubt that the damage done collectively by substances which do not occur naturally in the body, together with our high intake of refined foods, is largely responsible for the rapid increase in the incidence of this appallingly tragic disease. The fact remains, however, that just as all heavy cigarette smokers do not get lung cancer, millions of persons exposed to carcinogens do not develop malignancies. If given the raw material to work with, the body can detoxify most harmful substances (p. 171). One scientist puts it this way: "Prevention of liver injury is identical with prevention of the cancer disease."[23]

Diet and growing cancers. All types of experimental cancers grow more rapidly when the diet is high in calories,[8,61-63] regardless of whether the excessive calories are supplied by fats[44,61] or carbohydrates.[10] Conversely, low-calorie diets devoid of refined carbohydrate and hydrogenated fat retard cancer growth;[35,64] and rats kept on stock diets of natural foods are protected against cancer.[64] High-calorie diets of refined foods also accelerate the growth of human malignancies.[65]

Although excess protein is converted into calories, experimental cancers develop most rapidly on low-protein diets.[10] Cancer growth has not increased even when protein supplied 50 per cent of the calories; and the animals maintained far better general health than when the intake was low.[9] Yeasts rich in nucleic acid—which food yeast is—"significantly increased" the survival of rats given cancer-producing substances.[19] All yeasts are rich in protein and the B vitamins.

Tumor growth is inhibited by vitamin A,[4-6] which is not found in cancer cells unless stored in the parent tissue.[66] Vitamins B_1, B_{12}, inositol, and biotin appear neither to stimulate nor to retard cancer growth. Cancer cells have a much lower content of vitamin B_2 and pantothenic acid than do normal tissues, and giving these vitamins protects the body without stimulating the growth of malignancies.[67,68] Diets deficient in vitamin B_6 have caused certain types of experimental cancers to grow more slowly, but normal cells were so harmed that life was not prolonged.[69] Vitamin B_6-deficient diets given to patients with leukemia or cancer of the lymph glands caused several to develop convulsions but did not retard the cancers.[70] PABA has inhibited certain malignancies in humans,[71,72] whereas folic acid has caused some types of cancer to regress[56] and the growth of others to be accelerated.[73-75]

Application of experimental findings. With a few exceptions, there has been little attempt to apply the findings of cancer research. I myself have rarely planned diets for persons with malignancies because of fear that improved nutrition might prolong suffering or accelerate growth. Now that more information is available, however, I feel that an adequate diet is well worth while to protect normal tissues alone. When the will to live is strong, seeming miracles sometimes occur.

Several months ago I made out an antistress diet for a 24-year-old man with cancer of the lymph glands. A letter from his mother states: "Alan has surprised the doctors. Just last week they said they had thought he would not be living today. They also said it was miraculous how he had taken the cobalt with such little illness. They have x-rayed his lungs several times expecting to find the cancer had spread, but each time they have been clear.

"Alan is teaching, has picked up weight, his color is good, and to look at him, he appears in perfect health."

If the findings of nutritional research were consistently applied, such reports might be more numerous.

No case is hopeless. Dr. Charles W. Mayo has emphasized that no case of cancer is hopeless.[76] He tells of a 60-year-old woman upon whom he operated in 1950 for cancer of the descending colon. Because the malignancy had spread to the liver and other organs, her family was told that she could be expected to live only a few months. Yet she made a spontaneous recovery, and when reexamined at the Mayo Clinic in 1956, 1960, and 1962, no trace of cancer was found.

Dr. Mayo hazards no guess as to what may have brought about the recovery but, with the tenderness and compassion of a great man, he stresses that such a case is a blessing because it enables physicians to tell patients that there is always a chance.

Possibly everyone in the health field has seen similar recoveries. In 1946 I had a casual 15-minute conversation with a middle-aged nurse who told me that she had cancer throughout her body, was in constant pain, and probably had only two months to live. She showed me more huge swollen lymph glands than I even knew existed. Because I have long been especially interested in the effect of vitamin E on cancer growth, I remarked that if I had cancer I would take at least 600 units of vitamin E daily. Only five weeks later she stopped to see me on her way home from the cancer clinic. She had no swollen lymph glands, no pain, and, according to her doctors, no remaining signs of the disease. In addition to taking vitamin E, she had followed a diet I had planned for her brother, who had arthritis. For many years she invited me each summer to her ranch to pick apricots, and reported each time that physicians declared her health to be excellent.

Several similar cases have come to my attention. A number of people have also had skin cancers disappear after improving their diets, applying the contents of vitamin-E capsules directly to the growth, and using PABA ointment (p. 129) as protection from the sun.

Radiation. X-ray treatments and other radiation therapy destroy vitamins A, C, E, K, several B vitamins, and essential fatty acids.[41,77] The destruction of vitamin C is almost immediate, but that of vitamin A and fatty acids can be largely prevented if huge quantities of vitamin E are taken.[41] Simultaneously many harmful substances are formed from the destroyed malignant tissue; but the liver detoxifies these provided vitamins C, E, protein, and especially methionine are generously supplied (ch. 16). Severe radiation burns have been avoided, pain decreased, and scarring reduced when vitamin E has been taken internally and applied to the surface.[78-81]

The vomiting, diarrhea, headaches, hemorrhaging, and severe anemia that usually occur after therapy with radioactive cobalt, x-rays, mustard gas, or other mitotic poisons have been largely prevented by vitamins C, E, and the B vitamins provided generous amounts are started several days prior to treatment.[82-87] In most cases vitamin B_6 alone has prevented vomiting. At New York's Montefiore Hospital cancer patients given 3 tablespoons of yeast daily starting a week before receiving "heavy irradiation" remained symptom-free, whereas patients not given yeast had severe vomiting and developed marked anemia.[110]

Because of the stress of radiations, large amounts of vitamin C, pantothenic acid, and protein—the antistress formula (p. 31) and pep-up containing many egg yolks—should be taken around the clock after each treatment.

Cancer and stress. Probably malnutrition invariably precedes all malignancies; hence large nutritional debts have already been incurred. The shock and terror resulting from a diagnosis of cancer, worry over family and perhaps financial problems, and treatments such as radiation and/or surgery, all add stresses of enormous magnitude. The body requirements are, therefore, so tremendously high that it may be impossible to meet them.

As I see it, the diet need be no different from that outlined on pages 330–331. The six small daily meals should be high in adequate protein, low in calories, moderate in fat, and supply generous amounts of all antistress factors and all nutrients that appear to inhibit malignant growth. Particularly in Hodgkin's disease, or cancer of the lymph glands, the antistress formula (p. 31) should be taken around the clock indefinitely.

Leukemia. Sound nutrition should certainly be applied the minute a diagnosis of leukemia is made. My experience has been, however, that usually death has seemed imminent before doctors have permitted parents to "try nutrition" if they wished. Outstanding leukemia specialists have approved diets I have planned for such patients, yet without exception these children have been far too ill to consume the food their bodies needed. Nevertheless letters from parents contain such phrases as: "Mary has not needed a transfusion for 18 months"; "Tom is full of pep and back in school"; "The doctors are completely baffled by this case"; "Everyone says it's a miracle," and a dozen similar remarks. Many of these children have now died, but their last months seem to me to have been less miserable than most; and in a few cases, parents have felt the improved nutrition gave them an extra year of life. If an adequate diet were started early enough and continued consistently, particularly during remissions, perhaps lives could be saved.

I cannot but believe that a lack of vitamin E may be a cause of leukemia; and that the toxicity of fats oxidized rapidly by x-rays in the absence of vitamin E[41,42] may explain why many children whose mothers have been x-rayed prior to their birth later succumb to this disease. Rats lacking vitamin E develop too many white blood cells, which decrease when the vitamin is given;[88] and vitamin E causes the blood platelet count, usually low in leukemia, to increase.[89] Furthermore, a deficiency of vitamin E allows human bone marrow to become abnormal;[90] and giving this vitamin to anemic infants has quickly improved the bone marrow.[91] Supplements of this vitamin are rarely given to persons with leukemia, yet foods furnish only a fraction of the amount needed by healthy individuals.[38,92]

Because folic acid has at times accelerated the development of leukemia,[73-75] folic-acid antagonists are currently used as a treatment.[93-96] These substances take the place of the vitamin in the cells, and cause a severe deficiency to be produced. Many physicians believe that the replacement of folic acid damages the normal tissues much more quickly than it does the cancer cells.[97-105] Others have found that giving folic acid itself has not made leukemia worse, but that it has improved the general well-being without affecting the disease.[106,107]

A folic-acid deficiency prevents dozens of important physiological functions: it decreases appetite, interferes with the utilization of sugar and amino acids, stops all cell division and healing, and causes the hair, eyebrows, and eyelashes to fall out.[73,108,109] Furthermore, the antagonist is so toxic that it usually produces vomiting, diarrhea, and at times such severe hemorrhaging as to be fatal.[93] When it is used, all nutrients known to help prevent toxicity (ch. 16) should be given in as large amounts as possible, and vitamins C, E, and the "bioflavonoids" (p. 316) increased the minute any bleeding is detected.

Every bite of food offered should build health and be served in any form or combination that is readily taken. Children two to five years old often get far more nourishment if allowed to drink milk and juices from a nursing bottle without ridicule. The diet itself need not vary from that outlined on pages 330–331. Regardless of the age of the child, I feel that the antistress formula should be given with fortified milk and 100 units of vitamin E six times daily; that a vitamin-B syrup should be given in addition to yeast and wheat germ; and, except for vitamin D, folic acid, and calories, that one should err by giving too many nutrients rather than too few. Though companies are no longer permitted to grow yeasts rich in folic acid or to add more than a tiny amount to any supplement, a physician must determine whether or not liver, the richest source, can be served.

Neither parents nor doctors need be fearful that improved nutrition will in any way harm the patient. Whether or not such a program can sustain life cannot be known until every nutrient is given daily from the onset.

Nutrition and cancer prevention. Hospital records of Seventh-day Adventists, who avoid highly refined foods, show that they suffer far less from cancer than the same number of persons whose diets are more inadequate.[59] Similar reports have come from other peoples living on natural foods: the Latter-day Saints, the Navajo Indians, and many formerly isolated groups throughout the world.[111]

When doctors with the Sloan-Kettering Institute for Cancer Research injected living cancer cells into the forearms of volunteers with advanced incurable cancer, the implantations grew and later had to be removed.[112]

In some of these patients, these cancers returned and were excised again, though normal cells, similarly injected under the skin of volunteers with growing cancers, did not multiply. Before injected cancer cells would develop in experimental animals, their bodies first had to be depleted by a combination of x-ray and cortisone. Cancer implants in healthy volunteers of different ages from the Ohio Penitentiary caused prompt inflammation, but the injected cells quickly degenerated and disappeared. These men produced antibodies, the complement, and other defenses (ch. 11) which cancer patients were unable to form. Such studies indicate that anyone who keeps his resistance consistently high can be relatively sure of not contracting cancer.

Most cancer could probably be prevented if the nutritional knowledge now available were applied; and active cancer might be inhibited in some cases were a highly adequate diet adhered to. Dr. Roger J. Williams, of the University of Texas, has pointed out that there is extreme difference in the incidence of cancer in various strains and even families of animals; and that some animals are susceptible because they have unusually high hereditary requirements for certain nutrients.[113] These facts may be equally true of humans. In referring to cancer patients, Dr. Williams states, "There has never been a serious attempt to provide all nutritional requirements in quantities adequate to meet genetrophic needs that may be several times above those considered normal."

Unfortunately, our national diet becomes progressively worse each year; and the number of cancer-producing substances in our foods and environment steadily increases. It seems to me, therefore, that every form of malignancy can be expected to become more numerous, though the incidence of this disease in the United States is now greater than in any nation throughout all history.

When cancer is suspected, under no circumstances should nutrition be tried as a "home remedy" instead of seeking a physician's help. Consult a doctor immediately. After a diagnosis has been made the best nutrition possible in conjunction with the best medical help available may save your life.

32
The Two Unvarying Rules

There are two unvarying rules that apply to all diets for all diseases and all abnormalities. The first is to improve nutrition the minute the initial symptom is noticed; an enormous amount of suffering could be prevented were this simple rule followed. The second is to see that each of the 40 body requirements is adequately supplied, erring on the side of taking too much rather than too little of the nutrients that meet the needs of stress. Our culture is so oriented to the medical, aspirin-for-a-headache approach that this rule is continuously violated. Most medications are effective alone, whereas no nutrient is of value unless accompanied by 39 others. To add large amounts of some while ignoring the rest is like trying to remodel a house with nothing except hundreds of doorknobs and shingles.

The body requirements include essential fatty acids, carbohydrates, complete proteins, and every known vitamin and mineral. If only unrefined foods are eaten, nutrients still unknown will probably be furnished. Hundreds of thousands of animal experiments have shown that if a single nutrient or any combination of nutrients is omitted, disease is produced. There can no longer be doubt but that people produce illnesses in themselves by selecting diets as faulty as those that cause disease in animals. Yet, provided injury is not irreparable, a diet including all nutrients in ample amounts can restore health. Because this fact has been repeatedly proved beyond question, no person—not even a physician, in my opinion—has the right to impose an inadequate diet on another individual. There are times, of course, when these rules cannot be applied, but during such periods health is being torn down rather than built up.

In planning any diet, each of the body requirements discussed in the remainder of this chapter should be carefully checked.

Proteins come first. During severe stress ((illness) as

much as 135 grams of body protein—the amount in seven steaks or 4 quarts of milk—may be destroyed in a single day;[1] and the body cannot synthesize the "non-essential" amino acids rapidly enough to meet the demand; hence persons hoping for a speedy recovery would do well to count protein grams (p. 405). Literally hundreds of persons who have an egg at breakfast and meat at dinner have assured me that they eat a "high-protein diet," when they have actually obtained approximately 25 grams daily. During mild illnesses, 80 to 120 grams daily is sufficient, but more is often advantageous.

Foods supplying complete proteins of the highest biological value are, in descending order: eggs; milk and milk products; liver and other glandular meats; muscle meats, fish, and fowl; yeast, wheat germ, soy flour, and a few nuts. Because the proteins in cereal grains, legumes, and most nuts lack some of the essential amino acids, they are of value as proteins only when eaten with eggs, milk, or meat or with each other so that all essential acids are furnished. The most rapid recovery from illness occurs if protein is supplied largely by eggs, milk, cheese, and glandular meats.

When rats are given half of the essential amino acids during the day and the other half only at night, they develop symptoms of a severe protein deficiency.[2] Moreover, if an essential amino acid is lacking or a nonessential one is supplied in excess, a dangerous imbalance occurs, causing large amounts of the essential amino acids to be lost in the urine.[3-8] Gelatin, for example, lacks so many essential amino acids and supplies such an excess of glycine that it inhibits healing and can be toxic when added to an otherwise adequate diet.[4-8]

It is almost impossible to meet the protein needs of an ill individual unless a reasonably palatable drink is taken prepared with fresh milk fortified with foods supplying all the amino acids. Because yogurt and acidophilus milk are largely digested during the culturing process, they are particularly well tolerated by ill and elderly persons. When prepared at home and fortified with non-instant powdered milk, they can contain twice the amount of protein, calcium, and vitamin B_2 at a fraction of the price as do the commercial products; hence an electric yogurt maker— not of glass—is a good investment.

The protein intake can be tremendously increased by fortifying such foods as cereals, hotcakes, waffles, muffins, and cookies with wheat germ, soy flour, and non-instant powdered milk.* Instant powdered milk is excellent to add to fresh milk for drinking, but it makes foods gummy when used in cooking. Instantized foods, like puffed wheat compared with the natural product, are bulky; ½ cup of non-instant powdered milk, available at health-food stores, equals a quart of fresh milk, compared with 1⅓ cups of the instant variety. Any form of powdered milk, however, has been somewhat harmed by heat and should not be substituted for fresh milk.

Carbohydrates, or starches and sugars. Superior carbohydrates are supplied by root vegetables, whole-grain breads and cereals, and fresh fruits and juices. Though all starch is easily changed into sugar in the intestine, this conversion is sufficiently gradual that sugar is released slowly and can thus give a sustained energy pickup. Refined sugar overstimulates the production of insulin (p. 74) and alkaline digestive juices (p. 259), interferes with the absorption of proteins, calcium, and many other minerals,[9] and retards the growth of valuable intestinal bacteria (p. 145); hence it should be used sparingly and only to increase palatability.

If sufficient calories are not obtained, body protein and/or the proteins supplied in foods are used for calories. When the calorie needs are high, such foods as bananas, dried fruits, baked yams, cooked whole-grain cereals, root vegetables, and a variety of breadstuffs made of nutritious ingredients can be emphasized. Frozen undiluted fruit juices served over yogurt as a sundae or added to milk drinks can supply natural sugar as well as other nutrients in concentrated form.

To decrease the destruction of body protein and prevent acidosis (p. 123), some carbohydrate should be obtained six times daily, though the amount need not be large. The more ill the person, the more important it becomes to give a little carbohydrate every hour or two, otherwise vomiting, headache, and the unpleasant symptoms of acidosis occur. If vomiting has already set in, a few teaspoons of concentrated fruit juice or honey taken every 15 minutes, preferably with vitamin B_6 (p. 141), usually rectify the situation.

Fats. The 2 tablespoons of vegetable oil needed daily to supply essential fatty acids can be obtained from salad

---

* See *Let's Cook It Right,* by Adelle Davis, Harcourt, Brace & World, Inc., Revised Edition, 1962.

dressings, mayonnaise, nuts, sunflower seeds, avocados, and "old-fashioned" (unhydrogenated) peanut butter or other nut butters, most of which average ⅓ to ½ fat. Because oil can be used for cooking and seasoning vegetables, it seems to me ridiculous to take it directly from the spoon or to purchase linoleic-acid capsules.

Safflower, sunflower-seed, sesame-seed, walnut, and soy oils contain more linoleic acid than corn, peanut, or cottonseed oil, and many times more than olive oil. Other essential fatty acids can be made in the body from linoleic acid provided several minerals and vitamins are present. Because peanut oil is a rich source of arachidonic acid (p. 52), safflower oil of linoleic, and soy of linolenic, I use a mixture of equal parts of these three oils for salads and cooking.

Since even slight rancidity can destroy many nutrients (p. 188), oils, salad dressings, and lecithin should be kept refrigerated after being opened. It is said that margarines, hydrogenated cooking fats, and highly refined commercial vegetable oils—usually extracted with hexane, or a sort of cleaning fluid—are often prepared from rancid oils.[10] Though the unpleasant odor can be gotten rid of, deleterious chemical changes can never be reversed. The odor of rancidity can be detected for blocks around a vegetable-oil-refining company not far from our home. For this reason, I recommend only pressed unrefined oils and have become fearful of using margarines. Modified butter having an excellent flavor and more essential fatty acids than margarines or butter alone can be prepared as follows: Allow a pound of butter to warm to room temperature and blend it in a liquefier with 1 cup of pressed soy, safflower, or peanut oil, or of several oils combined; mold in an ice tray.

Fats are needed to improve the flavor of foods, to satisfy the appetite, and to stimulate bile flow. Butter, cream, gravies, rich cheeses, and other natural fats rarely need to be restricted provided weight permits and the diet includes all nutrients that assure adequate absorption and utilization.

Vitamin A. Cream, butter, whole milk, eggs, and liver supply vitamin A but are often avoided because of calories or cholesterol. Carotene, a substance in yellow and green vegetables and fruits that changes into vitamin A, is not well absorbed unless textures are unusually soft. Thus many individuals obtain too little vitamin A unless their diets are supplemented.

Excessive vitamin A can be toxic and cause such symptoms as thinning hair, sore lips, bruising, nosebleeds, headaches, blurred vision, flaky itching skin, painful joints and tenderness and swelling over the long bones.[11-13] These symptoms quickly disappear after the vitamin is withdrawn[14,15] or can be completely prevented by generous amounts of vitamin C.[16] Adults who have developed vitamin-A toxicity have usually taken 100,000 to 500,000 units daily for 15 months or longer before any symptoms became noticeable,[11-13,15] though they quickly appeared when a volunteer took 1 million units daily.[14] More than 25,000 units daily can be toxic to children.

Since such toxicity is unexpected, it has been difficult for physicians to diagnose. Because of a skin condition one woman took 500,000 units of vitamin A daily for almost eight years.[12] Before the resulting toxicity was pinpointed, she consulted innumerable doctors, was hospitalized eight times and given tentative diagnoses of brain tumor, meningitis, arthritis, and encephalitis; she was put in a cast because of back pains and underwent brain surgery in an attempt to relieve head pressure. After the vitamin A was stopped, all pain disappeared in two months.

The American Medical Association recommends that no more than 25,000 units of vitamin A be taken daily. Individual physicians, however, still give 50,000 units daily for periods of six months with excellent results and no signs of toxicity.[17] During illness the need is increased, absorption faulty, and storage impaired; hence 50,000 units daily may sometimes be desirable, especially for persons suffering from measles, acne, toxic thyroid, and kidney or sinus infections. Far more vitamin A is required when the diet is low in protein than when protein is adequate.[18] If lecithin is taken with vitamin A, absorption is so enhanced that 25,000 units daily is probably enough for most ill persons, but this 25,000 units daily should be continued throughout convalescence.[19] Infants should perhaps be given no more than 10,000 units, and small children, 20,000 units, even during illnesses, except possibly measles.

The B vitamins. The only good source of the B vitamins are liver, yeast, and wheat germ, though meats, seeds, nuts, a few vegetables, and whole-grain breads and cereals supply small amounts. Some foods are rich in individual B vitamins. The bacteria obtained from yogurt or acidophilus milk synthesize these vitamins in the intestine, but the quantities are not easily measured. The need for these vitamins, particularly pantothenic acid (sold as calcium pantothenate), increases tremendously during illness; hence it is usually impossible to rebuild health rapidly unless both natural sources and supplements are taken daily.

The B vitamins are so readily lost in the urine that almost no toxicity has been reported.[20-25] If one or more B vitamins is given during a multiple deficiency, however, symptoms of other B deficiencies become more severe.[26] In fact, because the sale of folic acid is restricted (p. 344), no B-vitamin preparation on the market at the present time is safe to use for a prolonged period. If supplements of B vitamins are taken daily without a good source of folic acid, such as liver or a cooked green leafy vegetable, a sore mouth, perhaps falling hair, anemia, and other symptoms of a folic-acid deficiency (p. 306) can easily occur. As a safeguard, natural sources furnishing the entire B complex should always be taken with supplements, which can then be used temporarily to great advantage.

During illnesses the need for certain B vitamins increases far more than for others. The therapeutic amounts suggested by the National Research Council have been criticized as supplying far too little.[28] Its recommendations, like most B-vitamin preparations on the market, completely lack cholin, inositol, PABA, and biotin, and are extremely low in folic acid, vitamins B_6 and B_{12}, and pantothenic acid. For these reasons I consider them to be dangerous.

To meet the increased demands of stress, I have obtained the best results by having ill persons take daily, when able to do so, the antistress formula at each meal and between each meal, or a tablet containing 500 and 100 milligrams respectively of vitamin C and pantothenic acid and smaller amounts of other B vitamins; a serving of fresh liver at one meal and a tablespoon of desiccated liver, or 15 tablets, at the other meals; ¼ to ½ cup of yeast fortified with calcium (p. 320); wheat germ as a cereal or used in cooking; 1 cup or more of yogurt or acidophilus milk or several tablespoons of culture; and 1 to 3 tablespoons of lecithin as a source of cholin and inositol as well as an aid to digestion (p. 185). When the patient is markedly improved, the antistress formula may be decreased to 1 tablet with each meal and finally to 1 daily; and, when health is attained, it should be discontinued. A tablet containing half the original quantities may be taken six times daily throughout convalescence. Recovery is more rapid when small quantitites are obtained frequently rather than a larger amount at one time.

When the requirements have decreased, I have used tablets supplying a daily total of 5 milligrams of vitamins B_1, B_2, and B_6; 30 milligrams of pantothenic acid, niacin amide, and PABA; 1,000 milligrams of cholin and inositol; and 15 and 25 micrograms respectively of vitamin B_{12} and biotin. Except for folic acid, these proportions are similar to those that maintain health in animals[29] and are found in normal human tissues.[27] Each member of our family takes 5 milligrams of folic acid daily in addition to these quantities, and I recommend that anyone using B-vitamin tablets obtain folic acid if possible, though it should never be taken without vitamin B_{12} (p. 344).

Unless a yeast or a B-complex supplement contains all of these vitamins in roughly the above proportion, I feel it should not be used. Some yeasts are "enriched" with so much vitamin B_1 that other B-vitamin deficiencies occasionally appear when much such yeast is taken. All varieties are high in protein and contain B vitamins; and torula yeast is extremely rich in trace minerals. In my opinion, torula yeast has much the better flavor, but brewers' yeast is sometimes better tolerated. Instant and flaked yeasts are so bulky and tablets such a nuisance that few people eat enough of them to do much good; 24 tablets, for instance, are required to equal a level tablespoon of yeast.

For those who do not wish to eat yogurt or drink acidophilus milk, fresh, dated acidophilus culture is available which contains the valuable bacteria in concentrated form. Because these bacteria grow only on milk sugar, the culture should be taken with milk. If milk is not tolerated, it can be added to juice with 1 teaspoon of milk sugar to each tablespoon of culture.

The vitamin-C requirements skyrocket. Animal experiments indicate that during severe stress the vitamin-C requirements increase fantastically, often as much as 70 times more than needed during health.[30] If a similar increase occurs in humans, approximately 5,000 milligrams would be needed daily during acute illnesses. This vitamin is non-toxic,[31] and taking massive quantities has sometimes resulted in amazing recoveries (ch. 11), but large amounts are rarely needed more than a few days.

Vitamin C is available in powder form and in tablets supplying 100, 250, and 500 milligrams each. During an acute infection, 500 milligrams every two or three hours taken in addition to the antistress formula is usually ample, though perhaps 250 milligrams extra are needed with each dose of medication. Should bruises, bleeding gums, or nosebleeds occur, the quantities of both vitamins C and E should be immediately increased. When health is fully achieved, 75 milligrams of vitamin C daily is considered adequate by the National Research Council.

The bioflavonoids. New laboratory methods have shown that the bioflavonoids, formerly thought to aid vitamin C, have no value in this respect.[32] Some still-unidentified nutrient associated with them—perhaps pectin—has apparently been responsible for improvement reported in hundreds of studies. The richest source of this unidentified nutrient appears to be the pulp of citrus fruit, and especially the white of orange rind; hence eating whole citrus fruits or unstrained juice is preferable to drinking strained juice.

Vitamin D. Though vitamin D is formed in the oil on the skin by summer sunshine, this oil is readily washed off even by cold water.[33] Winter sunshine produces no vitamin D; and this vitamin does not occur in ordinary foods. Healthy persons working indoors during the summer have been found to have no vitamin D in their blood.[34] Yet this vitamin is essential to maintaining well-mineralized teeth and bones. The only good natural sources are fish-liver oils, though synthetic vitamin D, known as irradiated ergosterol, is readily formed when vegetable oils are exposed to ultraviolet light.

Physicians have given patients with arthritis such excessive amounts of vitamin D—100,000 to 500,000 units daily—that weakness, vomiting, diarrhea, headaches, demineralization of bones, and calcification of soft tissues have resulted;[35] and in some instances, the toxicity has been fatal.[36] Women given 25,000 units daily because of porous bones have developed toxic symptoms, which disappeared within two weeks after the vitamin was withdrawn.[37] Toxicity has occurred in infants receiving approximately 4,000 units of synthetic vitamin D daily.[38,39] Even moderate amounts of synthetic vitamin D, or irradiated ergosterol, taken during pregnancy may damage the infant, though such harm can also result from a lack of vitamin E.[40,41]

Vitamin-D toxicity can be prevented if vitamin A, cholin, and particularly vitamin C are adequate.[38] Furthermore, the natural vitamin D obtained from fish-liver oils is much less toxic even in huge amounts than small quantities formed by irradiating oils; and any vitamin D is less toxic if given in oil rather than dispersed in water.[42] The fear of toxicity has become so great that I feel there is grave danger of getting too little rather than too much. The 400 units daily recommended by the National Research Council has been shown to be inadequate for adolescent girls (p. 247) and for persons with porous bones (p. 261); and during illness, the need for vitamin D is increased by stress.

The ideal vitamin-D intake is unknown. Research indicates that 2,500 units daily is advantageous for adults,[34,43] but this quantity should be supplied only by the natural vitamin D from fish-liver oil and never from the synthetic irradiated ergosterol. I now rarely recommend more than 2,500 units daily and that only from fish-liver oil supplying 25,000 units of vitamin A as well. Since vitamin C detoxifies excessive vitamin D, 1,000 milligrams or more of vitamin C might be taken at each meal in case too much vitamin D has been obtained. Capsules supplying more than 5,000 units of vitamin D are now sold only on prescription; hence danger of toxicity has become remote.

Vitamin E. Pressed vegetable oils, fresh or vacuum-packed wheat germ, and freshly ground whole-grain breads and cereals are our best sources of vitamin E.[44,45] Our average intake of 6 to 15 units daily is only a fraction of the amount needed[46,47] and that was obtained before foods were refined.[44,48]

Vitamin E is non-toxic.[49] As much as 3,000 units daily have been given to children for years.[40] Consistently better results, however, have been obtained from the natural vitamin, d-alpha tocopherol acetate, than from the synthetic one (p. 43). Mixed tocophcrols are said to be unstable.

Infants and small children should probably have about 30 units of vitamin E daily,[50] adolescents and adults no fewer than 100 units,[49] though more is required when oils are used liberally.[45,51,52] During illnesses, doctors have most frequently recommended 300 to 600 units daily, though 2,000 units or more have been taken with excellent results.[23,40]

Vitamin K. Green leafy vegetables, liver, and other unrefined foods contain vitamin K, but our most dependable source is supplied by intestinal bacteria. A deficiency, which may cause hemorrhages in any part of the body, often occurs when these bacteria are destroyed by oral antibiotics; hence, after such medication, yogurt or acidophilus should be obtained daily.

Newborn infants are particularly deficient in vitamin K. A resulting hemorrhage in the brain or spinal cord is considered to be a cause of cerebral palsy, preventable if only 1 milligram of vitamin K is given immediately after birth or 10 to 20 milligrams are allowed the mother during labor.[53] Because more than 10 milligrams can be toxic to infants, many physicians have tragically abandoned giving this vitamin.[53] A lack of vitamin E can also cause hemorrhage in newborn infants (p. 286) which may at times result in cerebral palsy.

The antistress factors. Fresh and desiccated liver, wheat germ, yeast, full-fat soy flour, and cooked green leafy vegetables, the only sources of the antistress factors (p. 28), should be taken daily during illness whenever possible. Creamed spinach is bland enough for any ulcer diet, and quickly steamed beet tops or chard, seasoned with oil and vinegar, are to my taste buds a pleasant way to restore health. These vitamin-like factors remain in green leaves and cannot be obtained from juices.

The taste of desiccated liver can be somewhat disguised if it is stirred into water, and vinegar or lemon juice added. Some brands, though expensive, are so mild flavored that the powdered liver can be added to any food.

Natural and synthetic vitamins. The advantage of natural sources of vitamins is that other nutrients are usually supplied simultaneously. Because synthetic vitamins are far more concentrated, however, they can be taken in amounts impossible to obtain from foods; hence they help to restore health quickly. There is no advantage in using natural vitamin C from rose hips, for example, over taking a less-expensive synthetic product. Both the natural and synthetic vitamins should be used as needed.

Potassium and sodium. Though potassium is supplied by vegetables and fruits, relatively few vegetables are now being eaten. In the days when most people had home gardens, three to five vegetables were usually served at every lunch and dinner. Potassium is readily lost in the urine during the alarm and resistance reactions to stress and/or when the salt (sodium) intake is high. Deficiencies of potassium, therefore, have become common, especially when illness increases the requirement and decreases retention. Equal parts of potassium chloride and ordinary salt can be used in foods (p. 216); and tablets supplying a gram of potassium chloride (15 grams) are available at drugstores.

Animal foods and table salt, or sodium chloride, furnish abundant sodium. During inflammations, when the adrenals are too exhausted to produce aldosterone, sodium rather than potassium is lost in the urine, and salty foods should be eaten. Conversely, sodium is retained at the onset of stress and when cortisone is given; during these periods, a low-salt diet should be adhered to and potassium taken, the amount depending on the quantity of water held in the tissues (p. 111).

Iron. Eggs, meats, green vegetables, and particularly yeast, wheat germ, and liver are all rich in iron. Any diet adequate in other respects will supply more than the 10 to 15 milligrams of iron recommended daily by the National Research Council. If additional iron is desired, ferrous fumarate appears to be the least toxic. Supplements containing ferrous sulfate or chloride should be strictly avoided (p. 33).

Magnesium. Hundreds of recent studies indicate that almost everyone, especially ill persons, is deficient in magnesium,[54-62] another mineral which has been largely discarded during refining. Furthermore, liming soils, a common farming practice, and the use of chemical fertilizers containing potassium (p. 342) prevent magnesium from being absorbed by plants; hence our foods are now particularly low in magnesium.[63-66] Probably no other single deficiency is so responsible for the widespread use of tranquilizers.[55,61,67,68]

The average diet furnishes approximately 300 milligrams daily, whereas 600 to 900 milligrams appear to be required for health;[69] thus supplementation is desirable. I use a tasteless magnesium oxide supplying 250 milligrams of magnesium per tablet or ¼ teaspoon. The magnesium intake, however, should be approximately half that of calcium.[69] If calcium is excessive in relation to magnesium, urinary losses can cause a magnesium deficiency to be produced.[70] Conversely, excess magnesium induces a calcium deficiency. The magnesium intake, therefore, must vary with the amount of calcium obtained. When extra calcium is needed, tablets or powder containing both calcium and magnesium in proper proportions are available.

Calcium and phosphorus. Most foods contain phosphorus; hence Americans have an extremely high intake. Except for minute amounts, calcium is supplied only by various forms of milk; even cheeses, unless made of sweet milk, contain little. When the phosphorus intake is too high in relation to calcium, both phosphorus and calcium are lost in the urine (p. 208). Such losses are greatly accelerated by the stress of illness. Probably no fewer than 2 grams of calcium, therefore, should be taken daily by an ill adult or a sick child. A quart of skim or whole milk, buttermilk, yogurt, acidophilus, or any combination thereof supplies a gram of calcium. The other gram can be obtained from calcium tablets and/or non-instant powdered milk added to milk drinks, cooked cereals, hotcakes, custards, eggnogs, and cream soups.

Unfortunately, such particularly nutritious foods as yeast, liver, wheat germ, and lecithin are all extremely high in phosphorus and low in calcium. Yeast and lecithin to which the proper proportions of calcium and magnesium have been added are now available. When these are not used, I recommend that ¼ cup of calcium lactate and 1 tablespoon of magnesium oxide be stirred or sifted into each pound of yeast and lecithin. Powdered milk can be mixed with wheat germ to be cooked as a cereal and added to breadstuffs containing wheat germ. Liver should be taken at the same meal with milk or a calcium tablet. Because bone meal is high in phosphorus, I feel it is not a satisfactory calcium supplement.

When milk cannot be tolerated, calcium gluconate, which dissolves easily and is sweet, can be stirred into foods or juices, but 7½ teaspoons are needed to supply 1 gram of calcium; therefore at least 1½ teaspoons should be taken at each meal and before bed. Calcium lactate contains twice as much calcium as gluconate, hence it is less bulky if tablets are used; 8 tablets or 3½ level teaspoons supply a gram of calcium. So little calcium is furnished by calcium pantothenate that it is not a source of this mineral.

Iodine. Fallout studies indicate that our iodine intake is far below ideal; and that if the thyroid gland is supplied with sufficient iodine, it will not absorb the dangerous radioactive material.[71,72] Yet Harvard physicians have found that Massachusetts children absorbed radioactive iodine avidly unless given a continuous daily supplement of iodine, a fact showing that their usual intake was markedly deficient.[73] These studies indicate that small children need 1 or 2 milligrams of iodine per day and adults 3 to 4 milligrams.

In Japan, where seaweed is used as food, abnormalities

of the thyroid are non-existent; and the average daily intake of iodine is approximately 3 milligrams. In contrast, hundreds of thousands of Americans have such underactive thyroids, caused in part by iodine insufficiency, that they must take thyroid medication. Unfortunately, our Food and Drug Administration has ruled that no daily supplement may contain more than 0.15 milligram of iodine, or approximately a twentieth of the amount that appears to be advantageous yet never toxic.

Adequate iodine is absolutely essential to health, and it, of all nutrients, is probably most easily lost in the urine. Iodized salt should be used exclusively, but to eat enough salt to supply 3 milligrams of iodine daily is certainly not advisable. In my opinion, the diet of every person, especially anyone who is ill, should be supplemented with 1 teaspoon of granular kelp daily unless a prescription for iodine can be obtained. Kelp tablets can be used advantageously only if the label is ignored and 15 to 25 swallowed each day. Because the Chinese are currently testing bombs and more testing can be expected, I obtained a prescription from my nutritionally minded dentist for 5-grain (325-milligram) tablets of potassium iodide; every member of our family takes one of these each week.

Trace minerals. Copper, manganese, zinc, cobalt, and other trace minerals are as essential to health as any of the vitamins. When commercial fertilizers are used, however, they saturate the soil solution to the extent that the trace minerals, which do not dissolve easily, are poorly absorbed. Seafoods, torula yeast, and kelp are dependable sources provided large quantities are taken daily. Green leafy vegetables and whole grains are also excellent if grown on mineral-rich soil without chemical fertilizers.

Unless one uses torula yeast liberally, the only way to be sure these nutrients are always included in the diet is to take a supplement of them. I often sift ¼ cup of mixed mineral powder into each pound of yeast. If yeast is not obtained regularly, 1 or 2 tablets of trace minerals can be taken after each meal.

An adequate diet. To build health, all of the foregoing nutrients must be supplied in adequate amounts. In addition, some 2 quarts of liquid—soups, milk, juices, other beverages, and water—are needed daily, and enough bulk, or cellulose, to support the growth of intestinal bacteria (p. 145). Whether well or ill, to omit a single nutrient is to invite eventual disaster.

33
Planning Your Nutrition Program

The more seriously ill the person, the poorer his appetite; hence the more important it is for food to taste delicious and to be attractively served. Fortunately, research has shown that any health-building food can be eaten during most sickness, and that "special diets," which ignore the increased needs of stress and the patient's individuality, are often 40 years behind scientific findings.

Verdict of highest authority. A combined committee of the American Medical Association and American Dietetic Association, made up of our country's most outstanding authorities, has summarized the work of thousands of experimenters in a critical review of diets for ill persons.[1] These authorities point out that such diets have been based on tradition rather than scientific fact, and that, like most folklore, the premises are often false. They emphasize that foods containing cellulose, or "roughage," are not rough; that no evidence substantiates the belief that bland, tasteless foods "soothe like a salve" or that refined breads and cereals should be used instead of nutritious whole-grain varieties; and that during illness there is no need for restricting pork, ham, spiced meats, fried foods, strong-flavored cheeses, turnips, cabbage, raw fruits, hot breads, spices, relishes, herbs, or dry beans, peas, and other legumes.

They state that distress is caused not by food itself but by eating too rapidly or too much, or by tensions, fears, or worries which interfere with digestion; and that foods blamed for heartburn, "hyperacidity," bloating, gas distention, and stomach pains are as "innocent as lambs." They point out that meals containing little residue, or cellulose, do not stop diarrhea; and that bulky foods and bran are not laxative, but that lactic-acid milks—yogurt and acidophilus—are.

Furthermore, the committee—bless them—stress that rules about diet should be flexible, and if a recommenda-

322

tion causes fear, worry, or pain, it should be quickly abandoned. They then emphasize the two factors vitally important for all ill persons: small, frequent meals; and the most nutritious foods possible.

Such a report can help persons relax and concentrate on foods that can build health. In other words, you prepare meals for an ill person exactly as you would for anyone you genuinely care for: select the best food available; prepare it with the least nutritive losses possible; and, if the patient desires, make it delicious by frying it or seasoning with condiments, spices, herbs, mustard, and pepper with the full permission of science.[2-4] While planning menus, glance through a cookbook for fresh ideas and interesting variations.

Search for quality. Health can usually be restored by carefully selected foods found in any market but the ill person is undoubtedly more harmed by nitrates, pesticide residues, food additives, and the nutritive losses caused by processing (ch. 34) than a well one. When possible, therefore, obtain medically certified raw milk and butter; fertile eggs; poultry grown on the ground rather than on wire; pressed vegetable oils; fresh, stone-ground flours and corn meal (or grind your own); and fruits and vegetables produced on humus-rich soils without chemical fertilizers and poison sprays. The flavor, texture, and keeping qualities of such fruits and vegetables far surpass ordinary market varieties. In communities where people have demanded these superior products, they have become available.

Much safe raw milk can be found if searched for; most persons of my generation grew up drinking it. Since some vitamin A is destroyed during homogenization, non-homogenized is preferable; whole milk is superior to skim, and any fresh milk to powdered milk. Yet all milk and natural milk products are excellent, though they vary in nutritive value with the food given the dairy animals. Goats' milk is unusually good and makes delicious yogurt.

Space thieves. If one earnestly desires to restore health, highly refined and overprocessed foods, which offer little nutritionally but take up stomach space, should be avoided. Such products, which my secretary calls "trash foods," include refined macaroni, spaghetti, noodles, and "enriched" white breads and cereals; refined bakery products and prepared mixes; packaged cereals; gelatin and gelatin desserts unless made with milk and eggs; precooked potatoes; all hydrogenated cooking fats, hydrogenated lard and peanut butter, processed cheeses, and possibly margarine (p. 312); jams, jellies, candies, and desserts prepared with refined products; imitation fruit juices; alcoholic beverages; all varieties of soft drinks; and coffee unless it has been decaffeinized. Such delicious foods can be prepared from fresh whole-grain products and oils that giving up refined ones need be no hardship. Because cancer has been produced in animals by feeding petroleum products (p. 298), fruits and vegetables sprayed with paraffin waxes should be avoided, and the use of these sprays prohibited by law.

"Raw" sugar is too low in nutrients to be of value, and nature herself did a remarkably good job of refining honey. To many people, however, desserts are symbols of the sweets of life, or love; and such individuals often become depressed and filled with anxieties if deprived of them. In such cases, occasional sweets are preferable to total restriction.

Small, frequent meals. Because malnutrition of years' standing often precedes the onset of any illness, digestion and absorption are usually below par and putrefactive bacteria thrive in the intestine. Sickness causes the digestion to become even more faulty. Simultaneously the need for body requirements skyrockets, and nutrients are often lost through vomiting, diarrhea, excessive fluid intake, and/or the use of diuretics. Furthermore, every cell in the body continuously needs nutrients, of which only a few can be stored. To escape this dilemma and to furnish an ever-flowing supply of nutrients, small, frequent meals, preferably containing 25 per cent of the calories as fat, are an essential part of every health-building program. These meals should supply only the amount of food that can be completely digested at one time.

The more ill the person, the more frequently food should be served and the smaller the meals should be, yet the greater are nutritional requirements. This situation is like having an overdrawn bank account when current bills are soaring; deposits must be large enough to cover both past overdrafts and present needs. Temporary aids to digestion such as enzymes, hydrochloric acid, and lecithin may be used; yogurt and acidophilus milk or culture can change the intestinal flora; and supplements, which require no digesting, should be heavily relied upon.

Supplements. Ideally, every nutrient should be furnished by foods alone, and when no food is refined and all are grown on excellent soils, supplements are not needed. The

Hunzas, who have been repeatedly investigated over the past 40 years,[5-7] have lived on such a diet and remained free from all diseases.

Nutritional supplements are expensive, yet they pay for themselves by reducing medical, dental, drug, and hospital bills. Although they are nothing more than nutrients that would normally be furnished in every mouthful of food were it of excellent quality, I never cease to be amazed at the number of persons afraid to use them during illnesses. This fear results from supplements being identified with dangerous drugs, largely because both are made up in capsule and tablet form. It is as logical to say that a cube of sugar becomes a drug when extracted from its natural source and pressed into a form as to hold that vitamin E, for example, is a drug after being distilled from oil and encapsulated.

Identifying supplements with drugs often causes laymen and even physicians to feel that taking them during an illness is "treating a disease." If a nutrient has been undersupplied, it should be generously added to a diet irrespective of the degree of health. To obtain that nutrient is no more "treating disease" than is the taking of supplements by an Olympic athlete to meet his increased requirements. Medicine is the study of disease, whereas nutrition is the study of health.

The discovery that an adequate diet at first appears to be complicated causes thousands of persons to write me each month wanting to know exactly what to eat. Since it is impossible to answer so many letters, I must emphasize that nutritional supplements are not medicines and that there are no exact rules. Doctors have given—not always wisely—hundreds of times more iodine, PABA, pantothenic acid, and other nutrients than the Food and Drug Administration and the National Research Council hold to be safe or advisable,[8 10] yet they have usually done no harm or less than has resulted from taking aspirin.

Before considering supplements, however, write down all foods eaten in one day on a wide sheet of shelf paper. Use the Tables of Food Composition (pp. 405–435), list the quantities of all nutrients obtained, and compare the day's total with the Recommended Daily Dietary Allowances (pp. 406–407). If your diet fails to meet this standard, study the Tables of Food Composition to see how your nutrition can be improved. After improvement, analyze your diet again, and then purchase supplements furnishing the nutrients you are not getting from foods.

Supplements kept in bottles are too often forgotten: hence I recommend that they be served from a divided plastic box or similar container sufficiently attractive to remain on the table. One friend keeps hers in a covered ceramic bowl, which she calls the "Davis cup." Because excessive fluids can wash water-soluble nutrients through the kidneys, supplements should be taken with milk during meals rather than later with water.

Anyone having difficulty in swallowing capsules or tablets can use potassium chloride as a salt, obtain all other minerals in powder form, get iodine from granular kelp or Lugol's solution, and take drops prepared for babies of vitamin A alone and of vitamins A and D. Vitamin-E capsules can be chewed or pierced with a needle and the contents squeezed into the mouth. B-vitamin syrups are available. Powdered vitamin C and the B vitamins may be added to milk or juices or made into a solution. Because the synthetic vitamins contain no enzymes and therefore are stable to heat, tablets can be crushed and dissolved in a cup of boiling water; if 50 tablets are used, a teaspoon of the resulting solution has the same potency as each original tablet; when sweetened, it tastes much like lemonade.

The amount of supplements needed depends on the previous diet and the size of the nutritional "debt." In the same way that a dry sponge requires much water to saturate it but little to keep it moist, starved cells absorb nutrients avidly at first but need smaller amounts later. A good rule to follow is to use caution in taking vitamins A and D, but err on the side of obtaining too much rather than too little of the other vitamins during illness. The amounts given by physicians in studies reported throughout this book can serve as guides.

Regardless of the value of supplements—and they should not be underestimated—they can never take the place of food.

Foods to emphasize. During illness, the limited stomach space should be used for foods with the most to offer. Emphasis should be placed on the following:

EGGS: 2 to 4 daily or more; use instead of most meats; boil, poach, or fry or scramble gently at moderate temperature with small amount of oil; serve in custards, eggnogs, soufflés, fondues, omelets, French toast; if not enjoyed otherwise, add to pep-up. They supply protein, iron, and vitamin A, but are especially needed as a source of methionine.

MILK: Obtain at least 1 quart daily including 1 cup or more of yogurt or acidophilus, preferably homemade; have cows' or goats' milk, whole or skim, or buttermilk; serve plain and in milk drinks, custards, and soups. Use non-instant powdered milk to fortify as many foods as possible. Milk supplies calcium, vitamin B_2, and excellent protein.

LIVER: Try to have ¼ pound of fresh liver daily, preferably at breakfast; broil, bake, or gently sautée with ½ teaspoon of oil; use any variety, such as lamb, pork, chicken, calves', or "baby" beef. Liver supplies superior protein, the B vitamins, the antistress factors, iron, other vitamins, and trace minerals.

YEAST: Both brewers' and torula yeasts are excellent. Sift or stir thoroughly into each pound ¼ cup of both calcium lactate and mixed trace minerals (optional); or purchase yeast to which calcium, magnesium, and perhaps trace minerals have been added. Yeast supplies B vitamins, antistress factors, and concentrated protein.

FULL-FAT SOY FLOUR: Use for making delicious hotcakes, waffles, or muffins; or add to milk or fruit juices. Purchase variety that is lightly toasted and keep refrigerated. Supplies antistress factors and concentrated starch-free protein.

CHEESES: Serve cottage cheese daily if enjoyed. When a high-calorie diet is desired, use other cheeses liberally in omelets and soufflés, on vegetables, or serve as rarebit or fondue; and do not overlook cheese blintzes. Cheeses supply excellent protein, but few are high in calcium.

MEATS, FOWL, FISH, AND SEAFOOD: Have daily if enjoyed but omit if sufficient eggs, milk, cheese, liver, and other proteins are obtained. All supply protein, iron, and phosphorus; seafood and ocean fish furnish iodine and trace minerals.

SOUPS: Cream soups, fortified with powdered milk, or delicious homemade vegetable soups may be served occasionally, but are usually too filling for ill persons unless a low-calorie diet is desired. Prepare a rich, flavorful broth, and cook the vegetables only until tender. Canned soups have been too overheated to be of much value. Nutrients supplied vary with the ingredients.

VEGETABLES: Serve daily a quickly cooked green leafy vegetable such as chard, spinach, kale, dandelions, mustard, or beet or turnip tops; season with oil and vinegar or lemon juice. Select other vegetables for their green or yellow color, such as broccoli, string beans, carrots, and yams; prepare without water. Use fresh when available, but frozen in preference to canned. Serve a vegetable at each lunch and dinner aside from potatoes. Green leafy vegetables supply an antistress factor; all furnish potassium, and, if grown on good soil and cooked with minimum losses, contribute small amounts of many minerals and vitamins.

FRUITS: Use fresh in preference to frozen, canned, and dried, and yellow, such as apricots and peaches, rather than colorless. Have a citrus fruit daily or fresh juice containing the pulp. Serve undiluted frozen juices over yogurt as a sundae, combine with yogurt to make popsicles, or add to milk drinks. Fruits supply potassium, natural sugar, carotene, vitamin C, and traces of several minerals.

WHOLEGRAIN BREADS AND CEREALS: Obtain fresh, stone-ground cereals, corn meal, and flours; keep refrigerated; select whole-grain breads made with stone-ground flour or prepare delicious homemade breads; use wheat germ and middlings as a cooked cereal; and add wheat germ to other cereals and to hotcakes, waffles, and muffins, which, if properly prepared, can serve as meat substitutes. These foods supply B vitamins, iron, some protein and vitamin E, and approximately 20 nutrients milled out of white flour.

VEGETABLE OILS: The 2 tablespoons needed daily can be obtained from avocado, mayonnaise, salad dressings, or non-hydrogenated nut butter; or from pressed soy, safflower, peanut, corn, sunflower-seed, or other oils; a mixture of several oils, such as equal parts of soy, peanut, and safflower, is preferable to one alone (p. 50); keep refrigerated. Use olive oil only as a flavoring. If more than 2 tablespoons are used daily, increase vitamin-E intake by 100 units for each additional tablespoon. Oils supply linoleic, linolenic, and arachidonic acids.

LECITHIN: Buy granular lecithin instead of the "liquid," which is mostly oil; keep refrigerated. Stir into milk or juices, or blend with peanut butter. It supplies cholin and inositol, aids digestion, and helps to absorb and utilize fats and fat-soluble vitamins.[11]

IODIZED SALT: Use exclusively. If few vegetables and fruits are eaten and a dependable source of iodine is available, the salt may be mixed with an equal amount of potassium-chloride salt substitute (p. 215). Supplies sodium, chlorine, and a small amount of iodine.

SALADS: For most ill persons, salads, which take up much stomach space, can be omitted in favor of cooked vegetables; or serve soft-textured salads such as cottage cheese with avocado, apricots, banana, or peach. Tossed green salads may be served during convalescence when low-calorie diets are desired.

Even with the most carefully selected foods, it is extremely difficult during illness to meet the protein and vitamin demands of stress unless a highly fortified milk is drunk frequently throughout the day.

Fortified milk, or pep-up. Tissues can rebuild at maximum speed only when all nutrients are supplied at one time; hence this drink—a friend calls it the sorcerer's potion—is an attempt to meet that need. It can be made with a variety of ingredients, however, and should be adjusted to your own taste buds. Combine and blend in a liquefier or with an electric mixer or egg beater:

> 2 egg yolks or whole eggs
> 1 tablespoon each lecithin and mixed vegetable oils
> 1½ teaspoons calcium lactate or 4 teaspoons
>   calcium gluconate
> ½ teaspoon magnesium oxide
> ¼ cup yogurt or 1 tablespoon acidophilus culture
> 1 teaspoon granular kelp (optional)

When thoroughly beaten, add:

> 1 to 2 cups whole or skim milk
> ¼ to ½ cup yeast fortified with calcium
> ¼ to ½ cup non-instant powdered milk
> ¼ cup soy flour or powder
> ¼ cup wheat germ (optional)
> Nutmeg or 1 teaspoon pure vanilla
> ½ cup frozen undiluted orange juice

Pour into a container and add the remainder of the quart of milk; cover and keep refrigerated. Stir each time before using.

Any ingredient may be decreased or omitted provided it is obtained in some other manner. For instance, I prefer to take kelp and lecithin in buttermilk. When a high-calorie diet is desired, whole milk can be used and/or more oil, a banana, crushed pineapple, or any frozen undiluted fruit juice added. If the total day's phosphorus intake exceeds the calcium intake by more than one-third, the amount of calcium added to pep-up should be increased. Should milk be poorly tolerated, pineapple or grapefruit juice may be used as a base, powdered milk and yogurt omitted, 2 teaspoons of milk sugar included, and the amount of soy flour, acidophilus culture, and calcium doubled. In case much medication must be taken, no fewer than 3 or 4 eggs or egg yolks should be added to guard against liver damage. If calcium or powdered milk is omitted, the magnesium oxide should be decreased to ¼ teaspoon (p. 207), but if several members of a family share the drink, the magnesium allowance should be ¼ teaspoon for each. Vary the drink to meet individual requirements.

Ill persons and individuals subject to digestive disturbances should take only ¼ cup of pep-up at each meal and mid-meal with hydrochloric acid and digestive enzymes. Should gas prove to be no problem, larger amounts can be taken, but if distress does occur, the digestive aids and lecithin should be increased. As soon as digestion and absorption become efficient enough to permit, drinking the entire quart of pep-up daily, or 6 servings of ⅔ cup each, usually accelerates recovery. If little other food is desired, the pep-up and supplements can meet the nutritional needs.

Menu suggestions. When appetite, weight, and efficient digestion permit, an almost endless variety of delicious foods may be eaten by an ill person. Though meals and servings *must be kept small,* many foods are suggested to allow a freedom of choice.

BREAKFAST

Sliced orange or other citrus fruits or fresh, unstrained juice; or other fruit or juice, preferably fresh

omelet, or boiled, poached, scrambled, or fried eggs; ¼ pound liver, kidneys, lean ground beef, a chop, minute steak, ham, fish, or mixed grill; any whole-grain cereal, preferably fortified with powdered milk; whole-wheat toast or hotcakes, waffles, muffins, or French toast made with nutritious ingredients

modified butter (p. 312)

¼ to ⅔ cup of pep-up

decaffeinized coffee, preferably made with hot milk supplements

MORNING MID-MEAL

¼ to ⅔ cup of pep-up; or whole or skim milk, buttermilk, or yogurt; and/or citrus fruit or fresh juice, if none at breakfast, or other fruit; nuts; bouillon or weak tea if enjoyed, served after pep-up has been drunk; supplements

LUNCH

Eggs, liver, cheese, meat, fish, fowl, cream soup, or whole-grain-bread sandwich of cheese, meat, fowl, or non-hydrogenated peanut butter
cooked green leafy vegetable; and/or other vegetable or salad
¼ to ⅔ cup pep-up
whole or skim milk, buttermilk, or yogurt
whole-grain bread with modified butter
fruit, custard, junket, or milk pudding
supplements

AFTERNOON MID-MEAL

Pep-up and any food suggested for morning mid-meal; supplements

SUPPER *(should be the smallest meal of the day)*

Fish or fruit cocktail
cream soup or meat-and-vegetable soup forming a one-dish meal; or eggs, cheese, meat, fish, or fowl
cooked green leafy vegetable if none at noon; other cooked vegetable or salad if desired
whole-grain bread with modified butter
¼ to ⅔ cup of pep-up
whole or skim milk, buttermilk, or yogurt
fruit or custard
supplements

AT BEDTIME

¼ to ⅔ cup pep-up; or warm milk or a warm-milk drink; supplements

Supplementation schedule. During illness, supplements may be taken as follows:

WITH BREAKFAST: 1 capsule supplying 25,000 units of

natural vitamin A and 1,000 units or more of natural vitamin D; when additional vitamin A and/or D is desired, take with supper; vitamins A, D, and E are absorbed only when taken with some food containing fat.

WITH ANY MEAL OR MID-MEAL: 1 tablespoon desiccated liver stirred into water or juice; omit when fresh liver is served.

WITH EACH MEAL: 100 or more units of vitamin E; tablets supplying balanced B vitamins if full amounts of yeast, liver, and lecithin are not taken.

WITH EACH MEAL AND MID-MEAL DURING ACUTE ILLNESS: A single tablet or separate ones supplying the antistress formula of 500 milligrams of vitamin C, 100 milligrams of pantothenic acid (calcium pantothenate), and other B vitamins including 2 milligrams each of vitamins B_2 and B_6; for mild or chronic illness, half the foregoing potencies; and until digestion is normal, enzyme granules or enzyme tablets with bile and hydrochloric-acid tablets or liquid.

If calcium, magnesium, and trace minerals have not been added to yeast or pep-up, 1 or 2 tablets supplying trace minerals and a tablet furnishing calcium with magnesium could be taken at each meal and before bed.

Adjust the program to meet your individual needs by glancing through the chapter in which your problem is discussed, and emphasize the nutrients found to be most important in rebuilding your health. If your blood cholesterol is high, you may wish both to increase your lecithin intake and to use vitamin tablets high in cholin and inositol. Above all else, check and double-check to see that all body requirements are supplied, being careful not to get an excess of some while omitting others. To overlook a single nutrient is like trying to play Chopin with a piano key stuck.

Do not expect to rebuild in a few weeks what has taken years to tear down. Occasional off days and upsets are to be expected regardless of the food eaten. Patience and persistence are important.

After convalescence. As soon as digestion is normal, enzymes and hydrochloric acid may be discontinued. The body requirements decrease as the stress of illness passes, but to maintain health, the diet must furnish all essential nutrients every day throughout life.

Ideally, the following foods should be continued daily: 1 or 2 eggs; yeast, liver, and/or wheat germ; enough yogurt, buttermilk, and skim or whole milk to make a total of 1 quart; 2 servings of meat, fish, fowl, cheese, or meat substitute; 1 or 2 tablespoons of vegetable oil; 1 or 2 fresh cooked vegetables aside from potatoes; a tossed green salad; and supplements furnishing magnesium, iodine, the trace minerals (unless torula yeast is used liberally), and 25,000 units of natural vitamin A, 250 milligrams of vitamin C, 1,000 units or more of natural vitamin D, and 100 units or more of vitamin E. Insofar as possible, refined foods and hydrogenated fats should be permanently avoided.

Different age groups. Because the body requirements are particularly high during infancy, adolescence, and pregnancy, disease can attack swiftly and viciously. The diets of persons in these groups are appallingly deficient, especially in pantothenic acid, magnesium, iodine, and vitamins B_6 and E. The vitamin-A and -D needs of an infant are thought to be approximately one-fourth those of an adult. Sufficient iodine can be supplied by ½ teaspoon of kelp or a few drops of Lugol's solution. Other nutrients have been given temporarily to ill babies without toxic effects in quantities as large as those suggested for adults. Adolescent youngsters require the same foods and supplements during illness as do adults, and their nutritional "debt" is usually huge. The same is true during pregnancy, particularly when one pregnancy follows closely on another.

Persons over 65 years of age suffer 40 per cent of all illness in the United States, yet make up only 8 per cent of the population; and their diets have been found to be deficient in almost every nutrient except calories.[12-16] Loneliness, lack of money, ill-fitting dentures or none at all, ignorance of nutritional values, and loss of hope make their problem social and psychological as well as dietary. Yet tremendous improvements in health can occur when such foods as yogurt, wheat germ, an orange, eggs, pepup, and supplements are taken daily.

Repeatedly I have seen such simple alterations change oldsters from semi-invalids into vital individuals who still find life an exciting adventure. One woman of 93, whose hobby is calling on shut-ins, experienced such a lift after improving her diet that she has literally become a nutrition consultant in helping her contemporaries achieve better health. Another woman of 90 wrote me recently that she had regained her health after improving her diet at the age of 84. "I had to show my grandchildren that nutrition is worth-while," she stated. Thousands of persons could make their autumn years more colorful by doing what these women have done.

Your health is in your hands. Few diseases become a problem when the nutrition is improved the minute the first symptom is noticed; and an amazing degree of vitality, stamina, and youthfulness can be maintained if an adequate diet is adhered to thereafter.

As I see it, each of us is responsible for his own health. Others can make suggestions, but no one except ourselves can eat the foods of value to us. The health we enjoy or the amount of sickness we must endure, therefore, is largely of our own making. When one sincerely wants health and is willing to work patiently toward it, the rewards are usually forthcoming.

34
A Fortress Against Disease

While reviewing medical literature, I found the phrase "This disease is rapidly increasing" in discussions of allergies,[1] emphysema,[2] celiac disease,[3] cirrhosis,[4] myasthenia gravis,[5] diabetes,[6] hepatitis,[7] epilepsy,[8] muscular dystrophy,[1] cystic fibrosis,[9] and many other diseases. In the United States, influenza and pneumonia still rank as the sixth cause of death;[2] and as bacteria develop resistance to antibiotics, infections increase and some formerly not contagious become highly contagious.[10-13] Babies are being born with cancer, which, a rarity in children 30 years ago, now strikes 500,000 annually;[1,7] and cancer is increasing cruelly in all age groups.[2] New diseases are constantly appearing. "The most rapidly enlarging and surprisingly varied" are the inborn errors of metabolism[14] and the iatrogenic, or doctor-caused, diseases largely resulting from drug toxicity.[14,15] What will halt this increase in illness? A country whose citizens are unhealthy becomes a sick nation.

From June, 1963, to June, 1964, Americans suffered 387 million acute illnesses; 84 million reported one or more chronic diseases, a tremendous increase over 1961; and only 1.3 per cent of the entire population remained sufficiently well not to have consulted a doctor.[16] Other statistics give the registered chronically ill as 95,959,-534.[1] In 1964, sickness care cost approximately 33 billion dollars compared with 14 billion in 1950; and the drug bill soared to nearly 5 billion dollars.[17] The number of prescriptions increased 49 per cent in ten years,[18] approximately 48 million now being written annually for tranquilizers alone. Even the seemingly well are not in good condition. In two studies of 1,500 "healthy" adults, medical examinations showed that 77 per cent of one group had some abnormality, 52 per cent needing immediate treatment,[8] and that 87 per cent of the other had one or more illnesses.[1]

It is astonishing how difficult it is to find individuals with the basic attributes of health: excellent bone structure, erect posture, naturally pink cheeks, flawless skin, sparkling eyes, luxuriant glossy hair, rhythmical graceful movements, and buoyant energy; and a perfect set of teeth has become almost as rare as a dodo. Even our attitude toward health is so negative that persons interested in improvement are said to be on a "health kick" or "health binge" and are quickly labeled faddists or crackpots.

When young people are not healthy, there can be little hope for the future. Of American schoolchildren, 57.9 per cent failed a minimum muscular fitness test compared with only 9.5 per cent of European children.[19] Of men taken by the draft at the very height of physical fitness, 52 per cent were rejected during the Korean War compared with 21.3 per cent during World War I, though physical standards were drastically lowered.[20] Surveys show that 75 per cent of the diets of teen-agers do not meet the minimum daily requirements,[1] but that the food intake of girls, women of childbearing age, and especially pregnant women—the present and future mothers of America— is far more inadequate than that of boys.[21] This is the sand upon which America expects to maintain a strong and vigorous nation.

Are we watching a fall of Rome? Hundreds of informed people are convinced that we are, some believing that we have already passed the point of no return. The uninformed think such an idea is preposterous, but the situation is indeed highly critical.

The tremendous increase in ill-health has paralleled the ever-mounting consumption of sweets, refined foods, and soft drinks, and the corresponding decreased use of fresh vegetables, whole-grain breads and cereals, legumes, and potatoes.[18,22,23] Yet the intake of nutritionally barren foods skyrockets still more each year.

The multibillion-dollar refined-food industry has gained such power that it keeps people in ignorance and literally controls the health of our nation. Its relentless radio, television, newspaper, and magazine advertising reaches like the life-crushing tentacles of an octopus into every home. Half the space in our beautiful markets is given to health-destroying products which fill shoppers' baskets to a frightening degree. Hundreds of magazines and newspapers, depending on advertising income from the foodless food industry, have carried articles and syndicated columns—clever mixtures of truth, misinformation, and propaganda—particularly designed to prevent the slightest interest in nutrition from interfering with enormous profits.

The refined-food industry, by giving untold millions, also controls a vast amount of nutritional research. Much of it is valuable indeed, but information that might harm sales goes unreported and problems whose solution could decrease profits remain uninvestigated. Though most scientists are dedicated, scrupulously honest individuals, a few doctors, well paid by the vested interests, have become extremely vocal in proclaiming the excellence of the American diet. People attempting to alert the public are subjected to vicious sneer and smear campaigns, referred to as alarmists, and their books are widely publicized as "not recommended." The late Rachel Carson, author of *Silent Spring*, was thus shamefully attacked, her compassion for humanity damned as being "unscientific."

Invariably the propaganda articles state that America is the best-fed nation in the world, that our life expectancy is increasing, and that our diet is better than it was a generation ago, always implying that everyone enjoys maximum well-being. Americans are the most abundantly fed but their diet is far from the best nutritionally. Because fewer people die during childhood, millions are reaching the later years, but the life expectancy of a 40-year-old American is near the lowest in the world.[24] Government figures show how much our diet has "improved." Hydrogenation now causes the destruction of 850 million to 1 billion pounds of essential fatty acids annually,[22] a loss any nation clutching at a diseased heart can ill afford; and in only four years, the consumption of soft drinks increased 21 per cent; candy, 17 per cent; white flour, baked goods, macaroni, and packaged cereals 16 per cent each.[18] The national expenditure in one year alone for foods supplying almost no nutrients was over 13 billion dollars.[18] Though such foods produce disease rather than health, the misleading propaganda about them is believed by most of our citizens. Hard facts, however, are not altered in the slightest by anyone's desire to distort or ignore them or to keep them hidden.

How mercilessly the foodless food industry distorts truth is shown by a typical article extolling the "monumental success" of "enriched" white flour. A widely read woman's magazine of July, 1964, says, "Thanks to vitamin-enriched bread, white and whole wheat are now equally nutritious." Yet most of the pantothenic acid, folic acid, biotin, cholin, inositol, vitamins B_6 and E are discarded in the milling.[25,26] The "airy snow-white loaf" has been further damaged by being bleached.[27,28] Losses of iron, cobalt, potassium, magnesium, manganese, zinc, copper, and molybdenum range from 50 to 87 per cent.[29] The amounts of vitamins B_1, B_2, niacin, and iron returned to the ridiculously labeled "enriched" flour are far less than the quantity occurring naturally. Adding a few B vitamins can induce deficiencies of the B vitamins not supplied.[30-33,44] And a nation's health can improve, as did England's during both world wars, despite tremendous stress when refining of grains is prohibited.[35]

With callous indifference to suffering, the "health" value of packaged cereals is similarly extolled, yet the same nutritional losses occur as in the refining of flour but are even greater because of harm done by heat.[34,36] Numerous rapidly increasing diseases could be prevented by the nutrients discarded from wholesome grains, which cumulatively can be a tremendously rich source of nutrients, particularly for youngsters.

Another typical example of how ruthlessly the refined-food industry ignores the truth is the advertising of foods sweetened with cyclamate and saccharine as "dietary," implying such healthfulness that people believe them to be nutritious. The National Research Council warned against using these sweeteners in 1955 and again in 1962, saying their safety could not be guaranteed. Yet more than 100 "dietary" foods now contain them; and 200 million cases of nutrient-free soft drinks sweetened with cyclamate, many also high in caffeine and harmful acids, were sold last year. A person using such drinks may ingest as much as 5 grams—an entire teaspoonful—of cyclamate daily.[37] It is known to destroy vitamin C;[38] and some physicians believe that soft drinks cause serious liver damage.[39] The toxicity of artificial sweeteners has been studied,[40,41] but the maximum tolerance has not been found[40] and liver biopsies have not been taken before and after long-term use.

Articles and advertising that distort facts say in effect, "I care nothing about the health of your children or your right to know the truth." The tragedy is that millions of women would do anything to promote their family's health if often-repeated propaganda did not have the effect of mass hypnotism. I once intolerantly asked a woman whose child, given refined foods, had suffered for years from illnesses costing thousands: "How can you expect her to be well when you're feeding her such trash?" Tears came into the mother's eyes as she replied, "How can one know they're bad when the magazines say they're so good?" This case, multiplied by most of our population, shows something of the needless pain which results when financial gains are made at the expense of human health.

Articles singing profit-gaining lullabies have had so much to say about "food faddists" and "nutritional quackery" that even physicians are overemphasizing this problem. If faddism is defined as the use of diets that fail to meet body requirements, I know of no worse fads than the rice diet used for high blood pressure,[42] the elimination diet for allergies,[43] and the high-fat diet for epilepsy.[45] In a study at the Age Center of New England, customers of health-food stores were given a "high fad rating," yet their intake of essential nutrients was markedly superior to the group as a whole, which was "surprisingly low" in proteins, vitamins, and minerals.[46] As this study shows, health-food stores—in Germany they are called *Reformhäuser*—are doing much to help improve our diet; and when the University of California gave a nutrition course for college credit for owners and employees of health-food stores, these people were found to be particularly eager to stamp out fads, as is every intelligent person.

It has been my experience that fads and the exaggerated claims made by untrained persons are not nearly as dangerous as misinformation coming from the refined-food industry and from individuals of professional standing. Syndicated newspaper columns written by well-known physicians abound with such statements as "There is no evidence that humans need vitamin E," "Arthritis cannot be helped by diet," "Americans get all the vitamins they require from ordinary foods," and dozens of similar statements which have been proved untrue.

Repeatedly we are told that the "gullible public" annually "wastes" 400 million dollars[47] on "nutrition nonsense," which refers to money spent on stone-ground flours, whole-grain breads and cereals, pressed oils, unhydrogenated nut butters, mineral and vitamin supplements, and fresh fruits and vegetables grown without chemical fertilizers and insecticides. The 4 billion dollars spent each year on candy, 3 billion on soft drinks, and 11.5 billion on alcohol[48] have received little criticism. Foods that build health are paid for but once; foods lacking nutrients must be paid for again and again with each medical, dental, and drug expenditure. Everyone certainly has the right to spend his money as he wishes; and I doubt if any organization is concerned about how we "waste" money unless it wants that money to be spent for items on which it makes a profit.

The refined-food propagandists have particularly criticized money "wasted" on nutritional supplements, stressing the obvious fact that if a diet is adequate, additional vitamins and minerals are not needed. But how many Americans are obtaining adequate diets? Much criticism is valid: often supplements do not furnish nutrients their users lack;[49] usually numerous vitamins are omitted which are as important as those supplied; and many are shotgun preparations containing dozens of nutrients in insignificant amounts, "designed to impress the buyer and deceive the ignorant."[47] If wisely selected, however, they have much to offer.

Farmers are not criticized for routinely giving their stock supplements, the analysis of several of which I have before me: 32 supplements for dairy cows; 29 for "winning" race horses; 24 for "high-efficiency" laying hens; 22 for steers; 21 for hogs; and similar numbers for fox, mink, sheep, and goats. Without exception, each supplemental mixture, superior to any sold for humans, furnishes essential fatty acids, several concentrated, highly adequate proteins, and 12 or more minerals; and in addition to many natural sources of vitamins, they contain every known synthetic vitamin including those frequently omitted from human supplements—cholin, inositol, biotin, folic acid, PABA, and vitamins B_{12} and K. Since no farmer would give his animals candy, prepared mixes, packaged cereals, gelatin desserts, soft drinks, or hundreds of other empty-calorie foods even if obtainable at bargain prices, without supplements his animals are far better off than humans. I see little hope for a nation which values the health of its livestock more than that of its people.

Articles lulling Americans into complacency have also had much to say about the "nonsense" of the "organic cult," or people who wish to obtain foods grown on healthy soils. They claim that our soils are not worn out after 100 to 300 years of cultivation and that "evidence is lacking" that chemical fertilizers and pesticides might be detrimental to health. Without any criticism historians have frequently pointed out that early Virginia settlers moved westward because their soils were depleted after a few years of growing tobacco.

Nitrates from commercial fertilizers destroy or decrease the vitamin-C content of plants.[50-52] In the body, they can be changed to nitrates which have caused serious illnesses and fatalities in farm animals and babies.[52,53] After 33 infant deaths in Illinois were traced to nitrates, state authorities set ten parts per million as a maximum safety limit, but many foods contain more than 1,000 p.p.m., some as much as 5,400 and 6,600 parts.[54,55] Since nitrates are not destroyed by cooking,[56] strained baby foods are "especially high" in them.[57] These findings brought comments of "unjustified concern,"[53] though in experimental animals nitrates cause severe liver and kidney damage.[58]

Pesticide residues alter flavor, destroy various vitamins, and inhibit or stop the action of many enzymes.[59] The taste of peanuts raised on land previously dusted with benzene hexachloride was so unpleasant that they could not be made into peanut butter;[60] milk from cows getting traces of weed killer (toxaphene) has been too distasteful to be marketed;[61] and similar alterations in flavor cause millions of children to refuse vegetables.

A number of insecticides have induced fatal anemias and liver and kidney damage in laboratory and farm animals.[62,63] In rats, DDT and other pesticide residues are concentrated in the brain,[64] but their deposition in the human brain appears not to have been studied. Apparently the body fat of everyone in the United States, including that of a six-month-old bottle-fed baby,[65] contains DDT and other poison residues, and in far greater quantities than the fat of persons in other countries.[65-71] Single foods exceeding the so-called "level of safety" cannot be marketed, but the cumulative amounts of all pesticides ingested over prolonged periods can in no way be controlled. The argument that "evidence of toxicity is lacking" is not valid, because evidence of safety is even more lacking. The tremendous increase in cancer may in part be correlated with the 600 million pounds of pesticides added annually[73] to the billions of pounds already in the ground, bits of them carried by soil solution into every cell of our foods.

A few nutrients in foods are sometimes the same regardless of the type of fertilizer used;[74,75] and commercial fertilizers may increase the content of some vitamins over that in foods grown on worn-out soil.[76] Food plants from high-acre yields, forced by chemical fertilizers, contain more carbohydrates and are lower in protein and minerals than less luxuriant growth.[77] Potassium in the form of chemical fertilizers or liming the soil, unless done with a magnesium limestone or dolomite, both cause such a severe lack of magnesium in food plants[72,77] that magnesium deficiencies in humans have now become widespread (p. 220).

Vitamin B_{12}, usually occurring only in animal products, is found in leafy vegetables grown on manured soils;[78] and the calcium, magnesium, potassium, and iron contents of vegetables from mineral-rich ground have ranged from four to many hundreds of times higher than those grown on soil long under cultivation.[79] Foods from land rich in natural minerals and humus have a greater protein content[80,81] and they have repeatedly supported better health in farm animals than those from chemically fertilized soils.[82-85]

I remember an outbreak of hoof-and-mouth disease among cattle, which were then driven into massive trenches, shot, burned, and buried to prevent the contagion from spreading. Later I read how animals with this disease, turned into composted fields, quickly recovered and were not reinfected when rubbing noses with diseased animals across a fence.[83] Foods grown on healthy soils similarly appear to produce superior human health.[85] Furthermore, plants grown on well-mineralized, composted, and mulched land have a remarkable ability to remain healthy and are little bothered with pests. During the many years I gardened in rebuilt, humus-rich soil, no pest destruction occurred; certainly no pesticides or chemical fertilizers were needed, and the flavor of these foods was superior indeed. Thousands of organic gardeners have had the same experience; and one of the factors detrimental to American health has been the passing of the home garden.

On the vast commercial scale, where losses due to insects exceed 4 billion dollars annually[86] and no attempt is made to keep soils healthy, our food supply would at present be jeopardized without insecticides and chemical fertilizers. These facts, however, neither prove that nitrates and pesticides are harmless nor justify ridiculing individuals interested in sound farming practices. Were every city required to reclaim its sewage, and it was then returned to the land, our soils could be greatly enriched. If the boys and girls belonging to the 4-H garden clubs were taught composting, mulching, and natural soil mineralization, they could produce a tremendous amount of excellent food. I know of a girl who made $300 toward college expenses last summer by raising vegetables on composted soil and selling them to a health-food store. Millions of families could plant home gardens if they truly wanted health.

It is also called "nutritional quackery" to question the chemicals used in food processing, such as the 700 preservatives, stabilizers, emulsifiers, dyes, bleaching agents, and other food additives cleared as safe by the Food and Drug Administration and the approximately 3,000 more allowed as *probably* safe.[47] Yet butter yellow and nitrogen trichloride were permitted for twenty-five years before the dye was found to induce experimental cancer or the bleach known to cause convulsions.[87-89] Fumigating foods with ethylene oxide damages several essential amino acids[90] and, under certain circumstances, also vitamins B_1, B_2, B_6, niacin, and folic acid.[91-94] Traces of solvents left from extracting oils have been fatal to farm and laboratory animals;[94-96] and the chemical preventing decay in oranges (thioacetamide) causes severe liver damage in rats.[97] The "non-toxic" flour-bleaching agent chlorine dioxide harms several amino acids, oxidizes essential fatty acids, and destroys any remaining vitamin E.[27,28] If space permitted, dozens of similar examples could be given.[63,98]

Each chemical used in food processing has a slightly different pathological effect on experimental animals,[94] though all lower vitamin C in the blood.[99] Damage can be partially prevented if yeast is given and vitamins B_{12}, C, E, and protein, particularly methionine, are kept high.[98,100-102] Danger lies in the number of additives used, their cumulative amounts, and the reactions of one chemical with another.[103,104] Some foods, such as white bread, are said to contain no fewer than 30 different additives. The quantity of a particular chemical in any one food can be kept below the presumed level of toxicity, but the cumulative intake cannot be controlled. The soothing "no evidence for alarm" may well continue until irreparable damage has been done.

Another attempt to undermine nutrition, this time by suggesting that it may be dangerous, has been the widespread publicity concerning the toxicity of vitamin A. Physicians have given large amounts daily for varying periods with no recognized toxicity;[105-107] and to my knowledge, no fatalities have occurred. In contrast, no publicity has been given to the fact that aspirin annually kills dozens of children who apparently mistake it for candy, though Dr. Fredrick J. Stare has pointed out that this is no reason to discontinue using it.[108] That iron tablets have similarly caused many accidental deaths and far more severe poisoning than vitamin A[109-111] has been equally unpublicized. The overemphasis on vitamin-A toxicity appears to be part of a movement to limit the sale of most nutritional supplements to prescriptions, though, as far as I can learn, neither physicians nor the drug industry is urging this step.

The Food and Drug Administration has already ruled that no supplement sold without a prescription can contain more than 0.1 milligram of folic acid, 30 milligrams of PABA, and 0.15 milligrams of iodine,[112] causing people to assume these nutrients to be highly toxic. Physicians have given with no sign of toxicity 150 milligrams of folic acid daily to children[113] and 450 milligrams to adults,[113-115] or 1,500 to 4,500 times the amount now allowed. Folic-acid deficiencies have become prevalent, one study even showing that 45 per cent of hospitalized patients now suffer from a lack of this nutrient.[116] Its restriction was designed to protect the few people who eat no animal foods supplying vitamin B_{12}.[117,118] A vitamin-B_{12} deficiency may go undetected unless a simultaneous deficiency of folic acid causes anemia.[119-121] The restriction therefore says in effect: "Let everyone whose diet is not carefully selected develop anemia even if he takes supplements." Were 5 milligrams of folic acid added *with vitamin B_{12}* to supplements, vegetarians as well as most other persons could be protected, though some few require 20 milligrams of folic acid daily.[122]

PABA was put on prescription only because it makes the now little used sulfanilamide ineffective, again depriving many people for a few. Such large quantities as 20,000 milligrams of PABA have been given daily in treating numerous diseases, often with excellent results,[123-128] though this amount is needlessly high.[129] Placing PABA on prescription has stopped both its sale and all research concerning its value, yet only 300 to 600 milligrams daily help to restore the natural color of hair, often clear up eczemas and loss of pigmentation, and frequently alleviate the intense agony of burns. It may prevent skin cancers caused by overexposure to sun (p. 130) and perhaps old-age changes in the skin, found to be almost identical to changes in the skin of young people who work out of doors.[130] Certainly these problems are so worthy of further investigation that this vitamin should be sold without a prescription and perhaps 100 milligrams added to daily supplements.

Excessive iodine is toxic, yet doctors have given 2,400 milligrams daily to patients, including children, sometimes for as long as five years;[131-135] and physicians consider 300 milligrams daily a small quantity,[136,137] though it is 2,000 times the 0.15 milligram now allowed. Studies indicate that children should have 1 or 2 milligrams of iodine daily and adults 2 to 4 milligrams;[138] that adequate iodine not only promotes the health of the thyroid glands but also hastens the excretion of radioactive iodine from fallout already fixed in the glands;[139] and that Americans have been exposed to years of radioactive iodine without protection.[139] Because I have known many more people to have surgery for nodules on the thyroid during the past two years than during the previous three decades, I suspect that radioactive iodine from fallout is responsible, and that health has been harmed by the unnecessarily small iodine allowance. Since the Chinese are currently testing bombs and more testing can be expected, certainly all daily supplements should contain the tiny amount of 5 milligrams of iodine.

Obtaining supplements by prescriptions makes them prohibitively expensive. I recently paid the ridiculous price of $9.50 for 500 iodine tablets; and 100 tablets of folic acid of 5 milligrams each now costs me $6.65, whereas the same quantity and potency of folic acid with vitamin B_{12} formerly cost me $1.25. Such prices can prevent millions of people from achieving good health.

Restricting the sale of these nutrients shows a trend which can be far more disastrous. The last proposed revision of the dietary food laws would have made it impossible to obtain without a prescription any vitamins E, K, pantothenic acid, folic acid, cholin, inositol, biotin, PABA, magnesium, potassium, and several other minerals.[140] Vitamin A was to be restricted to a maximum of 7,500 units, vitamin B_6 to 2.4 milligrams, and vitamin C to 100 milligrams. Phosphorus, which Americans need the way Custer needed more Indians, and vitamin-E-destroying iron salts were to be allowed. Fortunately, protests prevented these proposals from being adopted, but revisions that may be almost as damaging are expected at any time.

Except for tiny amounts, iodine and potassium are already sold only on prescription. The healthy individual can apparently get enough iodine from the continuous use of iodized salt and sufficient potassium from eating generous amounts of fruits and vegetables, but an ill person cannot.

Dr. Roger J. Williams, of the University of Texas, has pointed out that many people have unusually high hereditary requirements for certain nutrients, which, if fully met, can prevent illness.[141] Thus "nutrition takes on new meaning and brings new hope," a hope thwarted by what he speaks of as "undue restrictions" on the sale of vitamin supplements.[142] Since bureaucratic edicts have the same effect as laws, I feel that every person interested in health should write his congressmen requesting that all non-toxic nutrients, including larger quantities of folic acid, PABA, iodine, and potassium, be sold without prescription.

Steps to improve the nutritional status of our nation should be made while much still exists on the positive side: children are taller than their parents; American athletes win medals at the Olympics; and millions of people enjoy reasonably good health. There is an awakening among some physicians and intelligent citizens, but not yet in enough numbers to turn the tide. The Physical Fitness Program is a constructive move, though rats on inadequate diets are not made stronger by exercise.[143] Just as in the past few decades atherosclerosis has increased from an unknown illness to one affecting almost every man, woman, and child in the United States, so can cirrhosis, cancer, and numerous other diseases become equally rampant in the next few decades, unless our national eating habits are changed.

If housewives once realized that they produce disease in their families in the same way that scientists do in experimental animals, and would select foods for their nutritive value and prepare them to be delicious with minimum losses, health would improve drastically; yet surveys have shown that homemakers lack the knowledge to plan adequate meals.[144] Nutritional education could largely rectify the situation, and should therefore be required in all elementary schools, junior and senior high schools, and universities; and it should be offered by adult-education classes, university extensions, and PTA groups. Women trained as hospital dietitians would be excellent for such teaching. Most state universities with an agricultural college offer training in nutrition. A few home-economics teachers are doing outstanding work, though my daughter's foods class in high school could be accurately entitled, "Lessons in how to produce disease."

Some doctors with whom I have talked believe that American health cannot be saved unless the advertising of the refined-food industry is curtailed. Others think that more and more research will cure our ills, but, despite its enormous value, unless scientific findings are applied, vast sums are wasted and the paper on which they are printed might well remain in a primeval forest. If the present degeneration is to be halted, the energies of every citizen are needed.

At the International Physiological Congress in Moscow in 1937, Dr. Agnes Fay Morgan, then professor of nutrition at the University of California, predicted what might be expected of nations by comparing the adequacy of their food intake. She said that because of the widespread use of white bread low in yeast and of wines containing almost no nutrients, France would become weaker; and that Germany, with its unrefined rye bread and beer, which, unlike ours, was high in B vitamins, would become stronger. Probably not one Frenchman would have agreed with her, yet only two years later her prophecy was realized.

If the United States and Russia were similarly compared today, how long may our world leadership be expected to continue? Prepared cereals, package mixes, hydrogenated fats, and hundreds of other refined foods are not advertised and are practically unknown in Russia. Their consumption of sugar, sweets, and soft drinks is extremely low. Insecticides and food additives are little used. Black bread and other wholesome foods make up their national diet. After spending months in their country, one doctor remarked, "I am not half so afraid of their bombs as I am of their *tremendous energy.*"

According to the British historian Arnold Toynbee, the fall of nations has usually been brought about by decay from within. If that be our destiny, we will not be the first destroyed by poor food, but certainly the first to degenerate while food is plentiful and the scientific knowledge of how to build health is available.

Physical health, which is the basis for mental, emotional, and spiritual development, cannot be maintained without adequate nutrition. Sound nutrition stands as a fortress against disease, a fortress whose gates are open and into which all may enter who wish. The strength of this fortress can help to protect our citizens and our nation.

Medical References

Chapter 1

1. Martin, W. C., J. Applied Nut. 10, 8, 1957
2. Nutrition Abstracts and Reviews, Aberdeen University Press, Scotland
3. Zöllner, N. J., Chron. Dis. 10, 6, 1959
4. Johnson, O. C., Nut. Rev. 21, 33, 1963
5. Editorial, Am. J. Clin. Nut. 10, 1, 1962
6. White, P. L., Nut. Rev. 21, 65, 1963
7. Sebrell, W. H., Jr., Am. J. Clin. Nut. 15, 111, 1964
8. J. Am. Med Assn. 183, 955, 1963
9. J. Am. Diet. Assn. 38, 425, 1961
10. Editorial, Am. J. Clin. Nut. 13, 254, 1963
11. Shank, R. E., Nut. Rev. 7, 1, 1949
12. Krehl, W. A., Borden's Rev. Nut. Res. 21, 75, 1960
13. Bean, W. B., Am. J. Clin. Nut. 13, 263, 1963
14. Wolf, S., Perspect Biol. Med. 4, 288, 1961
15. Lengemann, F. W., et al., J. Nut. 68, 443, 1959
16. Keys, A., et al., *The Biology of Human Starvation*, University of Minnesota Press, Minneapolis, Minn., 1950

Chapter 2

1. Hurley, L. S., et al., J. Biol. Chem. 195, 583, 1952
2. Ershoff, B. H., Nut. Rev. 13, 33, 1955
3. Ershoff, B. H., Metabolism 2, 175, 1953
4. Selye, H., J. Clin. Endocrinol. 6, 117, 1946
5. Selye, H., *The Stress of Life*, McGraw-Hill, New York, N.Y., 1956
6. Tui, C., J. Clin. Nut. 1, 232, 1953
7. Handler, P., et al., Am. J. Physiol. 162, 368, 375, 1950
8. Rosenkrantz, H., J. Biol. Chem. 223, 47, 1956; 224, 165, 1957
9. Verzár, F., Inter. Congress Vit. E, 1955
10. Wiswell, O. B., Aerospace Med. 33, 685, 1962
11. Dju, M. Y., et al., Am. J. Clin. Nut. 6, 50, 1958
12. Daft, F. S., et al., Pub. Health Rep. 55, 1333, 1940
13. Morgan, A. F., et al., J. Biol. Chem. 195, 583, 1952
14. Krehl, W. A., Am. J. Clin. Nut. 11, 77, 1962
15. West, H. F., Lancet 2, 877, 1958
16. Ershoff, B. H., et al., J. Nut. 50, 299, 1953

17. Guggenheim, K., et al., J. Nut. 48, 345, 1952
18. Nut. Rev. 18, 179, 1960
19. Peifer, J. J., et al., J. Nut. 70, 400, 1960
20. Wolf, G., et al., J. Biol. Chem. 230, 979, 1958
21. Nut. Rev. 20, 161, 1962
22. Wickson, M. E., et al., J. Biol. Chem. 162, 209, 1946
23. Glatzel, H., Nut. Abst. Rev. 34, 507, 1964
24. Merrill, J. M., Circul. Res. 7, 709, 1959
25. Willis, G. C., Canadian Med. Assn. J. 76, 1044, 1957
26. Nut. Rev. 15, 185, 1957
27. White, A., Ann. N.Y. Acad. Sci. 72, 79, 1958
28. Nut. Rev. 10, 217, 1952
29. Dugal, L. P., et al., Endocrinology 44, 420, 1945
30. Eisenstein, A. B., et al., Fed. Proc. 11, 207, 1952
31. Smolyanski, B. L., Fed. Proc. 22, T1173, 1963
32. Dumm, M. E., et al., Metabolism 2, 153, 1953
33. Ralli, E. P., Nut. Symposium Series 5, 78, 1952
34. Pollack, H., et al., *Therapeutic Nutrition,* Public. 234, Nat. Res. Council, 1952
35. Bean, W. B., et al., Proc. Soc. Exp. Biol. Med. 86, 693, 1954
36. Thornton, G. H. M., et al., J. Clin. Invest. 34, 1073, 1955
37. Jacobs, A. L., et al., J. Clin. Nut. 2, 155, 1954
38. Clark, I., et al., Endocrinology 56, 232, 1955
39. O'Dell, B. L., et al., Arch. Biochem. Biophys. 54, 232, 1955
40. Dryden, L. P., et al., J. Nut. 70, 547, 1960
41. Ershoff, B. H., et al., J. Nut. 62, 295, 1957; 65, 575, 1958
42. Ershoff, B. H., J. Dent. Med. 16, 71, 1961
43. Greenman, L., et al., J. Clin. Invest. 30, 644, 1951
44. Barter, F. C., Metabolism 5, 369, 1956
45. Egeli, E. S., et al., Am. Heart J. 59, 527, 1960
46. Bryant, J. M., Proc. Soc. Exp. Biol. Med. 67, 557, 1948
47. Womersley, R. A., et al., J. Clin. Invest. 34, 456, 1955
48. Moore, F. D., et al., Metabolism 4, 379, 1955
49. Rufenstein, E. C., Metabolism 7, 78, 1958
50. Pirani, C. L., et al., Fed. Proc. 11, 423, 1952
51. Nut. Rev. 17, 144, 1959
52. Zucker, T. F., Am. J. Clin. Nut. 6, 65, 1958
53. Conney, A. H., et al., Nature 184, Suppl. 6, 363, 1959
54. Meites, J., et al., Am. J. Clin. Nut. 5, 381, 1957
55. Robert, A., et al., Proc. Soc. Exp. Biol. Med. 98, 9, 1958
56. Ogawa, T., et al., Am. J. Physiol. 198, 619, 1960
57. Zimmerman, F., et al., Am. J. Clin. Nut. 4, 482, 1956
58. Welsh, A. L., Arch. Derm. Syph. 70, 181, 1954

Chapter 3

1. Nat. Health Fed. Bull. 10, 29, 1964
2. Goodman, L. S., and Gilman, A., *The Pharmacological Bases of Therapeutics,* Macmillan, New York, N.Y., 1941

3. Collins, E. N., et al., Cleveland Clin. Quart. 10, 105, 1943
4. Ershoff, B. H., J. Dent. Med. 16, 71, 1961
5. Ershoff, B. H., Proc. Soc. Exp. Biol. Med. 64, 500, 1947
6. Ershoff, B. H., J. Nut. 35, 269, 1948
7. Ershoff, B. H., Nut. Rev. 13, 33, 1955
8. Beyer, K. H., J. Pharmacol. Exp. Therap. 71, 394, 1941
9. Taylor, D. J., et al., Proc. Soc. Exp. Biol. Med. 90, 551, 1953
10. Bueding, E., et al., Proc. Soc. Exp. Biol. Med. 64, 111, 1949
11. Luttermoser, G. W., et al., Am. J. Trop. Med. Hygiene 10, 541, 1961
12. Millen, J. W., Lancet 2, 599, 1962
13. Kushner, D. S., Am. J. Clin. Nut. 4, 561, 1956
14. Smith, M. G. H., et al., Biochem. J. 57, 7, 1954
15. Manchester, K. L., et al., Brit. Med. J. 1, 1028, 1958
16. Quick, A. J., J. Food Nut. News 35, 2, 1964
17. Stare, F. J., Nut. Rev. 21, 1, 1963
18. Crichton, J. W., Canadian Med. Assn. J. 83, 1144, 1960
19. Kiser, J. R., Am. J. Dig. Dis. 8, 856, 1963
20. Gross, M., and Greenburg, L. A., *The Salicylates,* Hillhouse Press, New Haven, Conn., 1948
21. Reid, J., et al., Brit. Med. J. 2, 1071, 1957
22. Wolff, R. W., et al., J. Am. Med. Assn. 185, 102, 1963
23. Nut. Rev. 13, 46, 1955
24. Zucker, T. A., Am. J. Clin. Nut. 6, 65, 1958
25. Waddell, J., et al., J. Biol. Chem. 80, 431, 1928
26. Reissmann, K. R., et al., Blood 10, 35, 46, 1955
27. Mason, K. E., et al., Anat. Rec. 92, 33, 1945
28. Editorial, J. Pediat. 40, 141, 1952
29. Mattill, H. A., Nut. Rev. 10, 225, 1952
30. Verzár, F., Inter. Congress Vit. E, 1955
31. Bayer, R., Wien. Med. Wachschr. 109, 271, 1959
32. Tedeschi, C. G., et al., Am. J. Obst. Gynec. 71, 16, 1956
33. Horwitt, M. K., et al., Am. Med. Assn. Arch. Neurol. 1, 312, 1959
34. J. Am. Med. Assn. 184, 992, 1963
35. Hoppe, J. O., et al., Am. J. Med. Sci. 230, 558, 1955
36. Nut. Rev. 10, 299, 1952
37. Thompson, M. M., et al., Am. J. Clin. Nut. 7, 80, 1959
38. Ohlsson, W. T. L., et al., Lancet 2, 12, 1962
39. Parsons, W. B., Jr., J. Am. Med. Assn. 173, 1466, 1960
40. Parsons, W. B., Jr., Arch. Int. Med. 107, 653, 1961
41. Nut. Rev. 15, 185, 1957
42. Sulzberger, M. B., et al., Proc. Soc. Exp. Biol. Med. 32, 716, 1935
43. Cormia, F. E., Canadian Med. Assn. J. 36, 392, 1937
44. Cohen, M. B., J. Allergy 10, 15, 1938
45. Nut. Rev. 4, 259, 1946
46. Gabovich, R. D., et al., Fed. Proc. 23, T450, 1964
47. Holmes, H. N., et al., J. Lab. Clin. Med. 24, 1119, 1939
48. Ekman, B., Acta Pharmacol. Toxicol. 3, 261, 1947

49. Forssman, S., et al., Acta Med. Scand. 128, 256, 1947
50. Hove, E. L., Proc. Soc. Exp. Biol. Med. 77, 502, 1951
51. Hove, E. L., J. Nut. 50, 361, 609, 1953
52. Veddis, E. B., et al., J. Nut. 16, 57, 1938
53. Conney, A. H., et al., Nature 184, Suppl. 6, 363, 1959
54. Friend, F. J., et al., Proc. Soc. Exp. Biol. Med. 67, 374, 1948
55. Kinnunen, O., Acta Physiol. Scand. 17, 261, 1949
56. Keith, J. D., et al., Arch. Dis. Childh. 74, 125, 1938
57. Holmes, H. N., South. Med. Surg. 105, 393, 1943
58. Hawthorne, B. E., et al., Proc. Soc. Exp. Biol. Med. 67, 447, 1948
59. Spitzer, J. M., et al., Am. J. Dig. Dis. 15, 80, 1948
60. West, E. S., et al., J. Allergy 20, 344, 1949
61. Gosh, B., Ann. Biochem. Exp. Med. 2, 229, 1942
62. Beyer, K. N., et al., Surg. Gynec. Obst. 79, 49, 1944
63. Green, M. W., et al., J. Am. Pharmacol. Assn. 30, 613, 1941
64. Chapman, D. W., et al., Arch. Int. Med. 79, 449, 1947
65. McChesney, E. W., J. Pharmacol. Exp. Therap. 84, 222, 1945
66. Dainow, J., Ann. Derm. Syph. 10, 139, 1939
67. Kimball, O. P., J. Am. Med. Assn. 112, 1244, 1939
68. Frankel, S. I., J. Am. Med. Assn. 114, 1320, 1940
69. Beyer, K. H., Arch. Int. Med. 71, 315, 1943
70. Bicknell, F., and Prescott, F., The Vitamins in Medicine, Lee Foundation for Nutritional Research, Milwaukee, Wis., 1953
71. Jones, W. A., et al., Lancet 1, 1073, 1953
72. Dick, E. C., et al., Proc. Soc. Exp. Biol. Med. 104, 523, 1960
73. Portis, S. A., et al., J. Am. Med. Assn. 149, 1265, 1952
74. Ann. N.Y. Acad. Sci., 52, 63, 1949
75. Ditchburn, R. W., et al., Nature 147, 745, 1941
76. Patek, A. J., et al., Proc. Soc. Exp. Biol. Med. 46, 180, 1941
77. Shapiro, S., J. Am. Med. Assn. 125, 546, 1944
78. Young, G., et al., Am. J. Physiol. 131, 210, 1940
79. Biehl, J. P., et al., Proc. Soc. Exp. Biol. Med. 85, 389, 1954
80. Slinger, S. J., et al., J. Nut. 52, 75, 1954
81. Scudamore, H. H., Ann. Int. Med. 55, 433, 1961
82. Gabuzda, G. J., et al., Arch. Int. Med. 101, 476, 1958
83. Hutterer, F., et al., Brit. J. Exp. Path. 42, 187, 1961
84. Cohen, S. B., J. Am. Med. Assn. 186, 899, 1963
85. Wellman, J. S., et al., Lancet 1, 827, 1962
86. Josephson, E. M., The Thymus, Manganese, and Myasthenia Gravis, Chedney Press, New York, N.Y., 1961
87. Sumnar, J., J. Tubercul. 30, 62, 1949
88. Sarett, H. P., J. Nut. 47, 273, 1952
89. Harris, H. J., J. Am. Med. Assn. 142, 161, 1950
90. Kushner, D. S., Am. J. Clin. Nut. 4, 561, 1956

91. Nut. Rev. 16, 90, 1958
92. Nut. Rev. 13, 291, 1955
93. Smith, W. O., et al., J. Okla. State Med. Assn. 55, 248, 1962
94. Martin, H. E., et al., Med. Clin. No. Am. 36, 1157, 1952
95. Macht, D. I., J. Am. Med. Assn. 148, 265, 1952
96. Kay, J. H., et al., Surgery 28, 124, 1950
97. Zierler, K. I., et al., Am. J. Physiol. 153, 127, 1948
98. Cantin, M., et al., J. Exp. Med. Surg. 20, 318, 1962
99. Bentler, E., Blood 14, 103, 1959
100. Miller, Z., et al., J. Biol. Chem. 237, 968, 1962
101. Warkany, J., et al., Am. J. Dis. Child. 97, 36, 1959
102. Hillman, D. A., Canadian Med. Assn. J. 80, 200, 220, 1959
103. Prosperi, P., Inter. Congress Vit. E, 1955
104. Alexander, H. L., *Reactions with Drug Therapy*, W. B. Saunders, Philadelphia, Pa., 1955
105. Ames, S. R., et al., Inter. Rev. Vit. Res. 22, 401, 1951
106. Mason, K. E., Yale J. Biol. Med. 14, 605, 1942

Chapter 4

1. Cortesi, C., Bol. della Malattie dell'Orecchio, della Gola, del Naso 68, 343, 1950
2. Heinsen, H. A., et al., Deutsche Med. Woch. 76, 887, 1951
3. Nikolowski, W., Strahlentherapie 87, 113, 1952
4. Gibson, H. R. B., Brit. Med. J. 2, 446, 1952
5. Blaxter, K. L., et al., Brit. J. Nut. 6, 144, 1952
6. Piana, C., Acta Vitaminol. 6, 69, 1952
7. Bellanti, P., Rassegna Inter. Clin. e Terap. 29, 322, 1949
8. Aurig, G., et al., Strahlentherapie 89, 433, 1952
9. Riggiero, A., et al., Gior. Ital. di Chir. 8, 506, 1952
10. de Mello, A., Arquiv. Mineiros de Legrologia 11, 148, 1952
11. Lohel, H., Deutsche Gesundheirswesen 7, 1365, 1952
12. Dahl, O., Nord. Med. 50, 160, 1953.
13. Pult, H., Deutsche Med. Woch. 79, 471, 1954
14. Gartmann, H., et al., Derm. Woch. 128, 1213, 1953
15. Matoloy, G., Summary 15, 14, 1963
16. Nikolowski, W., Med. Welt. Syst. 29, 1634, 2042, 1962
17. Reuren, F., Lille Med. 7, 654, 1962
18. Scardino, P. O., et al., Ann. N.Y. Acad. Sci. 52, 390, 1949
19. Ross, J. A., Brit. Med. J. 2, 232, 1952
20. Steinberg, C. L., Arch. Surg. 63, 824, 1951
21. Steinberg, C. L., Ann. N.Y. Acad. Sci. 52, 380, 1949
22. Waller, J. I., et al., J. Urol. 68, 623, 1952
23. Van Duzen, R. E., et al., J. Urol. 65, 1033, 1951
24. Edgerton, M. T., Jr., et al., Plastic Reconstructive Surg. 8, 224, 1951
25. Shute, E. V., et al., J. Surg. Gynec. Obst. 86, 1, 1948

26. Shute, E. V., and Shute, W. E., *Alpha Tocopherol in Cardiovascular Disease*, Ryerson Press, Toronto, Canada, 1954
27. Green, J., Nature 177, 86, 1956
28. Butturini, W., Inter. Congress Vit. E, 1955
29. Harris, P. L., et al., Am. J. Clin. Nut. 13, 385, 1963
30. Harris, P. L., J. Nut. 40, 367, 1950
31. Muhlefluh, J., Nut. Abst. Rev. 33, 709, 1963
32. Vitamin E Symposium, Ann. N.Y. Acad. Sci. 52, 63, 1949
33. Mattill, H. A., Nut. Rev. 10, 225, 1952
34. Harris, P. L., et al., Inter. Congress Vit. E, 1955
35. Roderuck, D. H., et al., Ann. N.Y. Acad. Sci. 52, 156, 1949
36. Moore, T., J. Nut. 65, 185, 1958
37. Pazcek, P. L., et al., J. Biol. Chem. 146, 351, 1942
38. Beckman, R., Inter. Congress Vit. E, 202, 1955
39. Nitowsky, H. M., et al., Bull. Johns Hopkins Hosp. 98, 361, 1956
40. Bratzler, J. W., et al., J. Nut. 42, 59, 1950
41. Gerschman, R., et al., Fed. Proc. 14, 56, 1955
42. Telford, E. G., et al., Air Univ. Sch. Aviation Med. Rep. 4, Project 21, 1201, 1954
43. Steinberg, C. L., Med. Clin. No. Am. 30, 221, 1946
44. Sutro, C. J., et al., Arch. Surg. 42, 1065, 1941
45. Thomson, G. R., Brit. Med. J. 2, 1382, 1949
46. King, R. A., J. Bone Joint Surg. 31, 443, 1949
47. Annau, J. H., et al., Ann. Surg. 134, 186, 1951
48. Larsen, R. D., et al., J. Bone Joint Surg. 40A, 773, 1958
49. Scott, W. W., et al., South. Med. J. 41, 173, 1948
50. Kirk, J. E., et al., Proc. Soc. Exp. Biol. Med. 80, 565, 1952
51. Follis, R. H., Jr., Proc. Soc. Exp Biol. Med. 100, 203, 1959
52. Costa, A., et al., Inter. Congress Vit. E, 1955
53. Gresham, G. A., et al., Brit. J. Exp. Path. 43, 21, 1962
54. Editorial, J. Am. Med. Assn. 137, 1228, 1948
55. Editorial, J. Am. Med. Assn. 171, 1205, 1959
56. Auerbach, O., et al., New Engl. J. Med. 269, 1045, 1963
57. Passey, R. D., Great Britain Ministry of Health, Her Majesty's Stationery Office, London, Part 2, 48, 1958
58. Auerbach, O., et al., New Engl. J. Med. 265, 253, 1961
59. Leuchtenberger, C., et al., Cancer 13, 721, 1960
60. Tuchweber, B., et al., Am. J. Clin. Nut. 13, 238, 1963
61. Cantin, M., et al., Exp. Med. Surg. 318, 20, 1962

Chapter 5

1. Hirsch, E. F., et al., Physiol. Rev. 23, 185, 1943
2. Vannas, S., et al., Acta Ophthal. 36, 601, 1958
3. Parrish, H. M., J. Chron. Dis. 14, 339, 1961
4. Renaud, S., et al., J. Nut. 83, 149, 1964
5. Owren, P. A., Lancet 2, 975, 1964

6. Turpeinen, O., et al., Lancet 1, 196, 1960
7. McOsker, D. E., et al., J. Am. Med. Assn. 180, 380, 1962
8. Watanabe, N., Arch. Surg. 85, 136, 1962
9. Friedman, M., et al., Gerontology 10, 60, 1955
10. Kingsbury, K., J. Clin. Sci. 22, 161, 1962
11. Antonis, A., *Essential Fatty Acids,* Acadamic Press, New York, N.Y., 1958
12. Lewis, B., Lancet 2, 71, 1958
13. Scott, R. F., et al., Exp. Molec. Path. 1, 1, 1962
14. Mead, J. F., et al., J. Biol. Chem. 229, 575, 1957
15. Nut. Rev. 20, 220, 1962
16. Byers, S. O., Am. J. Clin. Nut. 6, 638, 1958
17. Zilversmit, D. B., et al., Am. J. Clin. Nut. 6, 235, 1958
18. Artom, C., Am. J. Clin. Nut. 6, 221, 1958
19. Adlersberg, D., et al., Clin. Chem. 1, 18, 1955
20. Thannhauser, S. J., et al., J. Biol. Chem. 129, 717, 1939
21. Horlick, L., Circulation 10, 30, 1956
22. Duff, G. L., et al., Am. J. Med. 11, 92, 1951
23. Adlersberg, D., et al., J. Nut. 25, 255, 1943
24. Davies, D. F., Clin. Sci. 17, 563, 1958
25. Ahrens, E. H., et al., J. Exp. Med. 90, 409, 1949
26. Leathes, J. B., Lancet 1, 1019, 1925
27. Hirsch, E. F., et al., Physiol. Rev. 23, 185, 1943
28. Downs, W. G., Am. Med. 41, 460, 1935
29. Kesten, H. D., et al., Proc. Soc. Exp. Biol. Med. 49, 71, 1942
30. Ladd, A. T., et al., Fed. Proc. 8, 360, 1949
31. Havel, R. J., J. Clin. Invest. 36, 848, 1957
32. Friedman, M., et al., Am. J. Physiol. 186, 13, 1956
33. Walker, W. J., Am. J. Med. 14, 654, 1953
34. Pilgeram, L. O., Fed. Proc. 14, 728, 1955
35. Friedman, M., et al., Proc. Soc. Exp. Biol. Med. 95, 586, 1957
36. Friedman, M., et al., Am. J. Physiol. 186, 13, 1956
37. Nath, N., et al., J. Nut. 74, 389, 1961
38. Wagner, A. L., et al., J. Lab. Clin. Med. 40, 324, 1952
39. Gross, K. L., et al., N.Y. State J. Med. 30, 2683, 1950
40. Sinclair, H. M., Lancet 2, 271, 381, 1956
41. Waddell, W. R., et al., Metabolism 7, 707, 1958
42. King, C. G., J. Am. Diet. Assn., 42, 199, 1963
43. Diller, E. R., et al., J. Nut. 73, 14, 1961
44. Morrison, L. M., Geriatrics 13, 12, 1958
45. Kuo, P. T., et al., Am. J. Med. 26, 68, 1959
46. Merigan, T. C., et al., J. Exp. Med. 113, 587, 1961
47. Adlersberg, D., et al., Clin. Chem. 1, 18, 1955
48. Brown, J. B., Nut. Rev. 17, 321, 1959
49. Lindgren, F. T., et al., Am. J. Clin. Nut. 9, 13, 1961
50. Swell, L., et al., Proc. Soc. Exp. Biol Med. 104, 325, 1960
51. Wilkens, J. A., et al., Canadian J. Biochem. Physiol. 40, 1079, 1091, 1962
52. Haust, H. L., et al., J. Nut. 81, 13, 1963
53. Ahrens, E. H., Jr., et al., Lancet 1, 115, 1959

54. Capeci, N. E., et al., Am. J. Med. 26, 76, 1959
55. Gordon, H., et al., Nature 180, 923, 1957
56. Hellman, L., et al., J. Clin. Invest. 36, 898, 1957
57. Deykin, D., et al., J. Biol. Chem. 237, 3649, 1962
58. Peifer, J. G., et el., J. Nut. 68, 155, 1959
59. Merrill, J. M., Circul. Res. 7, 709, 1959
60. Sebrell, W. H., Jr., et al., J. Am. Diet. Assn. 40, 403, 1962
61. Bernick, S., et al., Arch. Path. 72, 321, 1961
62. Peifer, J. G., et al., J. Nut. 70, 400, 1960
63. Jolliffe, N., et al., Postgrad. Med. 29, 569, 1961
64. Bjorntorp, P., et al., Am. J. Clin. Nut. 10, 217, 1962
65. Rosenfeld, B., et al., Canadian J. Biochem. Physiol. 35, 845, 1957
66. Nut. Rev. 10, 306, 1952
67. Ashworth, C. T., et al., Arch. Path. 72, 620, 1961
68. Hartroft, W. S., et al., Proc. Soc. Exp. Biol. Med. 81, 384, 1952
69. Clement, G., et al., Arch. Sci. Physiol. 11, 101, 1957
70. Wilgram, G. F., et al., Science 119, 842, 1954
71. Fillios, L. C., et al., Metabolism 3, 16, 1954
72. Barnes, R. H., et al., J. Nut. 69, 261, 269, 1959
73. Mann, G. V., et al., J. Exp. Med. 98, 195, 1952
74. Mann, G. V., Circul. Res. 9, 838, 1961
75. Labecki, T. D., Am. J. Clin. Nut. 6, 325, 1958
76. Williams, J. O., South. Med. J. 44, 369, 1951
77. Rawls, W. B., et al., J. Am. Geriat. Soc. 4, 89, 1956
78. Forbes, J. C., Endocrinology 35, 126, 1944
79. Katz, L. N., et al., J. Am. Med. Assn. 161, 536, 1956
80. Whittier, P. W., et al., Arch. Biochem. 41, 266, 1952
81. Blaxter, K. L., et al., J. Comp. Path. 64, 157, 176, 1954
82. Mushett, C. W., et al., Fed. Proc. 15, 526, 1956
83. Greenberg, L. D., et al., Am. J. Clin. Nut. 6, 635, 1958
84. Dam, H., et al., Acta Physiol. Scand. 36, 329, 1956
85. Jones, E. A., et al., J. Lab. Clin. Med. 52, 667, 1958
86. Steiner, A. J. Applied Nut. 16, 125, 1963
87. Bersohn, I., et al., Lancet 1, 1020, 1957
88. Malkiel, S. B., et al., Med. Proc. 2, 455, 1956
89. Barnett, L. B., Clin. Physiol. 1, 26, 1959
90. Bunce, G. E., et al., J. Nut. 76, 20, 1962
91. Vitale, J. J., J. Biol. Chem. 228, 573, 1957
92. Seelig, M. S., Am. J. Clin. Nut. 14, 342, 1964
93. Garcia, L. R., Am. J. Clin. Nut. 9, 315, 1961
94. McCollister, R. J., Am. J. Clin. Nut. 12, 415, 1963
95. Rosenkrantz, H., J. Biol. Chem. 223, 47, 1956; 224, 165, 1957
96. Gillman, T., et al., Lancet 2, 1117, 1957; 2, 901, 1958
97. Gresham, G. A., et al., Brit. J. Exp. Path. 41, 395, 1960
98. Gillman, T., et al., Am. Med. Assn. Arch. Path. 59, 733, 1955; 67, 624, 1959
99. Holman, R. L., et al., Am. J. Path. 34, 209, 1958
100. Nut. Rev. 18, 67, 1960

101. Josephson, E. M., *The Thymus, Manganese, and Myasthenia Gravis,* Chedney Press, New York, N.Y., 1961
102. Deuel, H. G., Jr., et al., Biochem. J. 61, 14, 1955
103. Quaife, M. L., J. Nut. 40, 367, 1950
104. Mattill, H. A., Nut. Rev. 10, 225, 1952
105. Telford, E. A., et al., Air Univ. Sch. Aviation Med. Rep. 4, Project 21, 1201, 1954
106. Zierler, M., et al., Ann. N.Y. Acad. Sci. 52, 180, 1949
107. Houchim, O. B. et al., J. Biol. Chem. 146, 309, 313, 1942
108. De Nicola, P., Inter. Congress Vit. E, 1955
109. Shute, E. V., Inter. Congress Vit. E, 1955
110. Jessen, K. E., et al., Acta Path. Microbiol. Scand. 29, 72, 1951
111. Shute, E. V., and Shute, W. E., *Alpha Tocopherol in Cardiovascular Disease,* Ryerson Press, Toronto, Canada, 1954
112. Tolgyes, S., et al., Canadian Med. Assn. J. 76, 730, 1957
113. Yudkin, J., Lancet 2, 155, 1957
114. Cohen, A. M., Am. Heart J. 65, 291, 1962
115. Fortman, O. W., et al., Proc. Soc. Exp. Biol. Med. 91, 321, 1956
116. MacDonald, I., J. Physiol. 160, 306, 1962
117. Antar, M. A., et al., Am. J. Clin. Nut. 14, 169, 1964
118. Macy, I. G., *Nutrition and Chemical Growth in Childhood,* Charles C. Thomas, Baltimore, Md., 1942, p. 84
119. Williams, R. J., et al., Quart. J. Studies Alcohol 16, 234, 1955
120. Wells, A. F., et al., J. Nut. 74, 87, 1961
121. Nut. Rev. 20, 213, 1962
122. Nath, M. C., et al., Proc. Soc. Exp. Biol. Med. 108, 337, 1961
123. Pallota, M. A., et al., Am. J. Clin. Nut. 13, 201, 1963
124. Kinley, L. J., et al., Proc. Soc. Exp. Biol. Med. 102, 353, 1959
125. Hammerl, H., et al., Nut. Abst. Rev. 31, 601, 1961
126. Beveridge, J. M. R., et al., J. Nut. 79, 289, 1963
127. Becker, R. R., et al., J. Am. Chem. Soc. 75, 2020, 1953
128. Booker, W., et al., Am. J. Physiol. 189, 75, 1957
129. Myaknikov, A. L., Circulation 17, 99, 1958
130. Brozěk, J., Nut. Rev. 19, 161, 1961
131. Borquin, A., Am. J. Dig. Dis. 20, 75, 1953
132. Calder, J. H., Lancet 1, 556, 1963
133. McCormick, W. J., Arch. Pediat. 69, 151, 1952
134. Pitt-Rivers, R., Ann. N.Y. Acad. Sci. 86, 362, 1960
135. Page, I. H., et al., Arch. Path. 19, 530, 1935
136. Pitel, N. Y., Fed. Proc. 22, T135, 1963
137. Cohn, C., Nut. Rev. 20, 321, 1962
138. Gwinup, G., et al., Am. J. Clin. Nut. 13, 209, 1963
139. Hashim, S. A., et al., Lancet 1, 1105, 1960
140. Guravich, J. L., et al., Fed. Proc. 21, 44, 1962
141. Nut. Rev. 14, 132, 1956
142. Horlick, L., Canadian Med. Assn. J. 83, 1186, 1960

143. Horlick, L., Canadian Med. Assn. J. 85, 1127, 1961
144. Albrink, M. J., Arch. Int. Med. 109, 345, 1962
145. Hand, D. B., J. Am. Med. Assn. 181, 411, 1962
146. Horlick, L., Lab. Invest. 8, 723, 1959
147. Haust, H. L., et al., Arch. Biochem. 78, 367, 1958
148. Lewis, B., Lancet 1, 1090, 1958
149. Reiser, R., et al., Circul. Res. 7, 833, 1959
150. Watanbe, M., et al., J. Clin. Invest. 42, 1619, 1963
151. Lambert, G. F., et al., Proc. Soc. Exp. Biol. Med. 97, 544, 1958
152. Siperstein, M. D., et al., J. Biol. Chem. 210, 181, 1954
153. Bremer, J., Biochem. J. 63, 507, 1956
154. Eastwood, G., et al., J. Am. Diet. Assn. 42, 518, 1963
155. Karvinen, E., et al., J. Applied Physiol. 11, 143, 1957
156. Gordon, H., Lancet 2, 244, 1958
157. Connor, W. E., et al., J. Lab. Clin. Med. 57, 331, 1961
158. Dock, W., Am. J. Clin. Nut. 5, 674, 1957
159. Dock, W., Am. J. Clin. Nut. 6, 171, 1958
160. Shaper, A. G., Am. Heart J. 63, 437, 1962
161. Lowenstein, F. W., Am. J. Clin. Nut. 15, 175, 1964
162. Field, H., Jr., et al., Circulation 22, 547, 1960
163. Heyman, A., et al., Arch. Neurol. 5, 264, 1961
164. Dock, W., J. Am. Med. Assn. 170, 2199, 1959
165. Schroeder, H. A., *Mechanisms of Hypertension*, Charles C. Thomas, Springfield, Ill., 1957
166. Kinsell, L. W., et al., Diabetes 3, 113, 1954
167. Beaumont, J. L., et al., J. Atherosclerosis Res. 3, 210, 1963
168. Vacca, J. B., et al., Ann. Int. Med. 51, 1019, 1959
169. J. Am. Med. Assn. 168, 1773, 1958
170. Peyman, M. A., Am. Heart J. 62, 676, 1961

Chapter 6

1. Jolliffe, N., et al., J. Chron. Dis. 9, 636, 1959
2. Field, H., Jr., et al., Circulation 22, 547, 1960
3. Wilbur, A. T., et al., Am. Heart J. 52, 581, 1956
4. Morrison, L. M., Geriatrics 13, 12, 1958
5. King, C. G., J. Am. Diet. Assn. 42, 199, 1963
6. Parrish, H. M., J. Chron. Dis. 14, 326, 1961
7. Anos, W. F., et al., J. Am. Med. Assn. 152, 1090, 1958
8. Steiner, A., et al., Circulation 5, 605, 1952
9. Morrison, L. M., J. Lab. Clin. Med. 39, 550, 1952
10. Dock, W., Am. J. Clin. Nut. 5, 674, 1957
11. Keys, A., J. Am. Med. Assn. 164, 1912, 1957
12. Groen, J., et al., Medicine 38, 1, 1959
13. Keys, A., et al., Ann. Int. Med. 48, 83, 1958
14. Grundy, S. M., et al., Circulation 19, 496, 1959
15. Rouser, G., Am. J. Clin. Nut. 6, 681, 1958
16. Horlick, L., Circulation 10, 30, 1954
17. Albrink, M. J., et al., Am. J. Med. 31, 4, 1961

18. Nut. Rev. 19, 100, 1961
19. Peyman, M. A., Am. Heart J. 62, 676, 1961
20. Segall, S., et al., Canadian Med. Assn. J. 83, 521, 1960
21. Kinsell, L. W., et al., Am. J. Clin. Nut. 6, 628, 632, 1958
22. Mashford, M. L., et al., Circul. Res. 9, 7, 1961
23. Brown, D. F., et al., Am. J. Clin. Nut. 13, 1, 1963
24. Kuo, P. T., et al., Am. J. Med. 26, 68, 1959
25. Albrink, M. J., et al., J. Clin. Invest. 39, 441, 1960
26. Kinsell, L. W., et al., Am. J. Clin. Nut. 9, 1, 1961
27. Montaye, H. J., et al., Am. J. Clin. Nut. 7, 139, 1959
28. Grell, D., et al., Am. J. Clin. Nut. 10, 471, 1962
29. Nut. Rev. 21, 178, 1963
30. Nut. Rev. 19, 221, 1961
31. Sebrell, W. H., Jr., et al., J. Am. Diet. Assn. 40, 403, 1962
32. Horlick, L., Canadian Med. Assn. J. 85, 1127, 1961
33. Peterson, J. E., et al., Circulation 22, 247, 1960
34. Adlersberg, D., et al., Clin. Chem. 1, 18, 1955
35. Rosenman, R. H., et al., J. Am. Med. Assn. 169, 1286, 1959
36. Labecki, T. D., Am. J. Clin. Nut. 6, 325, 1958
37. Keys, A., et al., Clin. Chem. 1, 34, 1955
38. Gertler, M. M., et al., Circulation 2, 205, 1950
39. Gofman, J. W., et al., Circulation 2, 161, 1950
40. Glazier, F. W., et al., J. Gerontol, 9, 395, 1954
41. Gofman, J. W., et al., Modern Med. 21, 119, 1953
42. Lyon, T. P., et al., Calif. Med. 84, 325, 1956
43. Hirsch, E. F., et al., Physiol. Rev. 23, 185, 1943
44. Cullen, C. F., et al., Circulation 9, 335, 1954
45. Cheng, S. H., et al., Proc. Soc. Exp. Biol. Med. 101, 223, 1959
46. Duff, G. L., et al., J. Exp. Med. 92, 299, 1950
47. Kritchensky, D., Am. J. Clin. Nut. 10, 269, 1962
48. Gresham, G. A., et al., Brit. J. Exp. Path. 41, 395, 1960
49. Adlersberg, D., et al., J. Nut. 25, 255, 1943
50. Holman, T. R., Nut. Rev. 16, 33, 1958
51. Nath, M. C., et al., J. Nut. 69, 403, 1959
52. Steiner, A., J. Applied Nut. 16, 125, 1963
53. Garcia, L. R., Am. J. Clin. Nut. 9, 315, 1961
54. Anstall, H. B., et al., Lancet 1, 814, 1959
55. Blaxter, K. L., et al., J. Comp. Path. 64, 157, 176, 1954
56. Renaud, S., et al., J. Nut. 83, 149, 1964
57. Brock, J. F., Nut. Rev. 13, 1, 1955
58. Gresham, G. E., Brit. J. Exp. Path. 42, 166, 1961
59. Owren, P. A., Lancet 2, 975, 1964
60. Robertson, W. B., Lancet 1, 44, 1959
61. Hellerstein, H. K., et al., Am. Heart J. 42, 271, 1951
62. Gale, E. T., et al., Geriatrics 8, 80, 1953
63. Willis, G. C., Canadian Med. Assn. J. 72, 500, 1955
64. Kay, J. H., et al., Surgery 28, 124, 1950
65. Zierler, K. L., et al., Am. J. Physiol. 153, 127, 1948
66. Crump, W. E., et al., Texas State J. Med. 48, 1, 1952
67. Ames, S. R., et al., Inter. Rev. Vit. Res. 22, 401, 1951

68. Mason, K. E., Yale J. Biol. Med. 14, 605, 1942
69. Wilson, M. G., et al., Lancet 2, 266, 486, 1951
70. Mattill, H. A., Nut. Rev. 10, 225, 1952
71. Telford, E. A., et al., Air Univ. Sch. Aviation Med. Rep. 4, Project 21, 1201, 1954
72. Zierler, M., et al., Ann. N.Y. Acad. Sci. 52, 180, 1949
73. Houchim, O. B., et al., J. Biol. Chem. 146, 309, 313, 1942
74. De Nicola, P., Inter. Congress Vit. E, 1955
75. Shute, E. V., Inter. Congress Vit. E, 1955
76. Jessen, K. E., et al., Acta Path. Microbiol. Scand. 29, 72, 1951
77. Goria, A., Nut. Abst. Rev. 24, 658, 1954
78. Bacigalupo, F. R., et al., Am. J. Vet. Res. 14, 214, 1953
79. Mason, K. E., et al., Anat. Rec. 92, 33, 1945
80. Follis, R. H., Am. J. Clin. Nut. 4, 107, 1956
81. Dju, M. Y., et al., Am. J. Clin. Nut. 6, 50, 1958
82. Gillman, T., et al., Lancet 2, 1117, 1957; 2, 901, 1958
83. Gwinup, G., et al., Am. J. Clin. Nut. 13, 209, 1963
84. Horwitt, M. K., et al., J. Am. Diet. Assn. 38, 231, 1961
85. Schottelius, B. A., et al., Am. J. Physiol. 193, 219, 1958
86. Govier, W. M., et al., J. Pharmacol. Exp. Therap. 88, 373, 1946
87. Spaulding, M. E., et al., J. Biol. Chem. 170, 711, 1947
88. Crump, W., et al., Texas State J. Med. 48, 11, 1952
89. Suffel, P., Canadian Med. Assn. J. 74, 715, 1956
90. Wilson, M. G., et al., Lancet 1, 486, 1954
91. Hillman, R. W., Am. J. Clin. Nut. 5, 597, 1957
92. Capeci, N. E., et al., Am. J. Med. 26, 76, 1959
93. Pastor, B. H., et al., J. Am. Med. Assn. 180, 747, 1962
94. Harvald, B., et al., Lancet 2, 626, 1962
95. Gumpert, T. E., Lancet 1, 399, 1962
96. Krohn, B. G., et al., Ann. West. Med. Surg. 6, 484, 1952
97. Vogelsang, A., et al., Med. Rec. 160, 1, 1947
98. Allardyce, J., et al., Am. J. Physiol. 164, 48, 1951
99. Shute, E. V., et al., Nature 159, 772, 1946
100. Shute, E. V., Med. Rec. 160, 279, 1947
101. Gubner, M. D., Nut. Rev. 15, 353, 1957
102. Brown, J. B., Nut. Rev. 17, 321, 1959
103. Harris, P. L., J. Nut. 40, 367, 1950
104. Quaife, M. L., J. Nut. 40, 367, 1950
105. McCollister, R. J., Am. J. Clin. Nut. 12, 415, 1963
106. Smith, W. O., et al., Am. J. Med. Sci. 237, 413, 1959
107. Adelson, S. F., et al., U.S. Dept. Agric., A. R. S. 18608, 11, 1962
108. Klatskin, G., et al., J. Exp. Med. 100, 605, 615, 1954
109. J. Am. Med. Assn. 188, 33, 1964
110. Paul, O., Food Nut. News 35, 1, 1964
111. Myaknikov, A. L., Circulation 17, 99, 1958
112. Haldi, J., et al., J. Nut. 34, 389, 1947
113. Briggs, M. E., et al., Proc. Soc. Exp. Biol. Med. 51, 59, 1942
114. Smith, W. O., et al., J. Am. Med. Assn. 174, 77, 1960

115. Martin, H. E., et al., J. Clin. Invest. 26, 217, 1947
116. Wohl, M. G., et al., Proc. Soc. Exp. Biol. Med. 83, 323, 1953
117. Nut. Rev. 13, 291, 1955
118. Nut. Rev. 18, 262, 1960
119. Gilbert, R. A., et al., Ann. Int. Med. 25, 928, 1946
120. Egeli, E. S., et al., Am. Heart J. 59, 527, 1960
121. Bryant, J. M., Proc. Soc. Exp. Biol. Med. 67, 557, 1948
122. McAllen, P. M., Brit. Heart J. 17, 5, 1955
123. Nut. Rev. 14, 94, 1956
124. Moon, H. D., Circulation 16, 263, 1957
125. Holman, R. L., Am. J. Clin. Nut. 9, 565, 1961
126. Hartroft, W. S., Am. J. Clin. Nut. 15, 245, 1964
127. Pickering, D., et al., Am. J. Dis. Child. 102, 42, 1961
128. Bersohn, I., et al., Am. J. Clin. Nut. 4, 117, 1956
129. Keys, A., et al., J. Nut. 59, 39, 1956
130. Rainton, C. R., et al., New Engl. J. Med. 268, 569, 1963
131. Herrick, J. B., J. Am. Med. Assn. 59, 2015, 1912; 72, 387, 1919
132. Antar, M. A., et al., Am. J. Clin. Nut. 14, 169, 1964

Chapter 7

1. Young, C. M., J. Am. Med. Assn. 186, 903, 1963
2. Bruch, H., Borden's Rev. Nut. Res. 19, 4, 1958
3. Stunkard, A. J., et al., Arch. Int. Med. 103, 79, 1959
4. McCann, M., et al., J. Am. Diet. Assn. 31, 1108, 1955
5. Young, C. M., N.Y. State J. Med. 59, 2215, 1959
6. Bruch, H., Psychosomatic Med. 14, 337, 1952
7. Joncs, R. J., Nut. Rev. 21, 193, 1963
8. Cheldelin, V. H., ct al., J. Am. Chem. Soc. 43, 5004, 1951
9. Editorial, J. Am. Med. Assn. 173, 1141, 1960
10. Kaplan, H. I., et al., J. Nerv. Ment. Dis. 125, 181, 1957
11. Nodine, J. H., and Moyer, J. H., *Psychosomatic Medicine,* Lea & Febiger, Philadelphia, Pa., 1962
12. Blair, D., Psychosomatics 5, 69, 1964
13. Carter, C. W., et al., Biochem. J. 49, 227, 1951
14. Kotake, Y., J. Vitaminol. 1, 73, 1955
15. Artom, C., Am. J. Clin. Nut. 6, 221, 1958
16. Nut. Rev. 12, 308, 1954
17. Alexander, H. D., et al., J. Nut. 61, 329, 1957
18. Albrink, M. J., Arch. Int. Med. 109, 345, 1962
19. Jolliffe, N., et al., Arch. Int. Med. 109, 566, 1962
20. Caldwell, A. B., et al., Am. J. Clin. Nut. 12, 401, 1963
21. Keys, A., Am. J. Pub. Health 44, 864, 1954
22. Zelman, S., Arch. Int. Med. 90, 141, 1952
23. Westwater, J. O., et al., Gastroenterology 34, 686, 1958
24. Leevy, C. M., et al., Arch. Int. Med. 92, 527, 1953
25. Guggenheim, K., Metabolism 3, 44, 1954
26. Diengott, D., et al., Endocrinology 65, 602, 1959
27. Hazlett, B. C., Canadian Med. Assn. J. 85, 677, 1961

28. Cohn, C., Nut. Rev. 20, 321, 1962
29. Gwinup, G., et al., Am. J. Clin. Nut. 13, 209, 1963
30. Hashim, S. A., et al., Lancet 1, 1105, 1960
31. Stunkard, A. J., et al., Am. J. Med. 19, 78, 1955
32. Peckham, S. C., et al., J. Nut. 77, 187, 1962
33. Peifer, J. G., et al., J. Nut. 68, 155, 1959
34. Merrill, J. M., Circul. Res. 7, 709, 1959
35. Deykin, D., et al., J. Biol. Chem. 237, 3649, 1962
36. Peifer, J. G., et al., J. Nut. 70, 400, 1960
37. Cederquist, D. C., et al., J. Am. Diet. Assn. 28, 113, 223, 1952
38. Fryer, J. H., et al., J. Lab. Clin. Med. 45, 684, 1955
39. Dole, V. P., et al., Am. J. Clin. Nut. 2, 38, 1954
40. Adam, D. J. D., et al., J. Nut. 66, 555, 1958
41. Yudkin, J., et al., Lancet 2, 939, 1960
42. Masoro, E. J., et al., J. Biol. Chem. 185, 845, 1950
43. Pilkington, T. R. E., et al., Lancet 1, 856, 1960
44. Hansberger, F. K., et al., J. Biol. Chem. 208, 431, 1954
45. Stunkard, A. J., et al., Proc. Soc. Exp. Biol. Med. 89, 258, 1955
46. Stunkard, A. J., et al., Fed. Proc. 13, 147, 1954
47. Davidson, C. S., Arch. Int. Med. 94, 463, 1954
48. Mellinkoff, S. M., et al., J. Applied Physiol. 8, 535, 1956; 9, 85, 1956
49. Hartsook, E. W., et al., J. Nut. 81, 209, 1963
50. Meyer, J. H., Am. J. Physiol. 193, 488, 1958
51. Mayer, J., New Engl. J. Med. 249, 13, 1953
52. Nut. Rev. 13, 115, 1955
53. Egeli, E. S., et al., Am. Heart J. 59, 527, 1960
54. Drenick, E. J., et al., J. Am. Med. Assn. 187, 100, 1964
55. Bloom, W. L., Metabolism 8, 214, 1959
56. Fineberg, S. K., Ann. Int. Med. 52, 750, 1960
57. Shank, R. E., Nut. Rev. 19, 289, 1961
58. Nut. Rev. 16, 292, 1958
59. Le Riche, W. H., et al., Canadian Med. Assn. J. 85, 673, 1961
60. Lowe, C. W., et al., Am. J. Dis. Child. 79, 91, 1950
61. Nut. Rev. 19, 289, 1961
62. Winters, R. W., et al., Endocrinology 50, 388, 1952
63. Ralli, E. P., et al., *Vitamins and Hormones*, Academic Press, New York, N.Y., 1953
64. Gordon, E. S., et al., J. Am. Med. Assn. 186, 50, 1963
65. Thompson, M. M., et al., Am. J. Clin. Nut. 7, 80, 1959

Chapter 8

1. Selye, H., *The Stress of Life*, McGraw-Hill, New York, N.Y., 1956
2. Wolf, S., et al., N.Y. State J. Med. 47, 2509, 1947
3. Wolf, S., et al., Gastroenterology 10, 251, 1948

4. Wolf, S., and Wolff, H. G., *Human Gastric Function*, Oxford University Press, New York, N.Y., 1947
5. Mittelmann, B., et al., Psychosomatic Med. 4, 5, 1942
6. Hale, E. H., et al., J. Lab. Clin. Med. 35, 249, 1950
7. Nut. Rev. 1, 396, 1943
8. Gubner, R., Arch. Derm. Syph. 64, 688, 1951
9. Li, T., et al., Gastroenterology 6, 140, 1946
10. Ogawa, T., et al., Am. J. Physiol. 198, 619, 1960
11. Robert, A., et al., Proc. Soc. Exp. Biol. Med. 98, 9, 1958
12. Shay, H., et al., Gastroenterology 5, 43, 1945
13. Nut. Rev. 5, 308, 1947
14. Am. J. Clin. Nut. 15, 240, 1964
15. Horwitt, M. K., Fed. Proc. 17, 245, 1958
16. Horwitt, M. K., Fed. Proc. 18, 530, 1959
17. Zucker, T. F., Am. J. Clin. Nut. 6, 65, 1958
18. Follis, R. H., et al., Arch. Path. 35, 579, 1943
19. Gray, S. J., et al., 5th Annual Report on Stress, M. D. Public, New York, N.Y., 1955-56, p. 138
20. Gray, S. J., et al., Gastroenterology 19, 658, 1951
21. Williams, R. J., *Biochemical Individuality*, Wiley, New York, N.Y., 1956
22. Treskunov, K. A., et al., Nut. Abst. Rev. 31, 611, 1961
23. Wissmer, B., Nut. Abst. Rev. 31, 972, 1961
24. Bicknell, F., and Prescott, F., *The Vitamins in Medicine*, Lee Foundation for Nutritional Research, Milwaukee, Wis., 1953
25. Sippy, B. W., J. Am. Med. Assn. 64, 1625, 1915
26. Tui, C., J. Clin. Nut. 1, 232, 1953
27. Thomson, T. J., Clin. Sci. 17, 701, 1958
28. Fitzgerald, M. G., et al., Clin. Sci. 15, 635, 1956
29. Feinberg, W. D., et al., Proc. Staff Meet. Mayo Clin. 32, 299, 1957
30. Adams, R. N., et al., Glasgow Med. J. 35, 64, 1954
31. Schneider, M. A., et al., Am. J. Gastroenterol. 26, 722, 1956
32. Osmon, K. L., et al., Am. J. Gastroenterol. 28, 432, 1957
33. J. Am. Diet. Assn. 38, 425, 1961
34. Dock, W., J. Am. Med. Assn. 131, 875, 1946
35. Morris, J. M., et al., Brit. Med. J. 2, 1485, 1958
36. Hartroft, W. S., Am. J. Clin. Nut. 15, 205, 1964
37. Thomas, W. A., et al., Circulation 20, 992, 1959
38. Briggs, P. D., et al., Circulation 21, 538, 1960
39. Thomas, W. A., et al., Circulation 19, 65, 1959
40. Laureta, H. C., et al., Am. J. Clin. Nut. 15, 211, 1964
41. Berkowitz, D., Am. J. Clin. Nut. 15, 218, 1964
42. Hock, C. W., Am. J. Clin. Nut. 15, 223, 1964
43. Cayer, D., et al., Am. J. Clin. Nut. 15, 227, 1964
44. McHardy, G., et al., Am. J. Clin. Nut. 15, 229, 1964
45. Sullivan, B. H., et al., Gastroenterology 26, 868, 1954
46. Sydenstricker, V. P., J. Am. Med. Assn. 118, 1199, 1942
47. Kaplan, I. J., Am. J. Med. 207, 733, 1944
48. Evans, P. R. C., Brit. Med. J. 1, 612, 1954

49. Doll, R., et al., Lancet 1, 5, 1956
50. Marshall, E. A., et al., J. Am. Geriat. Soc. 4, 499, 1956
51. Friedlander, P. H., et al., Clin. Sci. 16, 731, 1957
52. Czok, G., et al., Nut. Abst. Rev. 26, 387, 1956
53. Subrahmanyan, V., et al., Am. Biochem. Exp. Med. 19, 61, 1959
54. Strub, I. H., et al., J. Am. Med. Assn. 163, 1603, 1957
55. Weiss, S., et al., Am. J. Gastroenterol. 29, 629, 1958
56. Sporn, A., et al., Nut. Abst. Rev. 28, 477, 1958
57. Burnett, C. H., et al., New Engl. J. Med. 240, 787, 1949
58. Scholz, D. A., et al., Arch. Int. Med. 95, 460, 1955
59. Kessler, E., Ann. Int. Med. 42, 324, 1955
60. James, A. H., et al., Clin. Sci. 8, 181, 1949

Chapter 9

1. Medes, G., et al., J. Biol. Chem. 197, 181, 1952
2. Nut. Rev. 13, 115, 1955
3. Biehl, J. P., et al., Proc. Soc. Exp. Biol. Med. 85, 389, 1954
4. Olsen, N. R., et al., J. Nut. 53, 317, 329, 1954
5. Porter, C. C., et al., Arch. Biochem. 18, 339, 1948
6. Kotake, Y., et al., J. Biochem. 40, 287, 291, 1953
7. Kotake, Y., et al., J. Vitaminol. 1, 73, 1955
8. Gershoff, S. N., et al., J. Nut. 73, 308, 1961
9. Martin, H. E., et al., J. Clin. Invest. 26, 216, 1947
10. Nut. Rev. 10, 21, 1952
11. Carter, C. W., et al., Biochem. J. 49, 227, 1951
12. Albertson, V., Diabetes 2, 184, 1953
13. Dohan, F. C., et al., Fed. Proc. 6, 97, 1947
14. Keys, A., et al., Geriatrics 12, 79, 1957
15. Cohen, A. M., Am. Heart J. 65, 291, 1963
16. Vilter, R. W., et al., J. Lab. Clin. Med. 42, 335, 1953
17. Faber, S. R., et al., Am. J. Clin. Nut. 12, 406, 1963
18. Price, J. M., et al., J. Clin. Invest. 30, 1600, 1957
19. Miller, E. C., et al., J. Biol. Chem. 159, 173, 1945
20. Bessey, O. A., et al., Pediatrics 20, 33, 1957
21. Schreimer, A. W., et al., J. Lab. Clin. Med. 40, 121, 1952
22. Rosen, D. A., et al., Proc. Soc. Exp. Biol. Med. 88, 321, 1955
23. Chow, B. F., et al., Am. J. Clin. Nut. 5, 431, 1957
24. Wohl, M. G., et al., Proc. Soc. Exp. Biol. Med. 105, 523, 1960
25. Hillman, R. W., et al., Am. J. Clin. Nut. 10, 512, 1962
26. Nut. Rev. 21, 326, 1963
27. Barach, J. H., et al., Diabetes 1, 441, 1952
28. Adlersberg, D., et al., Diabetes 5, 116, 1956
29. Daughaday. W. H., et al., J. Clin. Invest. 33, 1075, 1954
30. McCollister, R., et al., J. Lab. Clin. Med. 52, 128, 1958
31. Emerson, K., Jr., Nut. Rev. 6, 257, 1948
32. Nut. Rev. 10, 163, 1952

33. Womersley, R. A., et al., J. Clin. Invest. 34, 456, 1955
34. Moore, F. D., et al., Metabolism 4, 379, 1955
35. Daughaday, W. H., Nut. Rev. 17, 289, 1959
36. Bortz, W. M., et al., Am. J. Clin. Nut. 3, 494, 1955
37. Slawson, P. F., et al., J. Am. Med. Assn. 185, 166, 1963
38. Osserman, K. E., et al., Ann. Int. Med. 34, 72, 1951
39. Nut. Rev. 9, 198, 1951
40. Hjörth, P., Acta Med. Scand. 105, 67, 1940
41. Banerjee, S., et al., J. Biol. Chem. 190, 177, 1951
42. Murray, H. G., Proc. Soc. Exp. Biol. Med. 69, 351, 1948
43. Nut. Rev. 4, 259, 1946
44. Diengott, D., et al., Endocrinology 65, 602, 1959
45. Schwarz, K., et al., Arch. Biochem. Biophys. 72, 515, 1957
46. Schwarz, K., et al., Arch. Biochem. Biophys. 85, 292, 1959
47. Mertz, W., et al., Am. J. Physiol. 196, 614, 1959
48. Gardner, L. I., J. Lab. Clin. Med. 35, 592, 1950
49. Meites, J., et al., Am. J. Clin. Nut. 5, 381, 1957
50. Cohn, C., Nut. Rev. 20, 321, 1962
51. Antoneades, H. N., et al., Diabetes 11, 261, 1962
52. Antoneades, H. N., et al., New Engl. J. Med. 267, 218, 1962
53. Vogelsang, A., Ann. N.Y. Acad. Sci. 52, 406, 1949
54. Butturini, U., Ann. N.Y. Acad. Sci. 52, 397, 1949
55. Gray, D. E., et al., Canadian J. Biochem. Physiol. 32, 491, 1954
56. Block, M. T., Clin. Med. 57, 112, 1950; 60, 1, 1953
57. George, N., Summary 3, 74, 1951
58. Day, R., South. Med. J. 44, 549, 1951
59. Coatsworth, R. C., Summary 3, 25, 1951
60. Tolgyes, S., et al., Canadian Med. Assn. J. 76, 730, 1957
61. Lee, P., Summary 8, 85, 1957
62. Dietrich, H. W., South. Med. J. 43, 743, 1950
63. Bicknell, F., and Prescott, F., *The Vitamins in Medicine*, Lee Foundation for Nutritional Research, Milwaukee, Wis., 1953
64. Nut. Rev. 13, 325, 1955
65. Sherman, W. C., Food Nut. News 35, 3, 1964
66. Harding, R. S., et al., J. Nut. 68, 323, 1959
67. Zucker, T. A., Am. J. Clin. Nut. 6, 65, 1958
68. Lamont-Havers, R. W., Borden's Rev. Nut. Res. 24, 1, 15, 1963
69. Oppenheimer, E. H., et al., Bull. Johns Hopkins Hosp. 107, 297, 1960
70. Krehl, W. A., Nut. Rev. 11, 225, 1953
71. Ershoff, B. H., et al., J. Nut. 50, 299, 1953
72. Thornton, G. H. M., et al., J. Clin. Invest. 34, 1073, 1955
73. Hodges, R. E., et al., J. Clin. Invest. 38, 1421, 1959
74. Guggenheim, K., Metabolism 3, 44, 1954
75. Hundley, J. M., J. Biol. Chem. 181, 1, 1949
76. Kimble, M. S., et al., Am. J. Med. Sci. 212, 574, 1946
77. Moore, T., Biochem. J. 31, 155, 1937
78. Vorhaus, M. G., et al., J. Am. Med. Assn. 105, 1580, 1935

79. Needles, W., Arch. Neurol. Psychiat. 41, 1222, 1939
80. Fein, H. D., et al., J. Am. Med. Assn. 115, 1973, 1940
81. Vorhaus, M. G., Am. J. Med. Sci. 198, 837, 1939
82. King, G., et al., J. Obst. Gynec. 52, 130, 1945
83. Thompson, M. M., et al., Am. J. Clin. Nut. 7, 80, 1959
84. Holler, J. W., J. Am. Med. Assn. 131, 1186, 1946
85. Bryant, J. M., Proc. Soc. Exp. Biol. Med. 67, 557, 1948
86. Nut. Rev. 18, 262, 1960
87. Gilbert, R. A., et al., Ann. Int. Med. 25, 928, 1946
88. Shils, M. E., Am. J. Clin. Nut. 14, 240, 1964
89. Egeli, E. S., et al., Am. Heart J. 59, 527, 1960
90. Holman, R. F., Nut. Rev. 16, 33, 1958
91. New, M. I., et al., Diabetes 12, 208, 1963
92. Kinsell, L. W., et al., New Engl. J. Med. 261, 431, 1959
93. Thomas, W. A., et al., Am. Heart J. 52, 581, 1956
94. Groen, J., et al., Am. J. Clin. Nut. 10, 456, 1962
95. Cochran, G. C., et al., J. Clin. Nut. 1, 295, 1953
96. Willis, G. C., Canadian Med. Assn. J. 76, 1044, 1957
97. Leevy, C. M., et al., Arch. Int. Med. 92, 527, 1953
98. Beckett, A. G., et al., Lancet 2, 14, 1960
99. Nut. Rev. 18, 182, 1960
100. Leevy, C. M., J. Med. Soc. N.J. 55, 151, 1958
101. Becker, B., et al., Diabetes 3, 175, 1954
102. Duncan, L. J. P., et al., Lancet 1, 822, 1958
103. Schneider, R. W., et al., Am. J. Med. Sci. 212, 462, 1946
104. Hartroft, W. S., Am. J. Path. 31, 381, 1955
105. Selye, H., et al., J. Urol. 56, 399, 1946

Chapter 10

1. Eising, L., J. Bone Joint Surg. 45a, 69, 1963
2. Silberberg, M., et al., J. Gerontol. 7, 24, 1952
3. Barboriak, J. J., et al., J. Nut. 63, 601, 1957
4. Morgan, A. F., J. Biol. Chem. 195, 583, 1952
5. Selye, H., Brit. Med. J. 2, 1129, 1949
6. Tuchweber, B., et al., Am. J. Clin. Nut. 13, 238, 1963
7. Hogan, A. G., et al., J. Nut. 41, 203, 1950
8. MacIntyre, I., et al., Biochem. J. 70, 456, 1958
9. Maynard, L. A., et al., J. Nut. 64, 85, 1958
10. Bunce, G. E., et al., J. Nut. 76, 23, 1962
11. Steiner, A. J., J. Applied Nut. 16, 125, 1963
12. Morgales, S., et al., J. Biol. Chem. 124, 767, 1938
13. Ames, S. R., J. Biol. Chem. 169, 503, 1947
14. Lamont-Havers, R. W., Borden's Rev. Nut. Res. 24, 1, 15, 1963
15. Abbasy, M. A., et al., Lancet 2, 181, 1937
16. Hall, M. G., et al., Ann. Int. Med. 13, 415, 1935
17. Hodge, R. E., et al., Am. J. Clin. Nut. 11, 180, 1962
18. Tui, C., J. Clin. Nut. 1, 232, 1953
19. Glatzel, H., Nut. Abst. Rev. 34, 507, 1964

20. Williams, R. J., *Biochemical Individuality*, Wiley, New York, N.Y., 1956
21. Bean, W. B., et al., Proc. Soc. Exp. Biol. Med. 86, 693, 1954
22. Wickson, M. E., et al., J. Biol. Chem. 162, 209, 1946
23. Dugal, L. P., et al., Endocrinology 44, 420, 1949
24. Nut. Rev. 15, 185, 1957
25. Ershoff, B. H., Nut. Rev. 13, 33, 1955
26. West, H. F., Lancet 2, 877, 1958
27. Selye, H., *Calciphylaxis*, University of Chicago Press, Chicago, Ill., 1962
28. Nut. Rev. 13, 46, 1955
29. Zucker, T. A., Am. J. Clin. Nut. 6, 65, 1958
30. Oppenheimer, E. H., et al., Bull. Johns Hopkins Hosp. 107, 297, 1960
31. Krehl, W. A., Nut. Rev. 11, 225, 1953
32. Ralli, E. T., Nut. Symposium Series 5, 78, 1952
33. Rufenstein, E. C., Metabolism 7, 78, 1958
34. Greenman, L., et al., J. Clin. Invest. 30, 644, 1951
35. Meites, J., et al., Am. J. Clin. Nut. 5, 381, 1957
36. Gardner, L. I., J. Lab. Clin. Med. 35, 592, 1950
37. Cantin, M., et al., Exp. Med. Surg. 318, 20, 1962

Chapter 11

1. Selye, H., *The Stress of Life*, McGraw-Hill, New York, N.Y., 1956
2. J. Am. Med. Assn. 140, 784, 1949
3. Seronde, J., et al., J. Inf. Dis. 97, 35, 1955
4. Clark, I., et al., Endocrinology 56, 232, 1955
5. Ludovici, P. P., et al., Proc. Soc. Exp. Biol. Med. 77, 526, 1951
6. Axelrod, A. E., Nut. Rev. 10, 353, 1952
7. Axelrod, A. E., et al., Ann. N.Y. Acad. Sci. 63, 202, 1955
8. Axelrod, A. E., J. Nut. 72, 325, 1960
9. Barboriak, J. J., et al., J. Nut. 63, 601, 1957
10. Williams, R. J., *Biochemical Individuality*, Wiley, Now York, N.Y., 1956
11. Hodges, R. E., et al., Am. J. Clin. Nut. 9, 244, 1961
12. Thornton, G. H., et al., J. Clin. Invest. 34, 1073, 1955
13. Bean, W. B., et al., Proc. Soc. Exp. Biol. Med. 86, 693, 1954
14. Hodges, R. E., et al., Am. J. Clin. Nut. 11, 187, 1962
15. Yamada, K., et al., J. Vitaminol. 5, 188, 1959
16. Vilter, R. W., et al., J. Lab. Clin. Med. 42, 335, 1953
17. Pinkerton, H., et al., Science 89, 368, 1939
18. Woolley, J. G., et al., Pub. Health Rep. 57, 149, 1942
19. Kligler, I. J., et al., J. Path. Bact. 46, 619, 1938
20. Jungeblut, C. W., et al., J. Immunol. 33, 203, 1937
21. Jungeblut, C. W., J. Exp. Med. 70, 315, 1939
22. Klenner, F. R., Tri-State Med. J. July 1954

23. Klenner, F. R., Tri-State Med. J. Sept. 1956
24. Klenner, F. R., Tri-State Med. J. June 1957
25. Klenner, F. R., Tri-State Med. J. Oct. 1958
26. Klenner, F. R., Tri-State Med. J. Feb. 1959
27. Klenner, F. R., Tri-State Med. J. Feb. 1960
28. Knight, C. A., et al., J. Exp. Med. 79, 29, 1944
29. Burkhaug, K. E., Acta Tubercul. Scand. 13, 45, 1939
30. Steinbach, M. M., et al., Am. Rev. Tubercul. 43, 401, 414, 1941
31. Cottingham, E., et al., J. Immunol. 47, 493, 1943
32. Banerjee, S., et al., J. Biol. Chem. 190, 177, 1951
33. Stefanini, M., et al., Proc. Soc. Exp. Biol. Med. 75, 806, 1950
34. Madison, R. R., et al., Proc. Soc. Exp. Biol. Med. 37, 402, 1937
35. Madison, R. R., et al., Proc. Soc. Exp. Biol. Med. 39, 545, 1938
36. Cameron, G. D. W., Canadian Pub. Health J. 29, 404, 1938
37. Cuttle, T. D., Quart. J. Med. 7, 575, 1938
38. Neander, G., Acta Med. Scand. 109, 453, 1942
39. Chu, F., et al., Proc. Soc. Exp. Biol. Med. 38, 679, 1938
40. Spink, W. N., et al., J. Immunol. 44, 289, 1942
41. Nut. Rev. 4, 259, 1946
42. Nungester, W. J., et al., J. Infect. Dis. 83, 50, 1948
43. Faulkner, J. M., New Engl. J. Med. 213, 19, 1935
44. Crandon, J. H., et al., New Engl. J. Med. 223, 353, 1940
45. Klenner, F. R., South. Med. Surg. 110, 36, 1948
46. Klenner, F. R., South. Med. Surg. 113, 101, 1951
47. Klenner, F. R., South. Med. Surg. 114, 194, 1952
48. Klenner, F. R., J. Applied Nut. 6, 274, 1953
49. Nut. Rev. 10, 217, 1952
50. Guggenheim, K., et al., J. Immunol. 58, 133, 1948
51. Wissler, R. W., J. Infect. Dis. 80, 250, 264, 1947
52. Nut. Rev. 16, 313, 1958
53. Ershoff, B. H., Nut. Rev. 13, 33, 1955
54. O'Dell, B. L., et al., Arch. Biochem. Biophys. 54, 232, 1955
55. Nut. Rev. 21, 170, 1963
56. Lahey, M. E., Pediat. Clin. No. Am. 9, 689, 1962
57. Wilson, J. F., et al., J, Pediat. 60, 787, 1962
58. Huizenga, K. A., et al., Am. J. Med. 31, 572, 1961
59. Lehman, E., et al. J. Am. Med. Assn. 114, 386, 1940
60. Wolf, J., Nut. Rev. 20, 161, 1962
61. Getz, H. R., et al., Am. Rev. Tubercul. 64, 381, 1951
62. Spector, S., et al., Am. J. Dis. Child. 66, 376, 1943
63. Brenner, S., et al., Arch. Int. Med. 71, 482, 1943
64. Popper, H., et al., Proc. Soc. Exp. Biol. Med. 68, 676, 1948
65. Jacobs, A. L., et al., J. Clin. Nut. 2, 155, 1954
66. Josephs, H. W., Am. J. Dis. Child. 65, 712, 1943
67. Green, H. N., et al., Brit. Med. J. 2, 595, 1931

68. Burn, C. G., et al., Yale J. Biol. Med. 14, 89, 1941
69. Simpson, J. W., et al., Am. J. Obst. Gynec. 32, 125, 1936
70. Kahn, R. H., Am. J. Anat. 95, 309, 1954
71. Porter, A. D., et al., Brit. J. Derm. 62, 355, 1950
72. Porter, A. D., Brit. J. Derm. 63, 123, 1951
73. Lewis, J. M., et al., J. Pediat. 31, 496, 1947
74. Abbott, O. D., et al., Am. J. Physiol. 126, 254, 1939
75. Moore, T., Biochem. J. 34, 1321, 1940
76. King, J. D., Brit. Dent. J. 74, 113, 141, 169, 1943
77. Smith, W. J., Brit. Dent. J. 72, 140, 1942
78. Hillman, R. W., et al., Am. J. Clin. Nut. 10, 512, 1962
79. Tompkins, E. H., Am. Rev. Tubercul. 33, 625, 1936
80. McCormick, W. J., Arch. Pediat. 68, 1, 1951; 69, 151, 1952
81. Dalton, W. L., J. Ind. State Med. Assn. 55, 1151, 1962
82. Calleja, H. B., et al., Ohio State Med. J. 56, 821, 1960
83. Baur, H., et al., J. Am. Med. Assn. 156, 565, 1954
84. Hoffer, A., Brit. Med. J. 1, 1342, 1962

Chapter 12

1. Sebrell, W. H., et al., Pub. Health Rep. 53, 2282, 1938; 54, 2121, 1939
2. Ramalingaswami, V., et al., Brit. J. Derm. 65, 1, 1953
3. Bicknell, F., and Prescott, F., *The Vitamins in Medicine,* Lee Foundation for Nutritional Research, Milwaukee, Wis., 1953
4. Zaraponetis, C. J. D., J. Invest. Derm. 15, 399, 1950
5. Shaw, C., Tenn. Med. Assn. J. 39, 329, 1946
6. Tuchweber, B., et al., Am. J. Clin. Nut. 13, 238, 1963
7. Zubiran, S., et al., *Vitamins and Hormones,* Academic Press, New York, N.Y., 1953
8. Herbert, V., Arch. Int. Med. 110, 649, 1962
9. Gough, K. R., et al., Quart. J. Med. 32, 243, 1963
10. Field, H., et al., Am. J. Dig. Dis. 12, 246, 1945
11. Sieve, B. F., Virg. Med. Month. 72, 6, 1945
12. Gross, P., et al., N.Y. State J. Med. 50, 2683, 1950
13. Vilter, R. W., et al., J. Lab. Clin. Med. 42, 335, 1953
14. Kritchevsky, D., Am. J. Clin. Nut. 10, 269, 1962
15. Lambert, G. F., et al., Proc. Soc. Exp. Biol. Med. 97, 544, 1958
16. Myaknikov, A. L., Circulation 17, 99, 1958
17. Lindberg, W. Q., Am. J. Clin. Nut. 6, 601, 1958
18. Spies, T. D., J. Am. Med. Assn. 167, 897, 1958
19. Vilter, R. W., et al., Nut. Symposium Series 5, 104, 1952
20. Holman, R. T., Nut. Rev. 16, 33, 1958
21. Holman, R. T., et al., Am. J. Clin. Nut. 14, 70, 1964
22. Wachstein, M., et al., J. Lab. Clin. Med. 40, 550, 1952
23. Horwitt, M. K., et al., J. Nut. 39, 357, 1949
24. Vakil, R. J., Nut. Rev. 4, 314, 1946
25. Hodges, R. E., et al., Am. J. Clin. Nut. 11, 180, 1962

26. Gershoff, S. M., et al., J. Nut. 73, 308, 1961
27. Porter, C. C., et al., Arch. Biochem. 18, 339, 1948
28. Mueller, J. F., et al., J. Clin. Invest. 29, 193, 1950
29. Schreiner, A. W., et al., J. Lab. Clin. Med. 40, 121, 1952
30. Hodges, R. E., et al., Am. J. Clin. Nut. 11, 187, 1962
31. Hubler, W. R., Arch. Derm. 79, 644, 1959
32. Morgan, A. F., J. Am. Med. Women's Assn. 6, 179, 1951
33. Mulholland, J. H., et al., Ann. Surg. 118, 1015, 1943
34. Lee, M., Brit. J. Derm. 65, 131, 1953
35. Burgess, J. F., et al., Canadian Med. Assn. J. 59, 242, 1948
36. Owing, J. C., Ann. Surg. 131, 652, 1950
37. Block, M. T., Clin. Med. 57, 112, 1950; 60, 1, 1953
38. Dowd, G. C., Ann. N.Y. Acad. Sci. 52, 365, 1949
39. Coatsworth, R. C., Summary 3, 1, 1951
40. Beattie, J., Brit. Med. J. 2, 813, 1947
41. Klenner, F. R., Tri-State Med. J. Dec. 1957
42. Klenner, F. R., Tri-State Med. J. July 1954
43. Babcock, M. J., J. Nut. 55, 323, 1955
44. Nut. Rev. 18, 112, 1960
45. Godwin, K. O., J. Nut. 69, 121, 1959
46. Bean, W. B., J. Invest. Derm. 20, 27, 1953
47. Sibinga, M. D., Pediatrics 24, 225, 1959
48. Nut. Rev. 15, 327, 1957
49. Snyderman, S. E., et al., Am. Med. Assn. J. Dis. Child. 97, 192, 1959
50. Maynard, L. A., et al., J. Nut. 64, 85, 1958
51. Poznanskaia, A. A., Biochemistry 23, 215, 1958
52. Kalz, F., Arch. Derm. 78, 740, 1958
53. Kinny, T. D., et al., J. Exp. Med. 102, 151, 1955
54. Gubner, R., Arch. Derm. Syph. 64, 688, 1951
55. Rogachefsky, H., N.Y. State J. Med. 64, 2988, 1964
56. Lamb, J. H., N.Y. State J. Med. 59, 59, 1959
57. Knox, J. M., et al., J. Am. Med. Assn. 179, 639, 1958

Chapter 13

1. Hodges, R. E., et al., Am. J. Clin. Nut. 11, 180, 187, 1962
2. Leevy, C. M., et al., Am. J. Clin. Nut. 10, 46, 1962
3. Merrill, A. G., et al., Am. J. Clin. Nut. 4, 497, 1956
4. Bicknell, F., and Prescott, F., *The Vitamins in Medicine,* Lee Foundation for Nutritional Research, Milwaukee, Wis., 1953
5. Vilter, R. W., et al., J. Lab. Clin. Med. 42, 335, 1953
6. Gubner, R., et al., Am. J. Med. Sci. 221, 176, 1951
7. Shils, M. E., Am. J. Clin. Nut. 15, 133, 1964
8. Abt, H. C., et al., Am. J. Med. Sci. 197, 229, 1939
9. Valberg, L. S., et al., Brit. J. Nut. 15, 473, 1961
10. Keuter, E. J. W., Nut. Abst. Rev. 29, 273, 1959
11. Foldes, F., et al., Brit. Med. J. 1, 317, 1941
12. Egana, E., et al., Am. J. Physiol. 137, 731, 1942
13. Williams, R. D., et al., Arch. Int. Med. 69, 721, 1942

14. Smith, S. C., et al., J. Nut. 36, 405, 1948
15. Bean, W. B., et al., Proc. Soc. Exp. Biol. Med. 86, 693, 1954
16. Nut. Rev. 14, 295, 1956
17. Thornton, G. H. M., et al., J. Clin. Invest. 34, 1073, 1955
18. Watson, J., et al., J. Am. Med. Assn. 129, 802, 1945
19. Goodhart, R. S., Am. J. Clin. Nut. 5, 612, 1957
20. Liener, I. E., Am. J. Clin. Nut. 11, 280, 1962
21. Irvin, J. L., et al., Am. J. Physiol. 132, 202, 1941
22. Thompson, S. Y., et al., Brit. J. Nut. 3, 50, 1945
23. Clausen, S. W., et al., Fed. Proc. 5, 129, 1946
24. Streeten, D. H. P., et al., J. Physiol. 118, 149, 1952
25. Black, D. A. K., et al., Lancet 1, 244, 1952
26. Tui, C., J. Clin. Nut. 1, 232, 1953
27. Ingelfinger, F. J., et al., J. Clin. Invest. 22, 699, 1943
28. J. Am. Diet. Assn. 38, 425, 1961
29. Krehl, W. A., Borden's Rev. Nut. Res. 20, 1, 1959
30. Slinger, S. J., et al., J. Nut. 52, 75, 1954
31. Keys, A., et al., J. Nut. 27, 165, 1944
32. Mass, W., et al., J. Bact. 60, 733, 1950
33. Najjar, V. A., et al., J. Am. Med. Assn. 126, 357, 1944
34. Nath, M. C., et al., Biochem. J. 81, 220, 1961
35. Elvehjem, C. A., et al., J. Agric. Food Chem. 5, 754, 1957
36. Barboriak, J. J., et al., J. Nut. 63, 601, 1957
37. Nut. Rev. 12, 245, 1954
38. Morgan, T. B., et al., Nature 180, 543, 1957
39. Luckey, T. D., et al., J. Nut. 57, 169, 1955
40. Nichol, C. A., Cancer Res. 22, 495, 1962
41. Yamaguchi, T., et al., J. Vitaminol. 5, 88, 1959
42. Walden, R. R., et al., Am. J. Med. 36, 269, 1964
43. Nut. Rev. 14, 166, 1956
44. Nut. Rev. 15, 65, 1957
45. Matsukawa, D., et al., J. Vitaminol. 1, 43, 1954; 2, 53, 1955
46. Smith, M. C., J. Nut. 20, 19, 1940
47. Becker, G. L., Am. J. Dig. Dis. 19, 344, 1952
48. Frazer, A. C., et al., Nature 148, 167, 1942
49. Editorial, J. Am. Med. Assn. 135, 512, 1947
50. Alvarez, W. C., Gastroenterology 9, 315, 1947
51. Curtis, A. C., et al., J. Am. Med. Assn. 113, 1785, 1939
52. Curtis, A. C., et al., Arch. Int. Med. 63, 54, 1939
53. Mahle, A. E., et al., Gastroenterology 9, 44, 1947
54. Javert, C. T., et al., Am. J. Obst. Gynec. 42, 409, 1941
55. Jackson, R. W., J. Nut. 7, 607, 1934
56. Elliott, M. C., et al., Proc. Soc. Exp. Biol. Med. 43, 240, 1940
57. Thiele, G. H., South. Med. J. 35, 920, 1942
58. J. Am. Med. Assn. 123, 967, 1943
59. Back, E. H., et al., Arch. Dis. Childh. 37, 106, 1962
60. Bunce, G. E., et al., J. Nut. 76, 23, 1962
61. Fernandez, J., et al., J. Clin. Invest. 41, 488, 1962

62. Nut. Rev. 10, 163, 1952
63. McAllen, P. M., Brit. Heart J. 17, 5, 1955

Chapter 14

1. Grace, W. J., et al., Gastroenterology 26, 462, 1954
2. Wolf, S., and Wolff, H. G., *Human Gastric Function,* Oxford University Press, New York, N.Y., 1947
3. Lahey, M. E., Pediat. Clin. No. Am. 9, 689, 1962
4. Uyeyama, K., et al., Gastroenterology 23, 143, 1953
5. Nut. Rev. 7, 349, 1949
6. Nut. Rev. 14, 295, 1956
7. Machella, T. E., Am. J. Med. 7, 191, 1949
8. Fernandez, J., et al., J. Clin. Invest. 41, 488, 1962
9. Butterworth, G. E., Jr., et al., Ann. Int. Med. 48, 8, 1958
10. Hand, D. B., J. Am. Med. Assn. 181, 411, 1962
11. Cooper, B. A., et al., Canadian Med. Assn. J. 85, 987, 1961
12. Crosby, W. H., J. Chron. Dis. 12, 583, 1960
13. Butterworth, C. E., et al., J. Lab. Clin. Med. 50, 673, 1957
14. Nut. Rev. 11, 261, 1953
15. Dju, M. Y., et al., Am. J. Clin. Nut. 6, 50, 1958
16. Adlersberg, D., et al., J. Nut. 25, 255, 1943
17. Nut. Rev. 10, 169, 1952
18. Sheldon, W., Pediatrics 23, 132, 1959
19. Boyer, P. H., et al., Am. J. Dis. Child. 91, 131, 1956
20. Gerrard, J. W., et al., Quart. J. Med. 24, 23, 1955
21. Bayless, T. M., et al., Arch. Int. Med. 111, 83, 1963
22. Mike, E. M., Am. J. Clin. Nut. 7, 463, 1959
23. Dicke, W. K., et al., Acta Pediat. 42, 34, 1953
24. Rubin, C. E., et al., Gastroenterology 38, 28, 1960
25. di Sant'Agnese, P. A., et al., J. Am. Med. Assn. 180, 308, 1962
26. Anderson, D. H., et al., Pediatrics 11, 207, 1953
27. Kowlessar, O. D., et al., J. Clin. Invest. 43, 894, 1964
28. Conrad, M. E., et al., J. Clin. Invest. 43, 963, 1964
29. Sakula, J., et al., Lancet 2, 876, 1957
30. Bolt, R. J., et al., Ann. Int. Med. 60, 581, 1964
31. Anderson, C. M., Arch. Dis. Childh. 35, 419, 1960
32. Yardley, J. H., et al., New Engl. J. Med. 267, 1173, 1962
33. Hendrix, T. R., et al., Gastroenterology 46, 203, 1964
34. Samloff, I. M., et al., Ann. Int. Med. 60, 673, 1964
35. Sheldon, W., Postgrad. Med. 15, 79, 1954
36. Levine, R. A., et al., Am. J. Clin. Nut. 14, 242, 1964
37. Adlersberg, D., et al., Gastroenterology 10, 822, 1948
38. Goldman, A. S., et al., Pediatrics 29, 448, 1962
39. Back, E. H., et al., Arch. Dis. Childh. 37, 106, 1962
40. Nut. Rev. 20, 335, 1962
41. Nut. Rev. 21, 195, 1963
42. Daynes, G., Proc. Roy. Soc. Med. 49, 391, 1956
43. Hogan, A. G., Nut. Abst. Rev. 19, 750, 1950

44. Watt, S. L., Am. J. Hygiene 39, 145, 1944
45. Cramer, W., et al., Brit. J. Exp. Path. 5, 300, 1924
46. Clausen, S. W., J. Am. Med. Assn. 101, 1384, 1933
47. McCance, R. A., Brit. J. Nut. 14, 59, 1960
48. Polachek, A. A., et al., Ann. Int. Med. 54, 636, 1961
49. Scudamore, H. H., Ann. Int. Med. 55, 433, 1961
50. Kinny, T. D., et al., J. Exp. Med. 102, 151, 1955
51. Beck, I. T., et al., Gastroenterology 43, 60, 1962
52. MacDonald, R. A., Arch. Int. Med. 110, 424, 1962
53. Davis, J. N. P., Lancet 1, 317, 1948
54. Holmes, E. G., et al., Lancet 1, 395, 1948
55. Duncan, L. J. P., et al., Lancet 1, 822, 1958

Chapter 15

1. Cooper, L. F., et al., *Nutrition in Health and Disease,* Lippincott, Philadelphia, Pa., 1958, ch. 26
2. Selye, H., *The Stress of Life,* McGraw-Hill, New York, N.Y., 1956
3. Selye, H., Canadian Med. Assn. J. 61, 553, 1949
4. Kaplan, H., et al., Ann. Allergy 21, 41, 1963
5. Berman, B. A., Ann. Allergy 21, 91, 1963
6. Pottenger, F. M., et al., Ann. West. Med. Surg. 6, 484, 1952
7. Tui, C., J. Clin. Nut. 1, 232, 1953
8. Goldfarb, A. A., et al., N.Y. State J. Med. 61, 2721, 1961
9. Smith, L. W., et al., Antibiotic Med. Clin. Therap. 4, 515, 1957
10. Annand, J. C., Practitioner 175, 725, 1955
11. Moll, H. H., Brit. Med. J. 1, 976, 1932
12. Yudkin, J., Brit. Med. J. 1, 1388, 1952
13. Simon, S. W., J. Allergy 22, 183, 1951
14. Ershoff, B. H., et al., J. Nut. 50, 299, 1953
15. Pudelkewicz, C., et al., J. Nut. 70, 348, 1960
16. Crook, W. G., et al., Pediatrics 27, 790, 1961
17. Moore, M. W., Ann. Allergy 16, 152, 1958
18. Moriarity, R. J., et al., Ann. Allergy 21, 424, 1963
19. Bean, W. B., et al., Proc. Soc. Exp. Biol. Med. 86, 693, 1954
20. Thornton, G. H. M., et al., J. Clin. Invest. 34, 1073, 1955
21. Hodges, R. E., et al., J. Clin. Invest. 38, 1421, 1959
22. Morgan, A. F., J. Am. Med. Women's Assn. 6, 179, 1951
23. Williams, R. J., *Biochemical Individuality,* Wiley, New York, N.Y., 1956
24. Seronde, J., et al., J. Infect. Dis. 97, 35, 1955
25. Wohl, M. G., and Goodhart, R. S., *Modern Nutrition in Health and Disease,* Lea & Febiger, Philadelphia, Pa., 1955
26. Irvine, W. T., Lancet 1, 1064, 1959
27. Irvine, W. T., et al., Lancet 1, 1061, 1959
28. Epps, H. M. R., Biochem. J. 39, 42, 1945
29. Wilson, C. W. M., J. Physiol. 125, 534, 1954

30. Bicknell, F., and Prescott, F., *The Vitamins in Medicine,* Lee Foundation for Nutritional Research, Milwaukee, Wis., 1953
31. Vilter, R. W., et al., J. Lab. Clin. Med. 42, 335, 1953
32. Noah, J. W., et al., J. Allergy 34, 203, 1963
33. Mitchell, R. G., et al., J. Applied Physiol. 6, 387, 1954
34. Sullivan, B. H., et al., Gastroenterology 26, 868, 1954
35. Roberts, H. J., New Engl. J. Med. 268, 562, 1963
36. Beall, G. N., J. Allergy, 34, 8, 1963
37. Van Arsdel, P. P., Jr., et al., Am. Med. Assn. Arch. Int. Med. 106, 714, 1960
38. Sircus, W., Quart. J. Exp. Physiol. 38, 25, 1953
39. Harris, P. L., et al., Inter. Congress Vit. E, 1955
40. Ames, S. R., et al., Inter. Rev. Vit. Res. 22, 401, 1951
41. Mason, K. E., Yale J. Biol. Med. 14, 605, 1942
42. Aitken, F. C., et al., Nut. Abst. Rev. 30, 341, 1960
43. Harris, P. L., Ann. N.Y. Acad. Sci. 52, 240, 1949
44. Pudelkewicz, C., et al., J. Nut. 70, 348, 1960
45. Nut. Rev. 4, 259, 1946
46. Klenner, F. R., Tri-State Med. J. July 1954
47. Nut. Rev. 6, 215, 1948
48. Nut. Rev. 15, 185, 1957
49. Brown, E. A., et al., Ann. Allergy 7, 1, 1949
50. Holmes, H. N., South. Med. Surg. 105, 56, 1943
51. Sulzberger, M. B., et al., Proc. Soc. Exp. Biol. Med. 32, 716, 1935
52. Cormia, F. E., Canadian Med. Assn. J. 36, 392, 1937
53. Cormia, F. E., J. Invest. Derm. 4, 81, 1941
54. Martin, G. J., et al., Exp. Med. Surg. 1, 38, 1943
55. McChesney, E. W., J. Pharmacol. Exp. Therap. 84, 222, 1945
56. Pelner, L., N.Y. State J. Med. 43, 1874, 1943
57. Hunt, H. B., Brit. Med. J. 1, 726, 1938
58. Crichton, J. W., Canadian Med. Assn. J. 83, 1144, 1960
59. Conn, J. W., et al., Lancet 1, 802, 1957
60. Womersley, R. A., et al., J. Clin. Invest. 34, 456, 1955
61. Moore, F. D., et al., Metabolism 4, 379, 1955
62. Greenman, L., et al., J. Clin. Invest. 30, 644, 1951
63. Freedman, S. S., Am. J. Dis. Child. 102, 76, 1961
64. Shannon, W. R., Am. J. Dis. Child. 24, 89, 1922
65. Korać, D., Nut. Abst. Rev. 30, 1458, 1960
66. Howard, W. A., South. Med. J. 52, 747, 1959.
67. Rowe, A. H., et al., J. Am. Med. Assn. 169, 1158, 1959
68. Rowe, A. H., *Elimination Diets and the Patient's Allergies,* Lea & Febiger, Philadelphia, Pa., 1958
69. Mormone, V., et al., Nut. Abst. Rev. 30, 1458, 1960
70. Fries, J. H., J. Am. Med. Assn. 165, 1542, 1957
71. Grogan, F. T., et al., J. Immunol. 87, 240, 1961
72. Crawford, L. V., Pediatrics 25, 432, 1960
73. Pediatrics 31, 329, 1963
74. Cochrane, W. R., et al., J. Pediat. 28, 771, 1961
75. Van Wyk, J. J., et al., Pediatrics 24, 752, 1959

76. Mann, G. V., Circul. Res. 9, 838, 1961
77. Sure, B., J. Nut. 36, 65, 1948
78. Snyderman, S. E., et al., J. Nut. 42, 31, 1950
79. Holt, L. E., Jr., Am. J. Dis. Child. 31, 427, 1956
80. Speer, F., Arch. Pediat. 75, 271, 1958
81. Bachman, K. D., et al., Pediatrics 20, 393, 1957
82. Lengemann, F. W., et al., J. Nut. 68, 443, 1959
83. Nut. Rev. 18, 182, 1960
84. Randolph, T. G., Ann. Allergy 3, 418, 1945
85. Winkelman, N. W., et al., J. Nerv. Ment. Dis. 93, 736, 1941
86. Schneider, W. F., J. Pediat. 26, 559, 1945
87. Clark, T. W., Ann. Allergy 8, 175, 1950
88. Davison, H. M., Quart. Rev. Allergy 6, 157, 1952
89. Speer, F., Inter. Arch. Allergy 12, 207, 1958

Chapter 16

1. Blond, K., *The Liver and Cancer,* John Wright and Sons, Bristol, England, 1960
2. Craig, J. M., et al., Am. J. Dis. Child. 90, 299, 1953
3. Portis, S. A., et al., J. Am. Med. Assn. 149, 1265, 1952
4. Kerner, I., et al., Am. J. Dis. Child. 99, 597, 1960
5. Hutterer, F., et al., Brit. J. Exp. Path. 42, 187, 1961
6. Zelman, S., Arch. Int. Med. 90, 141, 1952
7. Cooper, L. F., et al., *Nutrition in Health and Disease,* Lippincott, Philadelphia, Pa., 1958
8. Mitchell, K., et al., *Food in Health and Disease,* F. A. Davis, Philadelphia, Pa., 1958
9. Irvine, W. T., Lancet 1, 1064, 1959
10. Alexander, H. D., et al., J. Nut. 61, 329, 1957
11. Wohl, M. J., et al., *Modern Nutrition in Health and Disease,* Lea & Febiger, Philadelphia, Pa., 1955
12. Artom, C., Am. J. Clin. Nut. 6, 221, 1958
13. Eversole, W. J., et al., Endocrinology 45, 378, 1945
14. Ralli, E. P., et al., J. Clin. Invest. 24, 316, 1945
15. Diengott, D., et al., Endocrinology 65, 602, 1959
16. Kark, R. M., Am. J. Med. Sci. 222, 154, 1951
17. Tapley, D. F., Bull. Johns Hopkins Hosp. 96, 274, 1955
18. Krane, S. M., et al., J. Clin. Invest. 35, 874, 1958
19. Volpé, R., et al., Ann. Int. Med. 56, 577, 1962
20. Friend, D. G., New Engl. J. Med. 267, 1124, 1962
21. Thompson, W. O., et al., Arch. Int. Med. 45, 430, 1930
22. Bryson, M. J., et al., Endocrinology 47, 89, 1950
23. Nut. Rev. 18, 93, 1960
24. Hibbs, R. E., Am. J. Med. Sci. 213, 176, 1947
25. Jacobs, E. C., Ann. Int. Med. 28, 792, 1948
26. Guggenheim, K., Metabolism 3, 44, 1954
27. Leevy, C. M., Am. J. Clin. Nut. 7, 146, 1959
28. Cornfeld, D., et al., Pediatrics 10, 33, 1952
29. Maynard, L. A., et al., J. Nut. 64, 85, 1958

30. Nut. Rev. 8, 116, 204, 310, 1950
31. Hove, E. L., Arch. Biochem. 17, 467, 1948
32. Mattell, H. A., Nut. Rev. 10, 225, 1952
33. Nut. Rev. 12, 312, 1954
34. McLean, J. R., et al., J. Nut. 52, 499, 1954
35. Willis, G. C., Canadian Med. Assn. J. 76, 1044, 1957
36. Hartroft, W. S., Ann. N.Y. Acad. Sci. 57, 633, 1954
37. Leevy, C. M., et al., Arch. Int. Med. 92, 527, 1953
38. MacDonald, R. A., Arch. Int. Med. 110, 424, 1962
39. MacDonald, R. A., et al., Lab. Invest. 11, 544, 1962
40. Rabinovici, N., et al., Gastroenterology 40, 416, 1961
41. de la Huerga, J., et al., J. Clin. Invest. 31, 598, 1952
42. Davis, W. D., South. Med. J. 44, 577, 1951
43. Levy, J. S., et al., South. Med. J. 44, 571, 1951
44. Williams, J. O., et al., South. Med. J. 44, 369, 1951
45. Zieve, L., Ann. Int. Med. 48, 471, 1958
46. Kazantzis, F. V., et al., Quart. J. Med. 32, 165, 1963
47. Shils, M. E., et al., J. Indust. Hygiene Toxicol. 31, 175, 1949
48. Shils, M. E., et al., J. Nut. 41, 293, 1950
49. Klatskin, G., et al., J. Clin. Invest. 29, 1528, 1950
50. Popper, H., et al., J. Lab. Clin. Med. 34, 648, 1949
51. Stormont, J. M., et al., Am. J. Clin. Nut. 7, 206, 1959
52. Iver, F. L., et al., J. Lab. Clin. Med. 50, 417, 1957
53. Leevy, C. M., et al., Am. J. Clin. Nut. 10, 46, 1962
54. Stutzman, F. L., et al., J. Lab. Clin. Med. 11, 215, 1953
55. Flink, E. B., et al., J. Lab. Clin. Med. 43, 814, 1955
56. Colwell, A. R., Ann. Int. Med. 41, 963, 1954
57. Schwartz, R., et al., New Engl. J. Med. 251, 685, 1954
58. Plough, I. C., et al., Am. J. Med. Sci. 230, 182, 1955
59. Nefzger, M. D., et al., Am. J. Med. 25, 299, 1963
60. Dalton, W. L., J. Ind. State Med. Assn. 55, 1151, 1962
61. McCormick, W. J., Arch. Pediat. 68, 1, 1951; 69, 151, 1952
62. Baur, H., et al., J. Am. Med. Assn. 156, 565, 1954
63. Callejo, H. B., et al., Ohio State Med. J. 56, 821, 1960

Chapter 17

1. Wohl, M. G., et al., *Modern Nutrition in Health and Disease,* Lea & Febiger, Philadelphia, Pa., 1955.
2. Portis, S. A., et al., J. Am. Med. Assn. 149, 1265, 1952
3. *The Heinz Handbook of Nutrition,* McGraw-Hill, New York, N.Y., 1959
4. Litwak, L., et al., Borden's Rev. Nut. Res. 23, 45, 1962
5. Cooper, L. F., et al., *Nutrition in Health and Disease,* Lippincott, Philadelphia, Pa., 1958
6. Mitchell, K., et al., *Food in Health and Disease,* F. A. Davis, Philadelphia, Pa., 1958
7. Hand, D. B., J. Am. Med. Assn. 181, 411, 1962
8. Watanabe, N., et al., Arch. Surg. 85, 136, 1962

9. Bevans, M., et al., Am. Med. Assn. Arch. Path. 62, 112, 1956
10. Dam, H., et al., Acta Physiol. Scand. 36, 329, 1956
11. Okey, R., Proc. Soc. Exp. Biol. Med. 51, 349, 1942
12. Christensen, F., et al., Acta Physiol. Scand. 27, 315, 1952
13. Granados, H., et al., J. Dent. Res. 24, 197, 1945
14. Dam, H., et al., Acta Path. Microbiol. Scand. 30, 236, 1952
15. Christensen, F., et al., Acta Physiol. Scand. 31, 75, 1954
16. Duff, G. L., et al., Am. J. Med. 11, 92, 1951
17. Catalanie, E. L., et al., J. Am. Pharmacol. Assn. 34, 33, 1945
18. Duff, G. L., et al., J. Exper. Med. 92, 299, 1950
19. Horne, H. W., Jr., et al., Fertility and Sterility 3, 245, 1952
20. Nut. Rev. 16, 25, 1958
21. Nut. Rev. 14, 321, 1956
22. Miller, M. C., Gastroenterology 31, 588, 1956
23. Dwerken, M. G., Gastroenterology 38, 76, 1960
24. Lutton, R. G., et al., Surgery 42, 488, 1957
25. Johnston, C. G., et al., Am. Med. Assn. Arch. Surg. 75, 436, 1957
26. Selye, H., *The Stress of Life*, McGraw-Hill, New York, N.Y., 1956
27. Barker, M. H., et al., J. Am. Med. Assn. 128, 997, 1945
28. Merrill, J. M., Circul. Res. 7, 709, 1959
29. Mei, Y. D., et al., Am. J. Clin. Nut. 6, 50, 1958
30. Haust, H. E., et al., Arch. Biochem. 78, 367, 1958
31. Lewis, B., Lancet 1, 1090, 1958
32. Smith, A. L., et al., Am. J. Physiol. 193, 34, 1958

Chapter 18

1. Stetten, De W., Bull. N.Y. Acad. Med. 28, 664, 1952
2. Ralli, E. P., *Recent Advances in Nutrition Research*, National Vitamin Foundation, New York, N.Y., 1952, p. 95
3. Sorensen, L. B., Arch. Int. Med. 109, 379, 1962
4. Sorensen, L. B., Metabolism 8, 687, 1959
5. Selye, H., *The Stress of Life*, McGraw-Hill, New York, N.Y., 1956
6. Ralli, E. P., et al., *Vitamins and Hormones*, Academic Press, New York, N.Y., 1953
7. Drenick, E. J., et al., J. Am. Med. Assn. 187, 100, 1964
8. Vorhaus, M. G., et al., Acta Rheumatol. 10, 8, 1938
9. Birch, T. W., et al., Nature 138, 27, 1936
10. Callahan, E. J., et al., Med. Rec. 149, 167, 1939
11. Williams, R. J., *Biochemical Individuality*, Wiley, New York, N.Y., 1956
12. Nut. Rev. 21, 23, 1963

13. Zalkin, H., et al., Arch. Biochem. Biophys. 88, 113, 1960
14. Zalkin, H., et al., Fed. Proc. 26, 303, 1961
15. Tsen, C. C., et al., Canadian J. Biochem. Physiol. 38, 957, 1960
16. Benedict, J. D., et al., Metabolism 1, 3, 1952
17. Zalkin, H., et al., J. Biol. Chem. 237, 2678, 1962
18. Young, J. M., et al., J. Biol. Chem. 193, 743, 1951
19. Dinning, J. S., J. Biol. Chem. 212, 735, 1955
20. Horwitt, M. K., et al., J. Am. Diet. Assn. 38, 231, 1961
21. Vitamin E Symposium, Ann. N.Y. Acad. Sci. 52, 63, 1949
22. Quaife, M. L., J. Nut. 40, 367, 1950
23. Horwitt, M. K., et al., Fed. Proc. 17, 245, 1958
24. Nut. Rev. 16, 287, 1958
25. *The Heinz Handbook of Nutrition,* McGraw-Hill, New York, N.Y., 1959
26. Nut. Rev. 20, 287, 1962

Chapter 19

1. Eales, L., Am. J. Clin. Nut. 4, 529, 1956
2. Shils, M. E., Am. J. Clin. Nut. 15, 133, 1964
3. Streeten, D. H. P., et al., J. Physiol. 118, 149, 1952
4. Merrill, A. J., Am. J. Clin. Nut. 4, 497, 1956
5. Nut. Rev. 8, 189, 1950
6. Zimmerman, H. J., Am. J. Clin. Nut. 4, 482, 1956
7. Selye, H., *The Stress of Life,* McGraw-Hill, New York, N.Y., 1956
8. Griffith, W. H., et al., Proc. Soc. Exp. Biol. Med. 41, 188, 333, 1939; J. Biol. Chem. 131, 567, 1939; 132, 627, 639, 1940
9. Best, C. H., et al., Fed. Proc. 8, 610, 1949
10. Nut. Rev. 11, 123, 1953
11. Hartroft, W. S., Am. J. Path. 31, 381, 1955
12. Davies, J. N. P., Am. J. Clin. Nut. 4, 539, 1956
13. Klatskin, G., et al., J. Exp. Med. 100, 605, 615, 1954
14. Kagan, B. M., et al., J. Clin. Invest. 29, 141, 1950
15. Johnson, B. C., et al., J. Nut. 43, 37, 1951
16. Nut. Rev. 10, 306, 1952
17. Labecki, T. D., Am. J. Clin. Nut. 6, 325, 1958
18. Baxter, J. H., J. Exp. Med., 96, 401, 1952
19. Nut. Rev. 20, 297, 1962
20. Field, H., Jr., et al., Circulation 22, 547, 1960
21. Goldbloom, A. A., et al., Am. J. Gastroenterol. 22, 27, 1954
22. Ahrens, E. H., Jr., et al., J. Exp. Med. 90, 409, 1949
23. Adlersberg, D., et al., Clin. Chem. 1, 18, 1955
24. MacFarlane, M. G., et al., Biochem. J. 35, 884, 1941
25. Horlick, L., Circulation 10, 30, 1954
26. Forbes, J. C., Proc. Soc. Exp. Biol. Med. 54, 89, 1943
27. Christensen, A. P., Arch. Path. 34, 633, 866, 1942
28. Nut. Rev. 4, 345, 1946

29. Handler, P., J. Nut. 31, 141, 621, 1946
30. Griffin, W. H., et al., J. Nut. 19, 437, 1940; 21, 633, 1941
31. Leevy, C. M., et al., Arch. Int. Med. 92, 527, 1953
32. Nishizawa, Y., et al., J. Vitaminol. 3, 106, 1957
33. Holman, R. T., Nut. Rev. 16, 33, 1958
34. Burr, G. O., Fed. Proc. 1, 224, 1942
35. Borland, V. G., et al., Arch. Path. 11, 687, 1931
36. Moore, T., et al., J. Nut. 65, 185, 1958
37. Hodgkinson, A., Proc. Roy. Soc. Med. 51, 970, 1958
38. Randall, R. E., Jr., et al., Ann. Int. Med. 50, 257, 1959
39. Vitale, J. J., et al., J. Lab. Clin. Med. 53, 433, 1957
40. Maynard, L. A., et al., J. Nut. 64, 85, 1958
41. MacIntyre, I., et al., Biochem. J. 70, 456, 1958
42. Gershoff, S. N., et al., J. Nut. 73, 308, 1961
43. Crawhall, J. C., et al., Lancet 2, 806, 1959
44. Gershoff, S. N., et al., Am. J. Med. 27, 72, 1959
45. Archer, H. D., et al., Lancet 2, 320, 1957
46. Hogan, A. G., et al., J. Nut. 41, 203, 1950
47. Moore, T., et al., Biochem. J. 49, 77, 1951
48. Herrin, R. C., Proc. Soc. Exp. Biol. Med. 42, 695, 1939
49. Herrin, R. C., Am. J. Physiol. 125, 786, 1939
50. Steck, I. E., et al., Ann. Int. Med. 10, 951, 1937
51. Thornjarnason, T., et al., Biochem. J. 32, 5, 1938
52. Harris, A. D., Brit. Med. J. 1, 553, 1947
53. Herrin, R. C., J. Clin. Invest. 19, 489, 1940
54. Martin, A. J. P., et al., J. Hygiene 39, 643, 1939
55. Raverdino, E., Inter. Congress Vit. E, 1955
56. Nut. Rev. 18, 271, 1960
57. Cantin, M., et al., Exp. Med. Surg. 318, 20, 1962
58. O'Conner, V. R., et al., Summary 8, 24, 1956; 11, 71, 1959
59. Accornero, S. R., Inter. Congress Vit. E, 452, 1955
60. Emmel, V. M., J. Nut. 61, 51, 1957
61. Choudbury, A. K. R., et al., Calcutta Med. J. 53, 414, 1956
62. Mervyn, L., et al., Biochem. J. 72, 106, 1959
63. Shute, W. E., Summary 5, 2, 1953
64. Shute, E. V., Canadian Med. Assn. J. 82, 72, 1960
65. Telford, I. R., et al., Proc. Soc. Exp. Biol. Med. 87, 162, 1954
66. Holman, R., Proc. Soc. Exp. Biol. Med. 66, 307, 1947
67. Allardyce, J., et al., Am. J. Physiol. 164, 48, 1951
68. Krohn, B. G., et al., Ann. West. Med. Surg. 6, 484, 1952
69. Greenman, L., et al., J. Clin. Invest. 30, 644, 1951
70. Kolff, W. J., Nut. Rev. 11, 193, 1953
71. Sargent, F., et al., Am. J. Clin. Nut. 4, 466, 1956
72. Ralli, E. P., Nut. Symposium Series, 5, 78, 1952
73. Kushner, D. S., Am. J. Clin. Nut. 4, 561, 1956
74. Bronsky, D., et al., J. Lab. Clin. Med. 44, 774, 1954
75. Bloom, W. L., Arch. Int. Med. 109, 26, 1962
76. Calloway, D., U.S. Armed Forces Med. J. 11, 403, 1960
77. Gaunt, R., et al., Endocrinology 38, 127, 1946

78. Chapman, D. W., et al., Arch. Int. Med. 79, 449, 1947
79. Chow, B. F., Nut Symposium Series 5, 1, 1952
80. Kolff, W. J., Ann. N.Y. Acad. Sci. 56, 107, 1953
81. Lahey, M. E., Pediat. Clin. No. Am. 9, 689, 1962
82. Jeejeebhoy, K. N., Lancet 1, 343, 1962
83. Wilson, J. F., et al., J. Pediat. 60, 787, 1962
84. Schubert, W. K., et al., Pediatrics 24, 710, 1959
85. Nut. Rev. 21, 170, 1963
86. Davis, J. O., et al., Am. J. Med. 3, 704, 1947
87. Shroeder, H. A., Circulation 1, 481, 1950
88. Shaffer, C. F., et al., Am. J. Med. Sci. 219, 674, 1950
89. Anderson, W. F., Glasgow Med. J. 31, 114, 1950
90. Abbasy, M. A., Biochem. J. 31, 339, 1937
91. Evans, W., Lancet 1, 308, 1938
92. Shaffer, C. F., J. Am. Med. Assn. 124, 700, 1944
93. Bing, R. J., Am. J. Physiol. 140, 240, 1943
94. Meneely, G. R., et al., Ann. Int. Med. 39, 991, 1953
95. Womersley, R. A., et al., J. Clin. Invest. 34, 456, 1955
96. Moore, F. D., et al., Metabolism 4, 379, 1955
97. Conn, J. W., et al., Am. J. Clin. Nut. 4, 523, 1956
98. Wohl, M. G., et al., Proc. Soc. Exp. Biol. Med. 83, 329, 1953
99. Youmans, J. B., et al., Trans. Assn. Am. Phys. 55, 141, 1940
100. Williams, R. H., et al., Arch. Int. Med. 73, 203, 1944
101. McCollister, R. J., Am. J. Clin. Nut. 12, 415, 1963
102. Martin, H. E., et al., Med. Clin. No. Am. 36, 1157, 1952
103. Smith, W. O., et al., J. Okla. State Med. Assn. 55, 248, 1962
104. Daughaday, W. H., et al., J. Clin. Invest. 33, 1075, 1954
105. Bicknell, F., and Prescott, F., *The Vitamins in Medicine*, Lee Foundation for Nutritional Research, Milwaukee, Wis., 1953
106. Gorrie, D. B., Lancet 1, 1005, 1940
107. Ames, S. R., et al., Inter. Rev. Vit. Res, 22, 401, 1951
108. Nut, Rev. 16, 329, 1958
109. Wohl, M. G., et al., *Modern Nutrition in Health and Disease*, Lea & Febiger, Philadelphia, Pa., 1955
110. Schinaki, R. T., J. Biol. Chem. 237, 459, 1921, 1962
111. Mason, G., et al., J. Lab. Clin. Med. 34, 925, 1949
112. Caldwell, E. F., et. al., Arch. Biochem. Biophys. 44, 396, 1953
113. Vilter, R. W., et al., J. Lab. Clin. Med. 42, 335, 1953
114. Addis, T., et al., Arch. Int. Med. 77, 254, 1946
115. Nut. Rev. 8, 128, 1950
116. Schroeder, H. A., Am. J. Med. 4, 578, 1948
117. Odel, J. A., et al., Med. Clin. No. Am. 35, 1145, 1951
118. J. Am. Med. Assn. 156, 1081, 1171, 1252, 1954
119. Addis, T., J. Am. Diet. Assn. 16, 306, 1940
120. *The Heinz Handbook of Nutrition*, McGraw-Hill, New York, N.Y., 1963

Chapter 20

1. Wohl, M. G., and Goodhart, R. S., *Modern Nutrition in Health and Disease,* Lea & Febiger, Philadelphia, Pa., 1955
2. Krehl, W. A., Am. J. Clin. Nut. 11, 77, 1962
3. Hodgkinson, A., Proc. Roy. Soc. Med. 51, 970, 1958
4. Gershoff, S. N., et al., J. Nut. 73, 308, 1961
5. Gershoff, S. N., et al., Am. J. Med. 27, 72, 1959
6. Godwin, J. T., et al., New Engl. J. Med. 259, 1099, 1958
7. Sauberlich, G. E., et al., Am. J. Clin. Nut. 14, 240, 1964
8. Zinsser, H. H., et al., Am. J. Clin. Nut. 10, 357, 1962
9. Archer, H. D., et al., Lancet 2, 320, 1957
10. Faber, S. R., et al., Am. J. Clin. Nut. 12, 406, 1963
11. Gershoff, S. N., et al., Am. J. Clin. Nut. 8, 812, 1960
12. Archer, H. E., et al., Brit. Med. J. 1, 175, 1958
13. Crawhall, J. C., et al., Lancet 2, 806, 1959
14. Bicknell, F., and Prescott, F., *The Vitamins in Medicine,* Lee Foundation for Nutritional Research, Milwaukee, Wis., 1953
15. Hogan, A. G., et al., J. Nut. 41, 203, 1950
16. Kushner, D. S., Am. J. Clin. Nut. 4, 561, 1956
17. Long, H., et al., Brit. J. Urol. 11, 216, 1939
18. Erickson, W. J., et al., J. Am. Med. Assn. 109, 1706, 1937
19. Jewett, H. J., J. Am. Med. Assn. 121, 566, 1943
20. Womersley, R. A., et al., J. Clin. Invest. 34, 456, 1955
21. Black, D. A. K., et al., Clin. Sci. 11, 397, 1952
22. Blahd, W. H., et al., Metabolism 2, 218, 1953
23. Chen, P. S., Jr., et al., Am. J. Physiol. 180, 632, 1955
24. Crawford, J. D., et al., Am. J. Physiol. 180, 156, 1955
25. Steck, I. E., et al., Ann. Int. Med. 10, 951, 1937
26. Goormaghtigh, N., et al., Arch. Path. 26, 1144, 1938
27. Wyse, D. M., et al., Canadian Med. Assn. J. 71, 235, 1954
28. Deitrick, J. E., et al., Am. J. Med. 4, 3, 1948
29. Carr, C. W., Proc. Soc. Exp. Biol. Med. 89, 546, 1955
30. Sager, R. H., et al., Metabolism 4, 519, 1955
31. Shorr, E., et al., J. Am. Med. Assn. 144, 1549, 1950
32. Spellman, R. M., et al., J. Urol. 73, 660, 1955
33. Higgins, C. C., J. Urol. 68, 117, 1952

Chapter 21

1. Keys, A., et al., *The Biology of Human Starvation,* University of Minnesota Press, Minneapolis, Minn., 1951
2. Tui, C., J. Clin. Nut. 1, 232, 1953
3. Chazan, J. A., et al., Am. J. Med. 34, 350, 1963
4. Bicknell, F., and Prescott, F., *Vitamins in Medicine,* Lee Foundation for Nutritional Research, Milwaukee, Wis., 1953

5. Bean, W. B., et al., Proc. Soc. Exp. Biol. Med. 86, 693, 1954
6. Houchin, O. B., et al., J. Biol. Chem. 146, 309, 1942
7. Parrish, H. M., J. Chron. Dis. 14, 326, 1961
8. Selye, H., J. Clin. Endocrinol. 6, 117, 1946
9. Grollman, A., et al., Am. J. Physiol. 157, 21, 1949
10. Shenkin, H. A., et al., J. Clin. Invest. 32, 459, 1953
11. Handler, P., et al., Am. J. Physiol. 160, 30, 1950; 162 368, 1950
12. Olsen, N. S., et al., J. Nut. 53, 317, 329, 1954
13. Crawhall, J. C., et al., Lancet 2, 806, 1959
14. Hartroft, W. S., et al., Brit. Med. J. 1, 423, 1949
15. Best, C. H., et al., Fed. Proc. 8, 610, 1949
16. Nishizawa, Y., et al., J. Vitaminol. 3, 106, 1957
17. Osserman, K. E., et al., Ann. Int. Med. 34, 72, 1951
18. Steiner, A. J., J. Applied Nut. 16, 125, 1963
19. Belliveau, R., et al., Arch. Path. 71, 559, 1961
20. Meneely, G. R., et al., Ann. Int. Med. 39, 991, 1953
21. Dahl, L. K., et al., Fed. Proc. 13, 426, 1954; 15, 513, 1956
22. Dahl, L. K., et al., J. Am. Med. Assn. 164, 397, 1957
23. Selye, H., et al., Am. Heart J. 37, 1009, 1949
24. Sapirstein, L. A., et al., Proc. Soc. Exp. Biol. Med. 73, 82, 1950
25. Dahl, L. K., Am. J. Clin. Nut. 6, 1, 1958
26. Dahl, L. K., Nut. Rev. 18, 97, 1960
27. Schroeder, H. A., Circulation 1, 481, 1950
28. Schroeder, H. A., Am. J. Med. 4, 578, 1948
29. Chen, P. S., Jr., et al., Am. J. Physiol. 180, 632, 1955
30. Bronsky, D., et al., J. Lab. Clin. Med. 44, 774, 1954
31. Kimura, K., et al., J. Vitaminol. 4, 310, 1958
32. Womersley, R. A., et al., J. Clin. Invest. 34, 456, 1953
33. Darrow, D. C., et al., J. Clin. Invest. 27, 198, 1948
34. Black, D. A. K., et al., Clin. Sci. 11, 397, 1952
35. Blahd, W. H., et al., Metabolism 2, 218, 1953
36. Fourman, P., Clin. Sci. 13, 93, 1954
37. Egeli, E. S., et al., Am. Heart J. 59, 527, 1960
38. Bryant, J. M., Proc. Soc. Exp. Biol. Med. 67, 557, 1948
39. del Castillo, E. B., et al., Medicine 6, 471, 1945
40. Keith, N. M., et al., Am. Heart J. 27, 817, 1944
41. Keith, N. M., et al., Proc. Staff Meet. Mayo Clin. 21, 385, 1946
42. Sharpey-Schafer, E. P., Brit. Heart J. 5, 80, 85, 1943
43. Kempner, W., No. Carolina Med. J. 5, 125, 273, 1944; 6, 62, 117, 1945
44. Bishopric, G. A., et al., J. Clin. Endocrinol. Metabolism 15, 592, 1955
45. Bloom, W. L., Arch. Int. Med. 109, 26, 1962
46. Priddle, W. W., Canadian Med. Assn. J. 86, 1, 1962
47. Ruffin, J. M., Am. J. Clin. Nut. 15, 240, 1964
48. Hellerstein, E. A., et al., Am. Heart J. 42, 271, 1951
49. Dawber, T. R., et al., Am. J. Pub. Health 47, 4, 1957
50. Nut. Rev. 18, 262, 1960

51. Selye, H., et al., J. Urol. 56, 399, 1946
52. Levitt, L. M., et al., Am. J. Med. Sci. 215, 130, 1948
53. Shute, E. V., and Shute, W. E., *Alpha Tocopherol in Cardiovascular Disease,* Ryerson Press, Toronto, Canada, 1954
54. de Nicola, P., Inter. Congress Vit. E, 1955

Chapter 22

1. Tower, D. B., Nut. Rev. 16, 161, 1958
2. Hodges, R. E., et al., Am. J. Clin. Nut. 11, 180, 187, 1962
3. Bean, W. B., et al., Proc. Soc. Exp. Biol. Med. 86, 693, 1954
4. Bicknell, F., and Prescott, F., *The Vitamins in Medicine,* Lee Foundation for Nutritional Research, Milwaukee, Wis., 1953
5. Back, E. H., et al., Arch. Dis. Childh. 37, 106, 1962
6. Seelig, M. S., Am. J. Clin. Nut. 14, 342, 1964
7. Smith, W. O., et al., Am. J. Med. Sci. 237, 413, 1959
8. Fitzgerald, M. G., et al., Clin. Sci. 15, 635, 1956
9. Gellhorn, A., et al., Blood 4, 60, 1949
10. Spies, T. D., et al., J. Am. Med. Assn. 115, 292, 1940
11. Coursin, D. B., J. Am. Med. Assn. 154, 406, 1954
12. Bessey, O. A., et al., Pediatrics 20, 33, 1957
13. Hunt, A. D., Jr., et al., Pediatrics 13, 140, 1954
14. Tower, D. B., Am. J. Clin. Nut. 4, 329, 1956
15. Ralli, E. P., et al., *Vitamins and Hormones,* Academic Press, New York, N.Y., 1953
16. Livingstone, S., et al., Pediatrics 16, 250, 1955
17. Barnet, L. B., J. Clin. Physiol. 1, 25, 1959
18. Randall, R. E., Jr., et al., Ann. Int. Med. 50, 257, 1959
19. Ardill, B. L., et al., Clin. Sci. 23, 67, 1962
20. Snyderman, S. E., et al., Fed. Proc. 9, 371, 1950
21. Goldman, A. S., et al., Pediatrics 29, 948, 1962
22. Nut. Rev. 18, 72, 1960
23. Shils, M. E., Am. J. Clin. Nut. 15, 133, 1964
24. Martin, H. E., et al., Am. J. Clin. Nut. 7, 191, 1959
25. Stone, S., Dis. Nerv. Syst. 11, 131, 1950
26. Schwartzman, J., et al., J. Pediat. 19, 201, 1941
27. Nut Rev. 1, 15, 1942
28. Stone, S., Dis. Nerv. Syst. 11, 1, 1950
29. Jolliffe, N., Trans. Am. Neurol. Assn. 66, 54, 1940
30. Jolliffe, N., *Vitamins and Hormones,* Academic Press, New York, N.Y., 1943, pp. 1, 92
31. Baker, A. B., J. Am. Med. Assn. 116, 2484, 1941
32. Meller, C. L., Minn. Med. J. 25, 22, 1942
33. Rudesill, C. L., et. al., J. Ind. State Med. Assn. 34, 355, 1941
34. Barker, W. H., et al., Bull, Johns Hopkins Hosp. 69, 266, 1941
35. Vilter, R. W., et al., J. Lab. Clin. Med. 42, 335, 1953

36. Shute, E. V., and Shute, W. E., *Alpha Tocopherol in Cardiovascular Disease*, Ryerson Press, Toronto, Canada, 1954
37. McCormick, W. J., Arch. Pediat. 69, 151, 1952
38. Calder, J. H., Lancet 1, 556, 1963
39. Brown, M. R., J. Am. Med. Assn. 116, 1615, 1941
40. Shinagawa, T., et al., J. Vitaminol. 3, 135, 1957
41. Alexander, B., et al., J. Clin. Invest. 25, 294, 1946
42. Krehl, W. A., Nut. Rev. 11, 225, 1953
43. Hodges, R. E., et al., J. Clin. Invest. 38, 1421, 1959
44. Bean, W. B., et al., Am. J. Med. Sci. 220, 431, 1950
45. Ropert, R., Nut. Abst. Rev. 29, 273, 1959
46. Blankenhorn, M. A., et al., Trans. Assn. Am. Phys. 50, 164, 1935
47. Jones, W. A., et al., Lancet 1, 1073, 1939
48. Biehl, J. P., et al., Proc. Soc. Exp. Biol. Med. 85, 389, 1954
49. Vilter, R. W., et al., J. Am. Med. Assn. 115, 209, 1940
50. Clark, W. B., South. Med. J. 35, 489, 1942

Chapter 23

1. Kinney, T. D., et al., J. Exp. Med. 102, 151, 1955
2. Snyderman, S. E., et al., Fed. Proc. 9, 371, 1950
3. Hodges, R. E., et al., Am. J. Clin. Nut. 11, 180, 1962
4. Hines, J. D., et al., Am. J. Clin. Nut. 14, 137, 1964
5. Shils, M. E., Am. J. Clin. Nut. 15, 133, 1964
6. Marvin H. N., et al., Proc. Soc. Exp. Biol. Med. 105, 473, 1960
7. Butturini, U., Inter. Congress Vit. E, 1955
8. Prosperi, P., Inter. Congress Vit. E, 1955
9. Gordon, H. H., et al., Am. Med. Assn. J. Dis. Child. 90, 669, 1955
10. Nitowsky, H., et al., J. Pediat. 55, 315, 1959
11. Bishop, E. H., et al., J. Am. Med. Assn. 178, 812, 1961
12. Aitken, F. C., et al., Nut. Abst. Rev. 30, 341, 1960
13. Horwitt, M. K., Fed. Proc. 18, 530, 1959
14. Horwitt, M. K., et al., Fed. Proc. 17, 245, 1958
15. Friedman, L., et al., J. Nut. 65, 143, 1958
16. Marvin, H. J., Am. J. Clin. Nut. 12, 88, 1963
17. Nut. Rev. 20, 60, 1962
18. Horwitt, M. K., et al., Am. J. Clin. Nut. 12, 99, 1963
19. Greenberg, S. M., et al., J. Nut. 63, 19, 1957
20. Krehl, W. A., et al., Borden's Rev. Nut. Res. 24, 50, 1963
21. Day, P. L., et al., Fed. Proc. 15, 548, 1956
22. Harris, P. L., J. Nut. 40, 367, 1950
23. Telford, E. A., et al., Air Univ. Sch. Aviation Med., Rep. 4, Project 21, 1201, 1954
24. Zierler, M., et al., Ann. N.Y. Acad. Sci. 52, 180, 1949
25. Horwitt, M. K., et al., J. Am. Diet. Assn. 38, 231, 1961

26. Cooper, B. A., et al., Canadian Med. Assn. J. 85, 987, 1961
27. Vilter, R. W., et al., J. Lab. Clin. Med. 32, 1426, 1948
28. Thompson, R. B., et al., Quart. J. Med. 20, 187, 1951
29. Herbert, V., Arch. Int. Med. 110, 649, 1962
30. Gough, K. R., et al., Quart. J. Med. 32, 243, 1963
31. Herbert, V., Am. J. Clin. Nut. 12, 17, 1963
32. Herbert, V., Trans. Assn. Am. Phys. 75, 307, 1962
33. Chazan, J. A., et al., Am. J. Med. 34, 350, 1963
34. Scheid, A. S., et al., J. Nut. 47, 601, 1952
35. Lindenbaum, J., et al., New Eng. J. Med. 269, 875, 1963
36. Valberg, L. S., et al., Brit. J. Nut. 15, 473, 1961
37. Beutler, E., Blood 14, 103, 1959
38. Nut. Rev. 20, 52, 1962
39. Lahey, M. E., Pediat. Clin. No. Am. 9, 689, 1962
40. Wilson, J. F., et al., J. Pediat. 60, 787, 1962
41. Smith, S. C., et al., J. Nut. 36, 405, 1948; 45, 47, 1951
42. Schulman, M. D., et al., J. Biol. Chem. 226, 181, 1957
43. Williams, R. D., et al., Arch. Int. Med. 69, 721, 1942
44. Watson, J., et al., J. Am. Med. Assn. 129, 802, 1945
45. Beutler, E., Am. J. Med. Sci. 234, 517, 1957
46. Watson, W. C., et al., Brit. Med. J. 1, 971, 1963
47. Monto, R. W., et al., Am. J. Clin. Nut. 6, 105, 1958
48. Marsh, A., et al., Pediatrics 24, 404, 1959
49. Leonard, B. J., Lancet 1, 899, 1954
50. Whipple, G. H., et al., Am. J. Physiol. 72, 408, 1925
51. Taylor, K. B., et al., Brit. Med. J. 2, 1347, 1962
52. Waife, S. O., et al., Ann. Int. Med. 58, 810, 1963
53. Willis, M. D., et al., J. Am. Diet. Assn. 40, 111, 1962
54. Hartmann, A. M., et al., J. Am. Diet. Assn. 25, 929, 1949
55. Wokes, F., et al., Am. J. Clin. Nut. 3, 375, 1955
56. Prevost, E. W., et al., Acad. Sci. Med. 2, 453, 1946

Chapter 24

1. Shils, M. E., Am. J. Clin. Nut. 15, 133, 1964
2. Lubwak, L., et al., Borden's Rev. Nut. Res. 23, 45, 1962
3. Black, D. A. K., et al., Lancet 1, 244, 1952
4. Womersley, R. A., et al., J. Clin. Invest. 34, 456, 1955
5. Nut. Rev. 10, 163, 1952
6. Conn, J. W., et al., Lancet 1, 802, 1957
7. Gardner, L. I., J. Lab. Clin. Med. 35, 592, 1950
8. Editorial, J. Am. Med. Assn. 180, 775, 1962
9. Streeten, D. H. P., et al., J. Physiol. 118, 149, 1952
10. McAllen, P. M., Brit. Heart J. 17, 5, 1955
11. Moore, F. D., et al., Metabolism 4, 379, 1955
12. Nut. Rev. 16, 90, 1958
13. Ziegler, M. R., et al., Metabolism 1, 116, 1952
14. Poskanzer, D. C., et al., Lancet 2, 511, 1961
15. Oliver, C. P., et al., Am. J. Dis. Child. 68, 308, 1944
16. McQuarrie, I., et al., Metabolism 1, 129, 1952

17. Kunin, A. S., et al., New Engl. J. Med. 266, 228, 1962
18. Lown, B., et al., Am. J. Cardiol. 6, 309, 1960
19. Nut. Rev. 20, 132, 1962
20. Zalkin, H., et al., J. Biol. Chem. 237, 2678, 1962
21. Mattill, H. A., Nut. Rev. 10, 225, 1952
22. Friedman, L., et al., J. Nut. 65, 143, 1958
23. Marvin, H. N., et al., Proc. Soc. Exp. Biol. Med. 105, 473, 1960
24. Braunstein, H., Gastroenterology 40, 224, 1961
25. Nut. Rev. 21, 23, 1963
26. Houchin, O. B., et al., J. Biol. Chem. 146, 309, 1942
27. Roderuck, D. H., et al., Ann. N.Y. Acad. Sci. 52, 156, 1949
28. Wiessberger, L. H., et al., J. Biol. Chem. 151, 543, 1943
29. Pazcek, P. L., et al., J. Biol. Chem. 146, 351, 1942
30. Mason, K. E., et al., Anat. Rec. 92, 33, 1945
31. Nut. Rev. 6, 346, 1948
32. Morgules, S., et al., J. Biol. Chem. 124, 767, 1938
33. Ames, S. R., J. Biol. Chem. 169, 503, 1947
34. Waddell, J., et al., J. Biol. Chem. 80, 431, 1928
35. Waddell, J., et al., J. Nut. 4, 79, 1931
36. Aiyar, A. S., et al., Nature 190, 344, 1961
37. Jensen, H. P., Nut. Abst. Rev. 31, 1333, 1961
38. Nitowsky, H. M., et al., Am. J. Dis. Child. 92, 164, 1956
39. Nitowsky, H. M., Bull. Johns Hopkins Hosp. 98, 361, 1956
40. Del Giudice, A., Summary 12, 21, 1960
41. Desusclade, C., et al., Presse Med. 67, 855, 1959
42. Hillman, R. W., Am. J. Clin. Nut. 5, 597, 1957
43. Dyggve, H. V., et al., Acta Pediat. 146, 48, 1963
44. Dinning, J. S., et al., Am. J. Clin. Nut. 13, 169, 1963
45. Aitken, F. C., et al., Nut. Abst. Rev. 30, 341, 1960
46. Selye, H., *The Stress of Life,* McGraw-Hill, New York, N.Y., 1956
47. Faber, S. R., et al., Am. J. Clin. Nut. 12, 406, 1963
48. Hodges, R. E., et al., J. Clin. Invest. 38, 1421, 1959
49. Bean, W. B., et al., Proc. Soc. Exp. Biol. Med. 86, 693, 1954
50. Editorial, J. Am. Med. Assn. 167, 1806, 1958
51. Wechsler, I. S., Am. J. Med. Sci. 200, 765, 1940
52. Milhorat, A. T., Proc. Soc. Exp. Biol. Med. 58, 40, 1945
53. Meller, R. L., Journal-Lancet 61, 471, 1941
54. Rosenberger, A. I., Med. Rec. 154, 97, 1941
55. Steinberg, C. L., Ann. N.Y. Acad. Sci. 52, 419, 1949
56. Josephson, E. M., *The Thymus, Manganese, and Myasthenia Gravis,* Chedney Press, New York, N.Y., 1961
57. Denny-Brown, D., Medicine 26, 41, 1947
58. Feinberg, W. G., et al., Proc. Staff Meet. Mayo Clin. 32, 299, 1957
59. Zucker, T. A., Am. J. Clin. Nut. 6, 65, 1958
60. Cotzias, G. C., et al., J. Clin. Invest. 37, 1269, 1958

61. Hegde, B., et al., Proc. Soc. Exp. Biol. Med. 107, 734, 1961
62. Nut. Rev. 15, 80, 1957
63. Nut. Rev. 17, 25, 1959
64. Plumlee, M. P., et al., J. Animal Sci. 15, 352, 1956
65. Bentley, O. G., et al., Dairy Sci. 34, 396, 1951
66. Bicknell, F., and Prescott, F., *The Vitamins in Medicine*, Lee Foundation for Nutritional Research, Milwaukee, Wis., 1953
67. Hodges, R. E., et al., Am. J. Clin. Nut. 11, 187, 1965
68. Rinehart, J., et al., Blood 3, 1453, 1948
69. Hove, E. L., et al., J. Nut. 53, 377, 1954
70. Morgan, A. F., J. Am. Med. Women's Assn. 6, 179, 1951
71. von Muralt, A., *Vitamins and Hormones*, Academic Press, New York, N.Y., 1947, pp. 5, 93
72. Welsh, A. L., Arch. Derm. Syph. 70, 181, 1954
73. Mann, P. J. G., et al., Nature 145, 856, 1940
74. Hove, E. L., et al., J. Nut. 53, 396, 1954
75. Donovan, G. E., Lancet 2, 162, 1940
76. Goria, A., Nut. Abst. Rev. 24, 658, 1954
77. Holman, R., Proc. Soc. Exp. Biol. Med. 66, 307, 1947
78. Weil, A., J. Neuropath. Exp. Neurol. 7, 453, 1948
79. Baker, R. W. R., et al., Lancet 1, 27, 1963
80. Kurland, L. K., Am. J. Med. 12, 561, 1952
81. Swank, R. L., et al., New Engl. J. Med. 246, 721, 1952
82. Swank, R. L., Arch. Neurol. Phychiat. 69, 91, 1953
83. Fitzgerald, M. G., et al., Clin. Sci. 15, 635, 1956
84. Stone, S., Dis. Nerv. Syst. 11, 131, 1950
85. Cantin, M., et al., Exp. Med. Surg. 318, 20, 1962
86. Tuchweber, B., et al., Am. J. Clin. Nut. 13, 238, 1963
87. Krehl, W. A., Nut. Rev. 11, 225, 1953
88. Nut. Rev. 10, 235, 1952
89. Goettsch, M., et al., J. Exp. Med. 54, 145, 1931
90. Mackenzie, C. G., Ann. N.Y. Acad. Sci. 52, 161, 1949
91. Tsen, C. C., et al., Canadian J. Biochem. Physiol. 38, 957, 1960
92. Zalkin, H., et al., Arch. Biochem. Biophys. 88, 113, 1960
93. Zalkin, H., et al., Fed. Proc. 26, 303, 1961
94. Day, P. L., et al., Am. J. Clin. Nut. 4, 386, 1956
95. Williams, J. D., et al., Lancet 2, 464, 1957
96. Mackenzie, C. G., et al., J. Nut. 20, 399, 1940
97. Telford, I. R., et al., Proc. Soc. Exp. Biol. Med. 45, 135, 1940
98. Mackenzie, C. G., et al., J. Nut. 19, 345, 1940
99. Dinning, J. S., J. Nut. 55, 209, 1955
100. Williams, R. J., *Biochemical Individuality*, Wiley, New York, N.Y., 1956
101. Stone, S., Arch. Pediat. 66, 189, 1949
102. Minot, A., et al., Am. J. Dis. Child. 62, 423, 1941
103. Nattrass, E. J., Brain 77, 549, 1954
104. Machek, O., J. Applied Nut. 15, 210, 1962

105. Goldbloom, R. B., Canadian Med. Assn. J. 82, 114, 1117 1960

Chapter 25

1. Johnson, J. A., Am. J. Dis. Child. 67, 265, 1944
2. Whedon, G. D., Fed. Proc. 18, 1112, 1959
3. Selye, H., *The Stress of Life,* McGraw-Hill, New York, N.Y., 1956
4. Seelig, M. S., Am. J. Clin. Nut. 14, 342, 1964
5. Schofield, F. A., et al., Fed. Proc. 19, 1014, 1960
6. Smith, R. W., et al., Am. J. Clin. Nut. 14, 98, 1964
7. Nut. Rev. 9, 100, 1951
8. Zubiran, S., et al., *Vitamins and Hormones,* Academic Press, New York, N.Y., 1953, p. 97
9. Wokes, F., et al., Am. J. Clin. Nut. 3, 375, 1955
10. Monto, R. W., et al., Am. J. Clin. Nut. 6, 105, 1958
11. Sacks, M. S., et al., Ann. Int. Med. 32, 80, 1950
12. Ant, M., Ann. N.Y. Acad. Sci. 52, 374, 1949
13. Simpson, J. W., et al., Am. J. Obst. Gynec. 32, 125, 1936
14. Hesseltine, H. C., et al., J. Am. Med. Assn. 184, 1011, 1963
15. Hogan, A. G., Nut. Abst. Rev. 19, 750, 1950
16. Vakil, R. J., Nut. Rev. 4, 319, 1946
17. Nut. Rev. 8, 134, 1950
18. Kanichi, M., et al., J. Vitaminol. 1, 229, 1955
19. Shute, E. V., Canadian Med. Assn. J. 82, 72, 1960
20. Kahn, R. H., Am. J. Anat. 95, 309, 1954
21. Green, H. N., et al., Brit. Med. J. 2, 595, 1931
22. Lutwak, L., N.Y. State J. Med. 63, 590, 1963
23. Fuhr, R., et al., Ann. N.Y. Acad. Sci. 52, 63, 1949
24. McLaren, H. C., Brit. Med. J. 2, 1378, 1949
25. Finkler, R. S., J. Clin. Endocrinol. 9, 89, 1949
26. Nut. Rev. 15, 178, 1957
27. Homburger, F., and Fishman, W. H., *The Physiopathology of Cancer,* Paul B. Hoeber, New York, N.Y., 1953
28. Becker, G. L., Am. J. Dig. Dis. 19, 344, 1952
29. Twort, J. M., et al., J. Hygiene 39, 161, 1939
30. Platz, M., Am. J. Clin. Nut. 5, 618, 1957
31. J. Am. Med. Assn. 167, 1806, 1958
32. De Nicola, P., Inter. Congress Vit. E, 1955
33. Zierler, K. L., et al., Am. J. Physiol. 153, 127,, 1948
34. Zierler, K. L., et al., Ann. N.Y. Acad. Sci. 52, 108, 1949
35. Boyd, A. M., et al., J. Angiol. 14, 198, 1963
36. Williams, H. T., et al., Canadian Med. Assn. J. 87, 538, 1963
37. Dodd, H., Lancet 2, 809, 1964
38. Costa, A., Inter. Congress Vit. E, 1955

Chapter 26

1. Dallas, I., et al., Am. J. Clin. Nut. 11, 263, 1962
2. Dunning, G. M., J. Am. Diet. Assn. 42, 17, 1963
3. U.S. National Health Survey, Series B, No. 19, 1960
4. Grusin, H., et al., Am. J. Clin. Nut. 5, 644, 1957
5. Lutwak, L., et al., Borden's Rev. Nut. Res. 23, 45, 1962
6. Vinther-Paulsen, N., Geriatrics 8, 76, 1953
7. Grusin, H., et al., Am. J. Clin. Nut. 2, 323, 1954
8. Murray, P. D. E., et al., J. Anat. 83, 158, 205, 1949
9. Whedon, G. D., et al., J. Clin. Invest. 36, 966, 1957
10. Morgan, A. F., Calif. Agric. Exp. Stat. Bull. 769, 1959
11. Olson, M. A., et al., Fed. Proc. 18, 1075, 1959
12. MacIntyre, I., J. Chron. Dis. 16, 201, 1963
13. Barker, E. S., J. Chron. Dis. 11, 27, 1960
14. Wacker, W. E. C., et al., Med. Clin. No. Am. 44, 1357, 1960
15. Booth, C. C., et al., Brit. Med. J. 2, 141, 1963
16. MacIntyre, I., et al., Clin. Sci. 20, 297, 1961
17. Seelig, M. S., Am. J. Clin. Nut. 14, 342, 1964
18. Nut. Rev. 16, 148, 1958
19. Smith, R. W., Jr., et al., Am. J. Clin. Nut. 14, 98, 1964
20. Helmer, A. C., et al., Studies Institutum Divi Thomae 1, 83, 207, 1937
21. Walker, A. R. P., J. Am. Med. Assn. 145, 49, 1951
22. Smith, R. W., Jr., J. Lab. Clin. Med. 60, 1019, 1962
23. Nordin, B. E. C., Lancet 1, 1011, 1961
24. Whedon, G. D., Fed. Proc. 18, 1112, 1959
25. Nordin, B. E. C., Am. J. Clin. Nut. 10, 384, 1962
26. Bauer, G. C. H., et al., J. Bone Joint Surg. 40A, 171, 1958
27. Nordin, B. E. C., Clin. Orthoped. 17, 235, 1960
28. Harrison, M., et al., J. Endocrinol. 2, 197, 1960
29. McClendon, J. F., et al., Am. J. Roent. 82, 300, 1959
30. Thorangkin, D., et al., J. Am. Diet. Assn. 35, 23, 1959
31. Ackermann, P. G., et al., J. Gerontol. 8, 451, 1953; 9, 446, 1954
32. Roberts, P. H., et al., J. Am. Diet. Assn. 24, 292, 1948
33. Harrison, M., et al., Lancet 1, 1015, 1961
34. Nordin, B. E. C., Brit. Med. J. 1, 145, 1962
35. Smith, L. M., et al., J. Dairy Sci. 45, 581, 1962
36. Fraser, R., et al., Proc. Roy. Soc. Med. 50, 21, 1957
37. Vose, J. P., et al., J. Gerontol. 16, 120, 1961
38. Silberberg, M., et al., Anat. Rec. 80, 347, 1941
39. Aho, A. J., et al., Acta Endocrinol. 37, 63, 1961
40. Day, H. G., et al., Endocrinology 28, 83, 1941
41. Solomon, G. F., et al., Geriatrics 15, 46, 1960
42. Henneman, P. H., et al., Arch. Int. Med. 100, 715, 1957
43. Albright, F., et al., J. Am. Med. Assn. 116, 2465, 1941
44. Vaughan, K., Brit. Med. J. 2, 167, 1929

45. Krehl, W. A., Am. J. Clin. Nut. 11, 77, 1962
46. Krane, S. M., et al., J. Clin. Invest. 35, 874, 1956
47. Lengemann, F. W., et al., J. Nut. 61, 571, 1957
48. Atkinson, R. L., et al., J. Dairy Sci. 40, 1114, 1957
49. Fournier, P., et al., J. Physiol. 47, 351, 1955
50. Wasserman, R. H., et al., J. Nut. 62, 367, 1957
51. Lengemann, F. W., et al., J. Nut. 68, 443, 1959
52. Pettman, A. C., et al., J. Am. Diet. Assn. 40, 108, 1962
53. Willis, M. T., et al., J. Am. Diet. Assn. 40, 111, 1962
54. Crawford, J. D., et al., Am. J. Physiol. 180, 156, 1955
55. Bogdonoff, M. D., et al., J. Gerontol. 8, 272, 1953
56. Stevenson, F. H., J. Bone Joint Surg. 34, 256, 1952
57. Heaney, R. P., Am. J. Med. 33, 188, 1962
58. Dietrick, J. E., et al., Am. J. Med. 4, 3, 1948
59. Krehl, W. A., Borden's Rev. Nut. Res. 21, 86, 1960
60. Caldecott, R. S., et al., *Radioisotopes in the Biosphere,* University of Minnesota Press, Minneapolis, Minn., 1960, p. 256
61. Larson, B. L., J. Dairy Sci. 46, 759, 1963
62. Greenwood, J., Jr., Med. Ann. of D.C. 22, 48, 1963

Chapter 27

1. Stern, R. L., Am. J. Surg. 39, 495, 1938
2. Ochsner, A., et al., J. Am. Med. Assn. 114, 947, 1940
3. Nut. Rev. 17, 144, 1959
4. Pirani, C. L., et al., Fed. Proc. 11, 423, 1952
5. Kolff, W. J., Nut. Rev. 11, 193, 1953
6. Caldwell, E. F., et al., Arch. Biochem. Biophys. 44, 396, 1953
7. Nut. Rev. 12, 187, 1954
8. Howard, J. M., Am. J. Clin. Nut. 3, 456, 1955
9. Zucker, T. A., Am. J. Clin. Nut. 6, 65, 1958
10. Ershoff, B. H., Physiol. Rev. 28, 107, 1948
11. Streeten, D. H. P., et al., J. Physiol. 118, 149, 1952
12. Nut. Rev. 3, 253, 1945
13. Levenson, S. M., et al., Nut. Rev. 9, 257, 1951
14. Schlesinger, B., et al., Quart. J. Med. 24, 33, 1955
15. Henrikson, H. W., Am. J. Physiol. 164, 263, 1961
16. Nut. Rev. 14, 295, 1956
17. Leithauser, D. J., Surg. Gynec. Obst. 86, 543, 1948
18. Zintel, H. A., Am. J. Clin. Nut. 3, 501, 1955
19. Nut. Rev. 18, 212, 1960
20. Mecray, P., Jr., Am. J. Clin. Nut. 3, 461, 1955
21. Salmon, R. J., et al., J. Nut. 45, 515, 1952
22. Nut. Rev. 4, 259, 1946
23. Follis, R. H., et al., Arch. Path. 35, 579, 1943
24. Crandon, J. H., et al., New Engl. J. Med. 258, 105, 1958
25. Coon, W. W., Surg. Gynec. Obst. 114, 522, 1962
26. Pollack, H., et al., *Therapeutic Nutrition, Public.* 234, Nat. Res. Council, 1952

27. Sullivan, W. R., et al., J. Biol. Chem. 151, 477, 1943
28. Grusin, H., et al., Am. J. Clin. Nut. 2, 323, 1954
29. Roderuck, D. H., et al., Ann. N.Y. Acad. Sci. 52, 156, 1949
30. Holman, R. L., Proc. Soc. Exp. Biol. Med. 66, 306, 1947
31. Zierler, K. L., et al., Am. J. Physiol. 153, 127, 1948
32. Wilson, M. G., et al., Lancet 1, 266, 486, 1951
33. Kay, J. H., et al., Surgery 28, 24, 1952
34. Ochsner, A., et al., J. Am. Med. Assn. 144, 831, 1950
35. Ochsner, A., et al., Ann. Surg. 131, 652, 1950
36. Swanson, P. P., Fed. Proc. 10, 660, 1951
37. Nut. Rev. 9, 24, 185, 1951
38. O'Dell, B. L., et al., Proc. Soc. Exp. Biol. Med. 108, 402, 1961
39. Bosse, M. D., et al., Proc. Soc. Exp. Biol. Med. 67, 418, 1948
40. Horwitt, M. K., et al., J. Nut. 39, 357, 1949
41. Sacks, M. S., et al., Ann. Int. Med. 32, 80, 1950
42. Shank, R. E., J. Am. Diet. Assn. 40, 97, 1962
43. Gubner, R., et al., Am. J. Med. Sci. 221, 176, 1951
44. Mulholland, J. H., et al., Ann. Surg. 118, 1015, 1943
45. Tui, C., J. Clin. Nut. 1, 232, 1953
46. Barkhan, P., et al., Brit. J. Nut. 13, 389, 1959
47. Rouser, G., Am. J. Clin. Nut. 6, 681, 1958
48. Prosperi, P., Inter. Congress Vit. E, 1955
49. De Nicola, P., Inter. Congress Vit. E, 1955
50. Govier, W. M., et al., J. Am. Med. Assn. 126, 149, 1944
51. Nut. Rev. 10, 82, 1952
52. Lucas, B. G. B., Nature 148, 84, 1941
53. de Pasqualini, C. D., Am. J. Physiol. 147, 598, 1946
54. Werner, S. C., et al., Ann. Surg. 130, 688, 1949
55. Stewart, B. L., et al., J. Am. Med. Assn. 136, 1017, 1948
56. King, C. G., J. Am. Diet. Assn. 38, 223, 1961
57. Rapsky, H. A., et al., Geriatrics 2, 101, 1947
58. Bicknell, F., and Prescott, F., *The Vitamins in Medicine*, Lee Foundation for Nutritional Research, Milwaukee, Wis., 1953
59. Cox, W. M., et al., Pediatrics 11, 435, 1953
60. Williamson, M. B., et al., J. Biol. Chem. 212, 705, 1955
61. Deitrick, J. E., et al., Am. J. Med. 4, 3, 1948
62. Wyse, D. M., et al., Canadian Med. Assn. J. 71, 235, 1954
63. Cohn, C., Nut. Rev. 20, 321, 1962
64. Cope, O., et al., Ann. Surg. 137, 165, 1953
65. Shute, E. V., and Shute, W. E., *Alpha Tocopherol in Cardiovascular Disease*, Ryerson Press, Toronto, Canada, 1954
66. Beattie, J., Brit. Med. J. 2, 813, 1947
67. Lund, C. C., et al., Arch. Surg. 55, 557, 1942

Chapter 28

1. Mason, K. E., *Sex and Internal Secretions,* Williams & Wilkins, Baltimore, Md., 1939, p. 148
2. Gillman, J., and Gillman, T., *Perspective in Human Malnutrition,* Grune & Stratton, New York, N.Y., 1951
3. Griffith, W. H., et al., Proc. Soc. Exp. Biol. Med. 44, 333, 1939
4. Gasmami, M. N. D., et al., J. Chron. Dis. 16, 363, 1963
5. Harris, P. L., et al., Inter. Congress Vit. E, 1955
6. Verzár, F., Inter. Congress Vit. E, 1955
7. Beckman, R., Inter. Congress Vit. E, 1955
8. Costa, A., et al., Inter. Congress Vit. E, 1955
9. Nut. Rev. 10, 331, 1952
10. Keys, A., et al., *The Biology of Human Starvation,* University of Minnesota Press, Minneapolis, Minn., 1950
11. Zubirán, S., et al., *Vitamins and Hormones,* Academic Press, New York, N.Y., 1953, p. 97
12. Palmer, H. R., et al., J. Clin. Endocrinol. 10, 121, 1950
13. Kinny, T. D., et al., J. Exp. Med. 102, 151, 1955
14. Selye, H., *The Stress of Life,* McGraw-Hill, New York, N.Y., 1956, p. 176
15. Sillo-Seidl, G., Nut. Abst. Rev. 33, 812, 1963
16. Brožěk, J., et al., J. Personality 19, 246, 1951
17. Brožěk, J., Am. J. Clin. Nut. 3, 101, 1955
18. Brožěk, J., et al., J. Consult. Psychol. 12, 403, 1948
19. Randall, R. E., Jr., et al., Ann. Int. Med. 50, 257, 1959
20. Cleckley, H. M., et al., J. Am. Med. Assn. 112, 2107, 1939
21. Bowman, K. M., et al., Proc. Assn. Res. Nerv. Mental Dis. 22, 178, 1943
22. Williams, R. D., et al., Proc. Staff Meet. Mayo Clin. 14, 787, 1939
23. Egana, E., et al., Am. J. Physiol. 137, 731, 1942
24. Elsom, K., et al., Am. J. Med. Sci. 200, 757, 1940
25. Williams, R. R., et al., Arch. Int. Med. 66, 785, 1940; 69, 721, 1942
26. Brožěk, J., et al., Psychosomatic Med. 8, 98, 1946
27. Kreisler, E. S., et al., Am. J. Psychiat. 105, 107, 1948
28. Goodhart, R. S., Am. J. Clin. Nut. 5, 612, 1957
29. Williams, R. J., *Alcoholism: The Nutritional Approach,* University of Texas Press, Austin, Texas, 1959, p. 78
30. Hodges, R. E., et al., J. Clin. Invest. 38, 1421, 1959
31. Bean, W. B., et al., Proc. Soc. Exp. Biol. Med. 86, 693, 1954
32. Thornton, G. H. M., et al., J. Clin. Invest. 34, 1073, 1955
33. Hodges, R. E., et al., Am. J. Clin. Nut. 11, 181, 187, 1962
34. Hawkins, W. W., et al., Science 108, 2802, 1948
35. Monto, R. W., et al., Am. J. Clin. Nut. 6, 105, 1958
36. Sydenstricker, V. P., et al., J. Am. Med. Assn. 118, 1199, 1942

37. Shils, M. E., Am. J. Clin. Nut. 15, 133, 1964
38. Seelig, M. S., Am. J. Clin. Nut. 14, 342, 1964
39. Nut. Rev. 18, 110, 1960
40. Knox, W. E., Pediatrics 26, 1, 1960
41. Moriarty, J. D., Dis. Nerv. Syst. 12, 105, 1951
42. Beutler, E., Am. J. Med. Sci. 234, 517, 1957
43. Ralli, E. P., et al., *Vitamins and Hormones,* Academic Press, New York, N.Y., 1953, p. 147
44. Orent-Keiles, E., et al., U.S. Dept. Agric., Circular 827, 1949
45. Portis, S. A., J. Am. Med. Assn. 142, 1281, 1950
46. Winters, R. W., et al., Endocrinology 50, 388, 1952
47. Egeli, E. S., et al., Am. Heart J. 59, 527, 1960
48. Bryant, J. M., Proc. Soc. Exp. Biol. Med. 67, 557, 1948
49. Leak, D., et al., Am. Heart J. 63, 688, 1962
50. Thorn, G. W., et al., Ann. Int. Med. 18, 913, 1943
51. Abrahamson, E. M., and Pezet, A. W., *Body, Mind, and Sugar,* Holt, New York, N.Y., 1951
52. McCollister, R. J., Am. J. Clin. Nut. 12, 415, 1963
53. Ropert, R., Nut. Abst. Rev. 29, 273, 1959
54. Roberts, H. J., New Engl. J. Med. 268, 562, 1963
55. Brush, B. E., et al., J. Clin. Endocrinol. Metabolism 12, 380, 1952
56. Matovinovic, J., J. Am. Med. Women's Assn. 17, 427, 495, 1962
57. Saxena, K. M., et al., Science 138, 430, 1962
58. Matovinovic, J., J. Am. Med. Women's Assn. 17, 571, 646, 1962
59. Benson, J., et al., Cancer Res. 16, 135, 1956
60. Marek, G., et al., Am. Heart J. 63, 768, 1962
61. Danowski, T. S., Nut. Rev. 21, 225, 1963
62. Najjar, S. S., et al., Am. J. Clin. Nut. 13, 46, 1963
63. Follis, R. H., Jr., Proc. Soc. Exp. Biol. Med. 100, 203, 1959
64. Srinivasan, V., et al., J. Nut. 61, 87, 97, 1957
65. Nut. Rev. 8, 196, 1950
66. Van Wyk, J. J., et al., Pediatrics 24, 752, 1959
67. Thompson, W. O., et al., Arch. Int. Med. 45, 430, 1930
68. Volpé, R., et al., Ann. Int. Med. 56, 577, 1962
69. Tui, C., J. Clin. Nut. 1, 232, 1953
70. Forbes, J. C., Endocrinology 35, 126, 1944
71. Nut. Rev. 4, 259, 1946
72. Friend, D. G., New Engl. J. Med. 263, 1358, 1960
73. Falliers, C. J., et al., Am. Med. Assn. J. Dis. Child. 99, 428, 1960
74. Burrows, B., et al., Ann. Int. Med. 52, 858, 1960
75. Galina, M. P., et al., New Engl. J. Med. 267, 1124, 1962
76. Peacock, L. B., et al., Ann. Allergy 15, 158, 1957
77. Forbes, J. C., et al., J. Am. Pharmacol. Assn. 37, 509, 1948
78. Nut. Rev. 8, 141, 1950
79. Gibson, J. E., *This Week Magazine,* August 7, 1955

80. Taylor, R., *Hunza Health Secrets*, Prentice-Hall, Englewood Cliffs, N.J., 1964

Chapter 29

1. Bicknell, F., and Prescott, F., *The Vitamins in Medicine*, Lee Foundation for Nutritional Research, Milwaukee, Wis., 1953
2. Morgan, A. F., et al., Am. J. Clin. Nut. 10, 337, 1962
3. Nut. Rev. 20, 169, 1962
4. Josephson, E. M., *Nearsightedness Is Preventable*, Chedney Press, New York, N.Y., 1939
5. Campbell, D. A., et al., Brit. J. Ophthal. 46, 151, 1962
6. Spies, T., et al., J. Am. Med. Assn. 113, 931, 1939
7. Sydenstricker, V. P., et al., J. Am. Med. Assn. 114, 2437, 1940
8. Braun, K., et al., J. Obst. Gynec., Brit. Emp. 52, 43, 1945
9. Stannus, H. S., Trans. Ophthal. Soc. 62, 65, 1942
10. Métivier, V. M., Am. J. Ophthal. 24, 1265, 1941
11. Conners, C. A., et al., Arch. Ophthal. 29, 956, 1943
12. Bowles, L. L., et al., J. Nut. 37, 9, 1949
13. Vilter, R. W., et al., J. Lab. Clin. Med. 42, 335, 1953
14. Nut. Rev. 6, 244, 1948
15. Adamstone, F. B., et al., Arch. Path. 49, 173, 1950
16. Lerman, S., Arch. Ophthal. 65, 181, 1961
17. Dische, Z., et al., Arch. Ophthal. 55, 633, 1956
18. Lerman, S., et al., Am. J. Ophthal. 51, 1012, 1961
19. Isselbacker, K. J., Am. J. Clin. Nut. 5, 527, 1957
20. Patterson, J. W., Am. J. Physiol. 165, 61, 1951
21. Nut. Rev. 14, 246, 1956; 20, 274, 1962
22. Josephson, E. M., Science 82, 222, 1935
23. Maxwell, J. P., et al., Proc. Roy. Soc. Med. 33, 777, 1940
24. Kurinsky, I. A., Nat. Health Fed. Bull. 10, 25, 1964
25. Desusclade, C., et al., Presse Med. 67, 855, 1959
26. Vannas, S., et al., Acta Ophthal. 36, 601, 1958
27. Selye, H., *The Stress of Life*, McGraw-Hill, New York, N.Y., 1956
28. Josephson, E. M., *Glaucoma and Its Medical Treatment*, Chedney Press, New York, N.Y., 1962
29. Nut. Rev. 8, 116, 1950
30. Kinsey, V. E., et al., J. Am. Med. Assn. 139, 572, 1949
31. Owens, W. C., et al., Am. J. Ophthal. 32, 1631, 1949
32. Kinsey, V. E., Arch. Ophthal. 56, 481, 1956
33. Ashton, N., Ann. Rev. Med. 8, 441, 1957
34. Patz, A., Pediatrics 19, 504, 1957
35. Gyllensten, L. J., et al., Am. J. Ophthal. 41, 619, 1956
36. Aitken, F. C., et al., Nut. Abst. Rev. 30, 341, 1960
37. Gordon, H. H., et al., Am. Med. Assn. J. Dis. Child. 90, 669, 1955
38. Harris, P. L., et al., Proc. Soc. Exp. Biol. Med. 107, 381, 1961

39. Horwitt, M. K., et al., J. Am. Diet. Assn. 38, 231, 1961
40. Hodges, R. E., et al., Am. J. Clin. Nut. 11, 187, 1962
41. Goodhart, R. S., Am. J. Clin. Nut. 5, 612, 1957
42. Denny-Brown, D., Medicine 26, 41, 1947
43. Levitt, L. M., et al., Am. J. Med. Sci. 215, 130, 1948
44. Jeremy, R., Med. J. Australia 1, 302, 1950
45. Schneider, R. W., et al., Am. J. Med. Sci. 212, 462, 1946
46. Emerson, K., Jr., Nut. Rev. 6, 257, 1948
47. Demote, V., et al., Ophthalmology 101, 65, 1941
48. Lecoq, R., et al., Ann. N.Y. Acad. Sci. 52, 139, 1949
49. Hutschnecker, A., *The Will to Live,* Prentice-Hall, Englewood Cliffs, N.J., 1952

Chapter 30

1. Bean, W. B., Am. J. Clin. Nut. 13, 263, 1963
2. Shute, E. V., and Shute, W. E., *Alpha Tocopherol in Cardiovascular Disease,* Ryerson Press, Toronto, Canada, 1954
3. Martin, W. C., J. Applied Nut. 10, 3, 1957
4. Selfridge, G., Ann. Otol. Rhinol. Laryngol. 48, 419, 1939
5. Denny-Brown, D., Medicine 26, 41, 1947
6. Tuchweber, B., et al., Am. J. Clin. Nut. 13, 238, 1963
7. Matovinovic, J., J. Am. Med. Women's Assn. 17, 571, 646, 1962
8. Reid, J., et al., Brit. Med. J. 2, 1071, 1957
9. Hodges, R. E., et al., Am. J. Clin. Nut. 11, 187, 1962
10. Harris, H. E., et al., Med. Clin. No. Am. 24, 533, 1940
11. Atkinson, M., J. Am. Med. Assn. 116, 1753, 1941
12. J. Am. Med. Assn. 156, 1081, 1954
13. Goldman, H. B., Clin. Physiol. 5, 1, 1964
14. Houchin, O. B., et al., J. Biol. Chem. 146, 309, 1942
15. Hove, E. L., et al., Arch. Biochem. 8, 395, 1945
16. Hummel, J. P., et al., J. Biol. Chem. 101, 383, 1951
17. Telford, I. R., et al., Proc. Soc. Exp. Biol. Med. 87, 162, 1954
18. Nitowsky, H. M., et al., Bull. Johns Hopkins Hosp. 98, 361, 1956
19. Michelson, H. W., Proc. Staff Meet. Mayo Clin. 27, 433, 1952
20. Welsh, A. L., Arch. Derm. Syph. 70, 181, 1954
21. Bicknell, F., and Prescott, F., *The Vitamins in Medicine,* Lee Foundation for Nutritional Research, Milwaukee, Wis., 1953
22. Hagerman, G., Acta Derm. Venereal. 31, 225, 1951
23. Goldman, L., Med. Clin. No. Am. 35, 391, 1951
24. Selye, H., *Calciphylaxis,* University of Chicago Press, Chicago, Ill., 1962
25. Selye, H., *The Stress of Life,* McGraw-Hill, New York, N.Y., 1956
26. Cantin, M., et al., Exp. Med. Surg. 318, 20, 1962

27. Morgules, S., et al., J. Biol. Chem. 124, 767, 1938
28. Ames, S. R., J. Biol. Chem. 169, 539, 1947
29. Nut. Rev. 9, 336, 1951
30. Gordon, H. H., et al., Am. J. Dis. Child. 90, 669, 1955
31. Nitowsky, H. M., et al., Am. J. Dis. Child. 92, 164, 1956
32. Nut. Rev. 21, 195, 1963
33. di Sant'Agnese, P. A., et al., Pediatrics 12, 549, 1953
34. Oppenheimer, E. H., et al., Bull. Johns Hopkins Hosp. 107, 207, 1960
35. Duncan, L. J. P., et al., Lancet 1, 822, 1958
36. Nut. Rev. 15, 135, 1957
37. Bean, W. B., et al., Proc. Soc. Exp. Biol. Med. 86, 693, 1954
38. Kinny, T. D., et al., J. Exp. Med. 102, 151, 1955
39. Nut. Rev. 14, 183, 1956
40. Olsen, N. S., et al., J. Nut. 53, 317, 329, 1954
41. Porter, C. C., et al., Arch. Biochem. 18, 339, 1948
42. Kotake, Y., J. Vitaminol. 1, 73, 1955
43. Richards, M. B., Brit. J. Nut. 3, 109, 1949
44. Gershoff, S. N., et al., J. Nut. 73, 308, 1961
45. Editorial, J. Am. Med. Assn. 180, 322, 1962
46. Biehl, J. P., et al., Proc. Soc. Exp. Biol. Med. 85, 389, 1954
47. Davis, J. N. P., Lancet 1, 317, 1948
48. Holmes, E. G., et al., Lancet 1, 395, 1948
49. Blanc, W. A., et al., Pediatrics 22, 494, 1958
50. Nitowsky, H. M., et al., J. Pediat. 55, 315, 1959
51. Kerner, I., et al., Am. J. Dis. Child. 99, 597, 1960
52. Nitowsky, H. M., et al., Am. J. Clin. Nut. 4, 397, 1956
53. Lowe, C. W., et al., Am. J. Dis. Child. 79, 91, 1950
54. Adlersberg, D., et al., J. Nut. 25, 255, 1943
55. Adlersberg, D., et al., Gastroenterology 10, 822, 1948
56. Slanetz, A. S., et al., J. Nut. 30, 239, 1945
57. May, C. D., et al., J. Clin. Invest. 27, 226, 1948
58. Clausen, S. W., et al., Fed. Proc. 5, 129, 1946
59. Fernandez, J., et al., J. Clin. Invest. 41, 488, 1962
60. Williams, R. J., Nut. Rev. 8, 257, 1950
61. Williams, R. J., *Biochemical Individuality*, Wiley, New York, N.Y., 1956
62. Scrimshaw, N.S., et al., Am. J. Clin. Nut. 11, 539, 1962
63. Youman, J. B., J. Am. Med. Assn. 189, 672, 1964

Chapter 31

1. Homburger, F., and Fishman, W. H., *The Physiopathology of Cancer*, Paul B. Hoeber, New York, N.Y., 1953
2. Hartwell, J. L., U.S. Pub. Health Serv. Public. 149, 1951
3. Nut. Rev. 8, 184, 1950
4. Kuh, C., Yale J. Biol. Med. 5, 123, 1932
5. Dittmar, C., Am. J. Cancer 29, 746, 1936
6. Reinhold, H., Nut. Abst. Rev. 31, 601, 1961

7. Willherm, R., et al., Gastroenterology 23, 1, 1953
8. Nut. Rev. 4, 353, 1946
9. Allison, J. B., et al., J. Nut. 74, 176, 1961
10. Gilbert, C., et al., Brit. J. Cancer 12, 565, 1958
11. Griffin, A. C., et al., Cancer Res. 9, 82, 1949
12. Fenton, P. F., et al., J. Nut. 34, 273, 1947
13. Nut. Rev. 15, 178, 1957
14. Nut. Rev. 8, 86, 1950; 10, 55, 1952
15. Scott, G. M., Lancet 1, 102, 1949
16. Briggs, M. H., Australian J. Biol. Sci. 13, 196, 1960
17. Yamada, K., et al., J. Vitaminol. 5, 188, 1959
18. Tanaka, T., Nut. Abst. Rev. 30, 860, 1960
19. Salmon, W. D., et al., Ann. N.Y. Acad. Sci. 57, 664, 1954
20. Wilson, J. W., Ann. N.Y. Acad. Sci. 57, 678, 1954
21. Cerkes, L. A., et al., Nut. Abst. Rev. 30, 955, 1960
22. Leevy, C. M., Am. J. Clin. Nut. 7, 146, 1959
23. Blond, K., *The Liver and Cancer,* John Wright and Sons, Bristol, England, 1960
24. Ferenczi, A., Nut. Abst. Rev. 30, 247, 1960
25. Brock, J. F., Nut. Rev. 13, 17, 1955
26. Conney, A. H., et al., Nature 184, 363, 1959
27. Pirani, C. L., et al., Proc. Soc. Exp. Biol. Med. 75, 221, 1950
28. Clark, C. M., et al., Brit. J. Cancer 14, 327, 1960
29. Luhrs, W., et al., Nut. Abst. Rev. 30, 1278, 1960
30. Davidson, J. R., Canadian Med. Assn. J. 31, 486, 1934; 32, 364, 1935
31. Cater, D. B., J. Path. Bact. 63, 599, 1951
32. Adamstone, F. B., Am. J. Cancer 28, 540, 1936
33. Haber, S. I., et al., Proc. Soc. Exp. Biol. Med. 111, 774, 1962
34. Vitamin E Symposium, Ann. N.Y. Acad. Sci. 52, 63, 1949
35. Gardner, W. U., Cancer Res. 2, 468, 1942
36. Dobrovolskaia, Z. N., Cancer Res. Soc. Biol. 139, 551, 1945
37. Becker, G. L., Am. J. Dig. Dis. 19, 344, 1952
38. Horwitt, M. K., et al., J. Am. Diet. Assn. 38, 231, 1961
39. Tedeschi, C. G., Arch. Path. 47, 160, 1949
40. Voluter, G., et al., Nut. Abst. Rev. 30, 975, 1960
41. Lindberg, W. O., Am. J. Clin. Nut. 6, 601, 1958
42. Nut. Rev. 17, 351, 1959
43. Wynder, E. L., et al., Cancer 12, 1016, 1959
44. Benson, J., et al., Cancer Res. 16, 135, 1956
45. Najjar, S. S., et al., Am. J. Clin. Nut. 13, 46, 1963
46. Howell, J. S., Brit. J. Cancer 12, 594, 1958
47. Arffmann, E., J. Nat. Cancer Inst. 25, 893, 1960
48. Sugai, L. A., et al., Cancer Res. 22, 510, 1962
49. Haven, F. L., et al., Cancer Res. 4, 257, 1958
50. Hiegar, I., Brit. J. Cancer 3, 123, 1949
51. Lane, A., et al., Brit. J. Cancer 3, 1044, 1950
52. Poling, C. E., et al., J. Nut. 72, 100, 1960

53. Segaloff, A., et al., Endocrinology 34, 346, 1944; 38, 212, 1946
54. Ayre, J. E., et al., Science 103, 441, 1946
55. J. Am. Med. Assn. 123, 967, 1943
56. Greenstein, J. P., *Biochemistry of Cancer*, Academic Press, New York, N.Y., 1954
57. Farber, E., et al., Cancer Res. 18, 1209, 1958
58. Nut. Rev. 12, 344, 1954
59. Nat. Res. Council, Public. 749, 1960
60. Roe, F. J. C., Brit. J. Cancer 13, 92, 1959
61. Tannenbaum, A., Cancer Res. 2, 460, 1942
62. White, F. R., Cancer Res. 21, 281, 1961
63. Brown, C. E., et al., Cancer Res. 20, 329, 1960
64. Engel, R. W., et al., Cancer Res. 11, 180, 1951; 12, 211, 1952
65. Watkins, D. M., Am. J. Clin. Nut. 9, 446, 1961
66. Bicknell, F., and Prescott, F., *The Vitamins in Medicine*, Lee Foundation for Nutritional Research, Milwaukee, Wis., 1953
67. Mascitelli-Coriandoli, E., Nut. Abst. Rev. 30, 451, 1960
68. Pollock, M. A., et al., Cancer Res. 2, 739, 1942
69. Mihich, E., et al., Cancer Res. 19, 1244, 1959
70. Zellhorn, A., et al., Blood 4, 60, 1949
71. Zarafonetis, C. J. D., et al., Blood 3, 780, 1948
72. May, H. B., et al., Lancet 2, 607, 1948
73. Smith, C. H., et al., Am. J. Dis. Child. 79, 1031, 1950
74. Farber, S., et al., Cancer Chemotherapy Rep. 13, 159, 1961
75. Nichol, C. A., Cancer Res. 22, 495, 1962
76. Mayo, C. W., Cancer Bull. 15, 78, 1963
77. Nut. Rev. 13, 17, 1955
78. Block, M. T., Clin. Med. 57, 112, 1950
79. Block, M. T., J. Insurance Med. 5, 4, 1950
80. Pascher, F., et al., J. Invest. Derm. 17, 261, 1951
81. Shute, E. V., Ann. N.Y. Acad. Sci. 52, 358, 1949
82. Sokoloff, B., et al., J. Clin. Invest. 30, 395, 1951
83. Field, J. B., et al., Am. J. Med. Sci. 218, 1, 1949
84. Domokos, J., et al., Inter. Rev. Vit. Res. 21, 444, 1950
85. Wells, J. J., et al., Proc. Staff Meet. Mayo Clin. 22, 482, 1947
86. Wallace, W. S., South. Med. J. 34, 170, 1941
87. Bean, W. B., et al., Am. J. Med. Sci. 208, 46, 1944
88. Harris, P. L., et al., Inter Congress Vit. E, 1955
89. Di Nicola, P., Inter. Congress Vit. E, 1955
90. Krehl, W. A., et al., Borden's Rev. Nut. Res. 24, 50, 1963
91. Dinning, J. S., et al., Am. J. Clin. Nut. 13, 169, 1963
92. Harris, P. L., et al., Proc. Soc. Exp. Biol. Med. 107, 381, 1961
93. Skipper, H. E., et al., Cancer Res. 10, 510, 1950
94. Schoenback, E. B., et al., Cancer 2, 57, 1949
95. Skipper, H. E., et al., Blood 5, 358, 1950
96. Gunz, F. W., Blood 5, 161, 1950

97. Wilkinson, J. F., et al., Lancet 1, 325, 1951
98. Dameshek, W., et al., Blood 5, 898, 1950
99. Sacks, M. S., et al., Ann. Int. Med. 32, 80, 1950
100. Dacie, J. V., et al., Brit. Med. J. 1, 1447, 1950
101. Weber, E. J., et al., J. Pediat. 36, 69, 1950
102. Meyer, L. M., et al., J. Clin. Path. 19, 119, 1949
103. Thiersch, J. B., Cancer 2, 877, 1949
104. Berman, L., et al., Am. J. Clin. Path. 19, 127, 1949
105. Stickney, J. M., et al., Proc. Staff Meet. Mayo Clin. 24, 525, 1949
106. Wilkinson, J. F., Brit. Med. J. 1, 771, 1948
107. Dodds, E. C., Brit. Med. J. 2, 1191, 1949
108. Grubbs, R. C., et al., J. Applied Pharmacol. 2, 327, 1949
109. Davis, J. E., Am. J. Physiol. 147, 404, 1946
110. Samachson, J., et al., Arch. Biochem. Biophys. 88, 355, 1960
111. Price, W., *Nutrition and Physical Degeneration,* American Academy Applied Nutrition, Pasadena, Calif., 1945
112. *Immunological Studies,* Rep. 14, Sloan-Kettering Institute for Cancer Research, New York, N.Y., 1960
113. Williams, R. J., Nut. Rev. 8, 257, 1950

Chapter 32

1. Tui, C., J. Clin. Nut. 1, 232, 1953
2. Nut. Rev. 6, 244, 1948
3. Adamstone, F. B., et al., Arch. Path. 49, 173, 1950
4. Krehl, W. A., J. Biol. Chem. 162, 403, 1946
5. Nut. Rev. 14, 225, 1956
6. Crawhall, J. C., et al., Lancet 2, 806, 1959
7. Swendseid, M. E., et al., J. Nut. 78, 115, 1962
8. Hier, E. A., et al., Proc. Soc. Exp. Biol. Med. 56, 187, 1949
9. Harper, A. E., et al., Am. J. Physiol. 193, 483, 1958
10. Townsend, D. E., et al., *Rancidity in Oils,* Lee Foundation for Nutritional Research, Milwaukee, Wis., 1962
11. Caffey, J., Pediatrics 5, 672, 1950
12. Gerber, A., et al., Am. J. Med. 16, 729, 1954
13. Caffey, J., Am. J. Roent. Rad. Therap. 65, 12, 1951
14. Hillman, R. W., Am. J. Clin. Nut. 4, 603, 1956
15. Turtz, C. A., et al., Am. J. Ophthal. 50, 1, 1960
16. Vedder, E. B., et al., J. Nut. 16, 57, 1938
17. Pallotta, M. A., et al., Am. J. Clin. Nut. 13, 201, 1963
18. Williams, H. H., J. Nut. 76, 435, 1962
19. Adlersberg, D., et al., J. Nut. 25, 255, 1943
20. Traina, V., Arch. Path. 49, 278, 1950
21. Bean, W. B., et al., Proc. Soc. Exp. Biol. Med. 86, 693, 1954
22. Ralli, E. P., Nut. Symposium Series 5, 78, 1952
23. Welsh, A. L., Arch. Derm. Syph. 70, 181, 1954
24. Hodges, R. E., et al., Am. J. Clin. Nut. 11, 187, 1962

25. Vilter, R. W., et al., J. Lab. Clin. Med. 42, 335, 1953
26. Nut. Rev. 14, 186, 1956
27. Morgan, A. F., J. Am. Med. Women's Assn. 6, 179, 1951
28. Zintel, H. A., Am. J. Clin. Nut. 3, 501, 1955
29. Ershoff, B. H., J. Nut. 35, 269, 1948
30. Dugal, L. P., et al., Endocrinology 44, 420, 1949
31. Barboriak, J. J., et al., J. Nut. 63, 601, 1957
32. Lee, R. E., J. Nut. 72, 203, 1960
33. Helmer, A. C., et al., Studies Institutum Divi Thomae 1, 83, 207, 1937
34. Smith, R. W., et al., Am. J. Clin. Nut. 14, 98, 1964
35. Bauer, J. M., et al., J. Am. Med. Assn. 130, 1208, 1946
36. Eising, L., J. Bone Joint Surg. 45A, 69, 1963
37. Davies, P., Ann. Int. Med. 53, 1250, 1960
38. Buckley, G. F., et al., Am. J. Clin. Nut. 2, 396, 1954
39. Mitchell, R. G., Arch. Dis. Childh. 35, 385, 1960
40. Del Giudice, A., Summary 12, 21, 1960
41. Horwitt, M. K., et al., Am. Med. Assn. Arch. Neurol. 1, 312, 1959
42. Bicknell, F., and Prescott, F., *The Vitamins in Medicine*, Lee Foundation for Nutritional Research, Milwaukee, Wis., 1953
43. Johnson, J. A., Am. J. Dis. Child. 67, 265, 1944
44. Harris, P. L., et al., J. Nut. 40, 367, 1950
45. Horwitt, M. K., Am. J. Clin. Nut. 8, 451, 1960
46. Horwitt, M. K., et al., J. Am. Diet. Assn. 38, 231, 1961
47. Engel, C., Ann. N.Y. Acad. Sci. 52, 292, 1949
48. Vitamin E Symposium, Ann. N.Y. Acad. Sci. 52, 63, 1949
49. Steinberg, C. L., Arch. Surg. 63, 824, 1951
50. Gordon, H. H., et al., Am. J. Dis. Child. 90, 669, 1955
51. Moore, T., et al., J. Nut. 65, 185, 1958
52. Horwitt, M. K., Fed. Proc. 18, 530, 1959
53. Meyer, T. C., et al., Arch. Dis. Childh. 31, 212, 1956
54. Wallach, S., et al., J. Lab. Clin. Med. 59, 195, 1962
55. Horton, R., et al., J. Clin. Endocrinol. 22, 1187, 1962
56. MacIntyre, I., J. Chron. Dis. 16, 201, 1963
57. Barker, E. S., J. Chron. Dis. 11, 27, 1960
58. Wacker, W. E. C., et al., Med. Clin. No. Am. 44, 1357, 1960
59. Elkinton, J. R., Clin. Chem. 3, 309, 1957
60. Flink, E. B., J. Am. Med. Assn. 160, 1406, 1956
61. Hammersten, J. F., et al., New Engl. J. Med. 256, 897, 1957
62. Randall, R. E., Jr., et al., Ann. Int. Med. 50, 257, 1959
63. Nelson, G. Y., et al., J. Am. Diet. Assn. 38, 437, 1961
64. Stewart, J., et al., J. Comp. Path. 66, 1, 1956
65. Stevens, C. C., et al., J. Nut. 64, 67, 1958
66. Cohn, C., Nut. Rev. 20, 321, 1962
67. Hanna, S., et al., Lancet 2, 172, 1960
68. Editorial, J. Am. Med. Assn. 174, 69, 1960
69. Seelig, M., Am. J. Clin. Nut. 14, 342, 1964
70. Bunce, G. E., et al., J. Nut. 76, 23, 1962

71. Eisenbud, M., et al., Science 136, 370, 1962
72. Consumer Reports 27, 139, 1962
73. Saxena, K. M., et al., Science 138, 430, 1962

Chapter 33

1. J. Am. Diet. Assn. 38, 425, 1961
2. Wolf, S., and Wolff, H. G., *Human Gastric Function,* Oxford University Press, New York, N.Y., 1947
3. Brown, J. B., Nut. Rev. 17, 321, 1959
4. Platz, M., Am. J. Clin. Nut. 5, 618, 1957
5. McCarrison, R., *Studies in Deficiency Diseases,* Lee Foundation for Nutritional Research, Milwaukee, Wis., 1945
6. Raylor, R., *Hunza Health Secrets,* Prentice-Hall, Englewood Cliffs, N.J., 1964
7. Wrench, J. T., *The Wheel of Life,* Lee Foundation for Nutritional Research, Milwaukee, Wis., 1938
8. Siegal, S., J. Allergy 35, 252, 1964
9. Zarafonetis, C. J. D., et al., Blood 3, 780, 1948
10. Welsh, A. L., Arch. Derm. Syph. 70, 181, 1954
11. Adlersberg, D., et al., J. Nut. 25, 255, 1943
12. Moore, H. B., Am. J. Clin. Nut. 5, 77, 1957
13. Davidson, C. S., et al., Am. J. Clin. Nut. 10, 181, 1962
14. Hashin, S. A., Nut. Rev. 20, 1, 1962
15. Vinther-Paulsen, N., Geriatrics 7, 274, 1952
16. Bortz, W. M., et al., Am. J. Clin. Nut. 3, 494, 1955

Chapter 34

1. Martin, W. C., J. Applied Nut. 10, 3, 1957
2. Public Health Service, Public. 600, 1963
3. Sheldon, W., Pediatrics 23, 132, 1959
4. Portis, S. A., et al., J. Am. Med. Assn. 149, 1265, 1952
5. Josephson, E. M., *The Thymus, Manganese, and Myasthenia Gravis,* Chedney Press, New York, N.Y., 1963
6. *Diabetes Source Book,* U.S. Dept. HEW, Washington, D.C., 1964
7. Kahn, H. A., Pub. Health Rep. 66, 1246, 1951
8. Martin, W. C., Natural Food Farming 2, 6, 1956
9. Nitowsky, H. M., et al., Am. J. Dis. Child. 92, 164, 1956
10. Pub. Health Rep. 78, 1796, 1963; 79, 242, 1964
11. National Conference on Hospital-Acquired Staphylococcal Diseases, U.S. Dept. HEW, Communicable Disease Center, Atlanta, Georgia, 1958
12. Knight, V., et al., Ann. N.Y. Acad. Sci. 65, 206, 1956
13. Blair, J. E., et al., J. Am. Med. Assn. 166, 1192, 1958
14. Youman, J. B., J. Am. Med. Assn. 189, 672, 1964
15. Cartwright, G. E., J. Am. Med. Assn. 189, 30, 1964
16. Health Interview Survey, Series 10, No. 13, U.S. Dept. HEW, Washington, D.C., 1964

17. Harris, S. E., *The Economics of American Medicine,* Macmillan, New York, N.Y., 1964
18. Dilling, K., Nat. Health Fed. Bull. 10, 23, 1964
19. Kraus, H., et al., Institute Physic. Med. Rehabilitation, New York University, Bellevue Medical Center, New York, N.Y.
20. Registrant Examinations for Induction, D. A. Form 316, RCS-MED-66, Government Printing Office, Washington, D.C.
21. Morgan, A. F., et al., Yearbook of Agriculture, U.S. Dept. Agriculture, Washington, D.C., 1959, p. 187
22. Brown, J. B., Nut. Rev. 17, 321, 1950
23. Antar, M. A., et al., Am. J. Clin. Nut. 14, 169, 1964
24. Jolliffe, N., N.Y. State J. Med. 55, 2633, 1955
25. Muhlefluh, J., Nut. Abst. Rev. 33, 709, 1963
26. Jukes, T. H., J. Nut. 21, 193, 1941
27. Moran, F., et al., Nature 171, 103, 1955
28. Moore, R., et al., Brit. J. Nut. 12, 215, 1958
29. Czerniejewski, C. P., et al., Cereal Chem. 41, 65, 1964
30. Shinagawa, F., et al., J. Vitaminol. 3, 135, 1957
31. Alexander, B., et al., J. Clin. Invest. 25, 294, 1946
32. Richards, M. B., Brit. Med. J. 1, 433, 1945
33. Morrison, A. B., et al., J. Nut. 69, 111, 1959
34. Morgan, A. F., Food Technol. 18, 68, 1964
35. McCance, R. A., et al., Lancet 2, 205, 1955
36. Harris, R. S., et al., *Nutritional Evaluation of Food Processing,* Wiley, New York, N.Y., 1960
37. Consumer Reports, October, 1964
38. Thompson, M. M., et al., Am. J. Clin. Nut. 7, 80, 1959
39. Baker, H., et al., Nature 191, 78, 1961
40. Schoenberger, J. A., et al., Am. J. Med. Sci. 225, 551, 1953
41. *The Safety of Artificial Sweeteners for Use in Foods,* Nat. Acad. Sci., Nat. Res. Council, Public. 386, 1955
42. Kempner, W., No. Carolina Med. J. 5, 125, 273, 1944
43. Rowe, A. H., *Elimination Diets and the Patient's Allergies,* Lea & Febiger, Philadelphia, Pa., 1958
44. Morgan, A. F., Science 93, 261, 1941
45. Rudis, B. P., et al., Am. J. Dis. Child. 104, 506, 1962
46. Davidson, C. S., Am. J. Clin. Nut. 10, 181, 1962
47. Larrick, G. P., J. Am. Diet. Assn. 39, 117, 1961
48. Modern Nut. 17, 5, 1964
49. Leverton, R. M., Nut. Rev. 22, 321, 1964
50. Kilgore, L., et al., Am. J. Clin. Nut. 14, 52, 1964
51. Somers, G. F., et al., Plant Physiol. 26, 90, 1951
52. Walton, G., Am. J. Pub. Health 41, 986, 1951
53. Nut. Rev. 8, 230, 1950
54. Comly, H. H., J. Am. Med. Assn. 129, 112, 1945
55. Sci. News Letter 53, 275, 1948
56. Kilgore, L., et al., J. Am. Diet. Assn. 43, 39, 1963
57. Wilson, J. K., Agron. J. 41, 20, 1949
58. Holman, R., Proc. Soc. Exp. Biol. Med. 66, 307, 1947
59. Pank, G. L., J. Iowa Med. Soc. 54, 123, 1964

60. Reynold, H., et al., J. Agric. Food Chem. 1, 772, 1953
61. Bateman, G. Q., et al., J. Agric. Food Chem. 1, 332, 1953
62. Sikes, D., et al., J. Am. Vet. Med. Assn. 121, 337, 1952
63. Engel, R. W., Nut. Rev. 11, 97, 1953
64. Dale, W. E., et al., Science 142, 1474, 1963
65. Hayes, W. J., Jr., et al., J. Am. Med. Assn. 162, 890, 1956
66. Laug, E. P., et al., Arch. Indust. Hyg. 3, 245, 1957
67. Pearce, G. W., et al., Science 116, 254, 1953
68. Gannon, N., et al., J. Agric. Food Chem. 7, 824, 826, 829, 1959
69. Quinby, G. E., et al., J. Am. Med. Assn. 191, 109, 1965
70. Hoffman, W. S., et al., J. Am. Med. Assn. 188, 819, 1964
71. Fishbein, W. I., et al., J. Am. Med. Assn. 188, 819, 1964
72. Stewart, J., et al., J. Comp. Path. 66, 1, 1956
73. Kailin, E. W., Nat. Health Fed. Bull. 11, 10, 1965
74. Beeson, K. C., Plant Food J. 5, 7, 1951
75. Maynard, L. A., J. Am. Med. Assn. 161, 1478, 1956
76. Hunt, C. H., et al., Cereal Chem. 27, 79, 1950
77. Bear, F. E., Soil Crop Sci. Soc. Florida 17, 10, 1957
78. Nut. Rev. 18, 12, 1960
79. Bear, F. E., et al., Proc. Am. Soil Sci. Soc. 12, 380, 1958
80. Albrecht, W. A., Chem. Eng. News 21, 221, 1943
81. Sheldon, V. L., et al., Plant Soil 3, 33, 361, 1951
82. Picton, L. J., *Nutrition and the Soil*, Devin-Adair, New York, N.Y., 1949
83. Howard, A., *The Soil and Health*, Devin-Adair, New York, N.Y., 1947
84. Albrecht, W. A., *Soil Fertility and Animal Health*, Fred Hahne Printing Co., Webster City, Iowa, 1958
85. Gilbert, F. A., *Mineral Nutrition of Plants and Animals*, University of Oklahoma Press, Norman, Okla., 1953
86. Decker, G. C., Nut. Rev. 16, 289, 1958
87. Bentley, H. R., et al., Proc. Roy. Soc. Brit. 137, 402, 1950
88. Mellanby, E., Brit. Med. J. 2, 885, 1946
89. Reiner, L., et al., Arch. Biochem. 25, 447, 1950
90. Windmueller, H. G., et al., Fed. Proc. 15, 386, 1956
91. Phillips, C. R., et al., Am. J. Hyg. 50, 270, 1945
92. Windmueller, H. G., et al., J. Biol. Chem. 234, 895, 1959
93. Hawk, E. A., et al., Science 121, 442, 1955
94. Mickelson, O., J. Am. Diet. Assn. 33, 341, 1957
95. McKinney, L. L., et al., J. Agric. Food Chem. 3, 413, 1955
96. Pritchard, W. R., et al., J. Am. Vet. Med. Assn. 121, 1, 1952; 17, 430, 437, 448, 1956
97. Rather, L. J., Bull. Johns Hopkins Hosp. 88, 38, 1951
98. Hove, E. L., J. Nut. 50, 361, 1953; 51, 609, 1953
99. Pudelkervicz, C., et al., J. Nut. 70, 348, 1960
100. Shils, M. E., Am. J. Pub. Health 41, 417, 1951
101. Howe, E. L., et al., Proc. Soc. Exp. Biol. Med. 77, 502, 1951
102. Shils, M. E., et al., J. Indust. Hyg. Toxicol. 31, 175, 1949
103. Mulford, K. E., Arch. Envir. Health 2, 212, 1961
104. Hueper, W. C., Am. Med. Assn. Arch. Path. 62, 218, 1956

105. Porter, A. D., et al., Brit. J. Derm. 62, 355, 1950; 63, 123, 1951
106. Abramowitz, E. W., Arch. Derm. Syph. 45, 976, 1942
107. Kalz, F., Arch. Derm. 78, 740, 1958
108. Stare, F. J., Nut. Rev. 21, 1, 1963
109. Forbes, G., Brit. Med. J. 1, 367, 1947
110. Henderson, F., et al., J. Am. Med. Assn. 186, 1139, 1963
111. Santos, A. S., et al., Am. J. Dis. Child. 107, 424, 1964
112. Federal Register 29, 2557, 1964
113. Davis, P. L., Am. J. Med. 1, 634, 1946
114. Jacobson, L. D., et al., J. Lab. Clin. Med. 32, 1425, 1947
115. Cornatzer, L. E., et al., Proc. Soc. Exp. Biol. Med. 76, 552, 1957
116. Leevy, C. M., Med. World News 6, 53, 1965
117. Crosby, W. H., J. Chron. Dis. 12, 583, 1960
118. Crosby, W. H., Military Med. 125, 233, 1960
119. Conley, C. L., et al., New Engl. J. Med. 245, 529, 1951
120. Conley, C. L., et al., Ann. Int. Med. 43, 758, 1955
121. Schwartz, S. O., J. Clin. Lab. Med. 35, 894, 1950
122. Spies, T D., *Experiences with Folic Acid,* Year Book Publishers, Chicago, Ill., 1947
123. May, H. B., et al., Lancet 2, 607, 1948
124. Zarafonetis, C. J. D., et al., Blood 3, 780, 1948
125. Zarafonetis, C. J. D., Ann. Int. Med. 30, 1188, 1949
126. Snyder, J. C., Am. Assn. Advanc. Sci., Washington, D.C., 1948
127. Zarafonetis, C. J. D., Univ. Hosp. Bull. 8, 122, 1947
128. Zarafonetis, C. J. D., Am. J. Med. 5, 625, 1948
129. Cruickshank, A. H., et al., Bull. Johns Hopkins Hosp. 88, 211, 1951
130. Rogachefsky, H., N.Y. State J. Med. 64, 2988, 1964
131. Falliers, C. G., et al., Am. Med. Assn. J. Dis. Child. 99, 428, 1960
132. Burrows, B., et al., Ann. Int. Med. 52, 858, 1960
133. Galina, M. P., et al., New Engl. J. Med. 267, 1124, 1962
134. Siegal, S., J. Allergy 35, 252, 1964
135. Sheldon, J. M., et al., *A Manual of Clinical Allergy,* W. B. Saunders Co., Philadelphia, Pa., 1953, p. 93
136. Danowski, T. S., et al., J. Clin. Endocrinol. 10, 532, 1950
137. Slaughter, D., So. Dakota J. Med. Pharm. 1, 425, 1948
138. Saxena, K. M., et al., Science 138, 430, 1962
139. Borisov, V. P., Fed. Proc. 22, T1205, 1963
140. Federal Register 27, 5815, 1962
141. Williams, R. J., *Biochemical Individuality,* Wiley, New York, N.Y. 1956
142. Miller, C., Nat. Health Fed. Bull. 3, 5, 1962
143. Nut. Rev. 19, 221, 1961
144. Pub. Health Rep. 79, 242, 1964

Tables of Food Composition

Foods vary somewhat in composition; and the nutrients listed in the following tables are no more important than magnesium, cholin, pantothenic acid, and the many other items not listed. A comparison of nutrients obtained in one day with the Recommended Daily Dietary Allowances, however, often reveals many flaws in a diet. Since these allowances are designed for healthy individuals, ill ones should receive two or three times the amounts of all nutrients except sodium and possibly calories. Unfortunately, no data is available for the highly nutritious foods that can be prepared at home.

Because of people who must stay on low-sodium diets, foods are listed unsalted except when salt has been added during preparation, as in packaged cereals and canned soups. People who salt foods lightly should add 2,000 milligrams of sodium to a day's dietary, and those who enjoy well-salted foods, 6,000 milligrams. Normally the intake of potassium should be approximately the same as that of sodium; and the calcium intake should be two-thirds or more of that of phosphorus.

Both animal and vegetable fats contain large amounts of partially unsaturated oleic acid, a non-essential fatty acid that appears to be laid down in the walls of the blood vessels in atherosclerosis; therefore I have combined oleic acid with the saturated fatty acids in the following tables. When the total fat is greater than the sum of oleic acid, the saturated fatty acids, and linoleic acid, the difference represents the amount of linolenic and arachidonic acids present. The ideal amount of linoleic acid needed daily is not known, but it appears to be approximately 15 grams. To support the growth of valuable intestinal bacteria, the diet should also contain 15 grams or more of fiber.

RECOMMENDED DAILY

	Age Years from	to	Wgt. pounds	Hgt. inches	Calories	Protein gm.
MEN	18	35	154	69	2,900	70
	35	55	154	69	2,600	70
	55	75	154	69	2,200	70
WOMEN	18	35	128	64	2,100	58
	35	55	128	64	1,900	58
	55	75	128	64	1,600	58
	During last 6 months of pregnancy				+200	+20
	While nursing infant				+1,000	+40
CHILDREN	1	3	29	34	1,300	32
	3	6	40	42	1,600	40
	6	9	53	49	2,100	52
BOYS	9	12	72	55	2,400	60
	12	15	98	61	3,000	75
	15	18	134	68	3,400	85
GIRLS	9	12	72	55	2,200	55
	12	15	103	62	2,500	62
	15	18	117	64	2,300	58

Equivalents used in the following tables

1 quart = 4 cups

1 cup = 8 fluid ounces

= ½ pint

= 16 tablespoons

2 tablespoons = 1 fluid ounce

1 tablespoon (T.) = 3 teaspoons (t.)

1 stick butter or margarine = ½ cup

= 16 pats or squares

DIETARY ALLOWANCES[1]*

Calcium mg.	Iron mg.	VITAMINS					
		A units	B₁ mg.	B₂ mg.	Niacin mg.	C mg.	D units
800	10	5,000	1.2	1.7	19	70	
800	10	5,000	1	1.6	17	70	
800	10	5,000	.9	1.3	15	70	
800	15	5,000	.8	1.3	14	70	
800	15	5,000	.8	1.2	13	70	
800	10	5,000	.8	1.2	13	70	
+500	+5	+1,000	+.2	+.3	+3	+30	400
+500	+5	+3,000	+.4	+.6	+7	+30	400
800	8	2,000	.5	.8	9	40	400
800	10	2,500	.6	1	11	50	400
800	12	3,500	.8	1.3	14	60	400
1,100	15	4,500	1	1.4	16	70	400
1,400	15	5,000	1.2	1.8	20	80	400
1,400	15	5,000	1.4	2	22	80	400
1,100	15	4,500	.9	1.3	15	80	400
1,300	15	5,000	1	1.5	17	80	400
1,300	15	5,000	.9	1.3	15	70	400

[1] Report of Food and Nutrition Board, National Academy of Sciences, National Research Council, Public. 1146. Washington, D.C., Revised Edition, 1964.

* Intended to meet the needs of *healthy* individuals living in the United States.

TABLES OF FOOD COMPOSITION,

FOOD	Approximate Measure	Wgt. in grams	Calories	Protein grams	Carbohydrate grams	Fiber grams	Fat grams	Saturated fatty acid* grams
DAIRY PRODUCTS								
Cows' milk, whole	1 qt.	976	660	32	48	0	40	36
skim	1 qt.	984	360	36	52	0	8	8
Buttermilk, cultured	1 cup	246	127	9	13	0	5	4
Evaporated, undiluted	1 cup	252	345	16	24	0	20	18
Fortified milk, or pep-up†	6 cups	1,419	1,373	89	119	1.4	42	23
High-calorie pep-up†	⅔ cup	160	155	10	13	.2	5	2
Low-calorie pep-up‡	4½ cups	1,053	738	56	62	.2	28	12
Low-calorie pep-up‡	⅔ cup	200	148	11	12	8	5	2
Powdered milk, whole	1 cup	103	515	27	39	0	28	24
skim, instant	1⅓ cup	85	290	30	42	0	8	8
skim, non-instant	⅔ cup	85	290	30	42	0	8	8
Goats' milk, fresh	1 cup	244	165	8	11	0	10	8
Malted milk (½ cup ice cream)	2 cups	540	690	24	70	0	24	22
Cocoa	1 cup	252	235	8	26	0	11	10
Yogurt, of partially skim milk	1 cup	250	120	8	13	0	4	3
Milk pudding (cornstarch)	1 cup	248	275	9	40	0	10	9
Custard, baked	1 cup	248	285	13	28	0	14	11
Ice cream, commercial	1 cup	188	300	6	29	0	18	16
Ice milk, commercial	1 cup	190	275	9	32	0	10	9
Cream, light, or half-and-half	½ cup	120	170	4	5	0	15	13
Cream, heavy, or whipping	½ cup	119	430	2	3	0	47	42

SOURCES: Agriculture Handbook No. 8 and Home and Garden Bulletin No. 72; U.S. Dept. Agric., Washington, D.C.; Nutritional Data: H. J. Heinz Company, Pittsburgh, Pa., 1963.

EDIBLE PORTIONS

Lino-leic acid grams	Iron mg.	Cal-cium mg.	Phos-phorus mg.	Potas-sium mg.	Sodium mg.	A units	B₁ mg.	B₂ mg.	Niacin mg.	C mg.
				MINERALS				**VITAMINS**		
ϕ	.4	1,140	930	210·	450	1,560	.32	1.7	.8	.6
0	.4	1,192	940	215	480	0	.4	1.7	.8	6
ϕ	.1	298	270	52	250	180	.1	.4	.2	2
ϕ	.2	570	465	102	236	780	.1	.8	.5	ϕ
14.2	12.1	2,949	3,116	2,704	1,480	2,670	11.5	10.9	103.5	330
1.7	1.4	333	351	300	310	295	1.3	1.2	9.5	37·
11.2	7.4	1,792	2,040	1,015	1,290	0	10.4	11.4	100.8	6
2.5	1.5	358	408	203	300	0	2.1	2.3	20.1	1
ϕ	.4	968	2,160	200	810	2,160	.3	1.5	.7	ϕ
0	.4	1,040	940	210	793	ϕ	.2	1.4·	.7	ϕ
0	.4	1,040	940	.210	789	ϕ	.2	1.4	.7	ϕ
ϕ	.2	315	212	66	66	390	.2	.3	.7	2
ϕ	.8	270	615	60	398	670	.3	1.1	.2	2
ϕ	.9	280	212	50	120	390	.2	.5	.3	ϕ
ϕ	.1	295	270	50	262	170	.1	.4	.2	ϕ
ϕ	.1	290	260	48	258	360	.1	.4	.1	ϕ
1	1	278	370	100	158	870	.1	.5	.2	ϕ
1	.1	175	150	170	126	740	ϕ§	.3	.1	ϕ
ϕ	.1	290	250	54	136	390	.1	.4	.2	ϕ
ϕ	ϕ	130	90	95	55	550	ϕ	.2	ϕ§	ϕ·
1	0	82	70	65	50	1,900	ϕ	.1	ϕ	ϕ

ϕ Includes oleic acid. ϕ Indicates trace only.

† Made by recipe on p. 413 with 2 eggs, torula yeast fortified with calcium, and a 6-ounce can of frozen undiluted orange juice.

‡ Made by recipe on p. 86 with torula yeast fortified with calcium. Since lecithin and milk sugar are apparently not used for calories, the total calorie content is probably 425.

§ Contains less than .1 milligram.

FOOD	Approximate Measure	Wgt. in grams	Calories	Protein grams	Carbohydrate grams	Fiber grams	Fat grams	Saturated fatty acid* grams
DAIRY PRODUCTS (*Continued*)								
Cheese, cottage,								
creamed	1 cup	225	240	30	6	0	11	10
uncreamed	1 cup	225	195	38	6	0	1	1
Cheddar, or American	1-in. cube	17	70	4	1	0	6	5
Cheddar, grated	½ cup	56	226	14	1	0	19	17
Cream cheese	1 oz.	28	105	2	1	0	11	10
Processed cheese	1 oz.	28	105	7	1	0	9	8
Roquefort type	1 oz.	28	105	6	1	0	9	8
Swiss	1 oz.	28	105	7	1	0	8	7
Eggs, boiled, poached, or raw	2	100	150	12	1	0	12	10
Scrambled, omelet, or fried	2	128	220	13	1	0	16	14
Yolks only	2	34	120	6	1	0	10	8
OILS, FATS, AND SHORTENINGS								
Butter	1 T.	14	100	1	1	0	11	10
Butter	½ cup or ¼ lb.	112	800	1	1	0	90	80
Hydrogenated cooking fat	½ cup	100	665	0	0	0	100	88
Lard	½ cup	110	992	0	0	0	110	92
Margarine, ¼ pound or	½ cup	112	806	1	1	0	91	76
Margarine, 2 pats or	1 T.	14	100	1	1	0	11	9
Mayonnaise	1 T.	15	110	1	1	0	12	5
Oils								
Corn, soy, peanut‡ cottonseed	1 T.	14	125	0	0	0	14	5
Olive	1 T.	14	125	0	0	0	14	13
Safflower, sunflower seed, walnut	1 T.	14	125	0	0	0	14	3
Salad dressing								
French	1 T.	15	60	1	2	0	6	2
Thousand Island	1 T.	15	75	1	1	0	8	3
Salt pork	2 oz.	60	470	3	0	0	55	—

Lino-leic acid grams	Iron mg.	Calcium mg.	Phosphorus mg.	Potassium mg.	Sodium mg.	A units	B₁ mg.	B₂ mg.	Niacin mg.	C mg.
		MINERALS					VITAMINS			
ƒ	.9	207	360	170	625	430	.1	.6	.2	0
ƒ	.9	202	380	180	620	20	.1	.6	.1	0
ƒ	.1	133	128	30	180	230	ƒ	.1	ƒ	0
ƒ	.6	435	390	90	540	700	ƒ	.2	ƒ	0
ƒ	.1	18	170	25	180	440	ƒ	.1	ƒ	0
ƒ	.1	210	190	22	370	350	ƒ	.1	ƒ	0
ƒ	.2	122	100	22	284	350	ƒ	.2	.1	0
ƒ	.2	270	140	25	225	320	ƒ	.1	ƒ	0
1	2.3	54	205	129	122	1,180	ƒ	.3	ƒ	0
1	2.2	60	222	140	338	1,200	ƒ	.4	ƒ	0
1	1.8	48	175	33	9	1,180	ƒ	.1	ƒ	0
ƒ	ƒ	3	0	4	120	460	0	ƒ†	0	0
2	ƒ	22	0	28	990	3,700	0	ƒ	0	0
7	0	0	0	0	4	0	0	0	0	0
11	0	0	0	ƒ	ƒ	0	0	0	0	0
8	0	22	16	58	1,150	3,700	0	ƒ	0	0
1	0	3	2	9	144	460	0	0	0	0
6	.1	2	8	3	85	40	ƒ	ƒ	ƒ	0
7	0	0	0	0	0	0	0	0	0	0
1	0	0	0	0	0	0	0	0	0	0
9	0	0	0	0	0	0	0	0	0	0
3	.1	3	0	0	—	0	0	0	0	0
4	.1	2	ƒ	—	—	60	ƒ	ƒ	ƒ	0
—	.4	ƒ	ƒ	19	1,350	0	ƒ	ƒ	ƒ	0

* Includes oleic acid.
ƒ Indicates trace only.
† Contains less than .1 milligram.

‡ Richest source of arachidonic acid.
— No data available.

FOOD	Approximate Measure	Wgt. in grams	Calories	Protein grams	Carbohydrate grams	Fiber grams	Fat grams	Saturated fatty acid* grams
MEAT AND POULTRY, COOKED								
Bacon, crisp, drained	2 slices	16	95	4	1	0	8	7
Beef, chuck, pot-roasted	3 oz.	85	245	23	0	0	16	15
Hamburger, commercial	3 oz.	85	245	21	0	0	17	15
Ground lean	3 oz.	85	185	24	0	0	10	9
Roast beef, oven cooked	3 oz.	85	390	16	0	0	36	35
Steak, as sirloin	3 oz.	85	330	20	0	0	27	25
Steak, lean, as round	3 oz.	85	220	24	0	0	12	11
Corned beef	3 oz.	85	185	22	0	0	10	9
Corned beef hash, canned	3 oz.	85	120	12	6	8	8	7
Dried or chipped	2 oz.	56	115	19	0	0	4	4
Pot-pie, 4¼-inch diameter	1 pie	227	460	18	32	8	28	25
Stew, with vegetables	1 cup	235	185	15	15	8	10	9
Chicken, broiled	3 oz.	85	185	23	0	0	9	7
Fried, breast or leg and thigh	3 oz.	85	245	25	0	0	15	11
Chicken livers, fried	3 med.	100	140	22	2.3	0	14	12
Chicken, roasted	3½ oz.	100	290	25	0	0	20	16
Duck, domestic	3½ oz.	100	370	16	0	0	28	—
Lamb, chop, broiled	4 oz.	115	480	24	0	0	35	33
Leg, roasted	3 oz.	86	314	20	0	0	14	14
Shoulder, braised	3 oz.	85	285	18	0	0	23	21
Pork chop, 1 thick	3½ oz.	100	260	16	0	0	21	18
Ham, cured. pan-broiled	3 oz.	85	290	16	0	0	22	19
Ham, as luncheon meat	2 oz.	57	170	13	0	0	13	11
Ham, canned, spiced	2 oz.	57	165	8	1	0	14	12
Pork roast	3 oz.	85	310	21	0	0	24	21
Pork sausage, bulk	3½ oz.	100	475	18	0	0	44	40
Turkey, roasted	3½ oz.	100	265	27	0	0	15	—
Veal cutlet, broiled	3 oz.	85	185	23	0	0	9	8
Roast	3 oz.	85	305	23	0	0	14	13

Lino-leic acid grams	Iron mg.	Cal-cium mg.	Phos-phorus mg.	Potas-sium mg.	Sodium mg.	A units	B₁ mg.	B₂ mg.	Niacin mg.	C mg.
ƒ	.5	2	42	65	600	0	ƒ	ƒ	.8	0
ƒ	2.9	10	110	340	50	30	ƒ	.18	3.5	0
ƒ	2.7	9	145	320	100	30	ƒ	ƒ	5.1	0
ƒ	3	10	158	340	110	20	ƒ	ƒ	5.3	0
ƒ	2.1	7	105	350	60	60	ƒ	ƒ	3	0
ƒ	2.5	8	150	320	60	50	ƒ	ƒ	4	0
ƒ	3	11	180	300	62	20	ƒ	ƒ	4.8	0
ƒ	3.7	17	100	60	1,200	20	ƒ	.2	2.9	0
ƒ	1.1	20	125	180	540	10	ƒ	.1	2.4	0
0	2.9	10	60	190	30	ƒ	ƒ	.2	2.2	0
1	2.5	20	150	318	620	2,800	ƒ	.1	3	ƒ
ƒ	2.8	30	150	500	75	2,500	.1	.2	4.4	14
1	1.4	10	250	350	50	260	ƒ	.1	7	0
1	1.8	13	218	320	50	200	ƒ	.1	5	0
1	7.4	16	240	160	51	32,200	.2	2.4	11.8	20
4	1.9	10	220	280	58	960	ƒ	.2	7.4	0
—	2.4	9	170	285	74	—	ƒ	.4	7.9	0
1	3.1	10	140	275	75	0	.1	.2	4.5	0
0	2.8	9	190	270	70	0	.1	.2	5	0
1	2.4	8	170	260	60	0	.1	.2	4	0
1	2.2	8	250	390	30	0	.6	.2	3.8	0
1	2.2	8	240	370	1,000	0	.4	.1	3	0
1	1.5	5	170	290	700	0	.2	.1	1.6	0
1	1.2	5	170	280	800	0	.2	.1	1.8	0
1	2.7	9	240	360	40	0	.8	.2	4.4	0
1	2.4	7	165	270	958	0	.8	.3	3.7	0
—	3.8	23	320	320	60	0	ƒ	.1	8	0
ƒ	2.7	9	230	400	70	0	ƒ	.2	6	0
ƒ	2.9	10	200	390	70	0	.1	.3	6.6	0

* Includes oleic acid.
ƒ Indicates trace only.
— No data available.

FOOD	Approximate Measure	Wgt. in grams	Calories	Protein grams	Carbohydrate grams	Fiber grams	Fat grams	Saturated fatty acid* grams
VARIETY MEATS								
Brains, beef, calf, pork, sheep	3½ oz.	100	125	10	0	0	8	—
Chili con carne with beans	1 cup	250	325	19	30	1.2	15	14
Without beans	1 cup	255	510	26	15	ƒ	38	36
Heart, braised	3 oz.	85	160	26	1	0	5	4
Kidney, braised	3½ oz.	100	230	33	1	0	7	—
Liver, beef, sautéed with oil	3½ oz.	100	230	26	5	0	10	7
Calf, 1 large slice	3½ oz.	100	261	29	4	0	13	—
Lamb, 2 slices	3½ oz.	100	260	32	3	0	12	—
Pork, 2 slices	3½ oz.	100	241	29	3	0	11	—
Liver, desiccated see Supplementary foods								
Sausage, bologna	2 slices, ⅛ × 4"	50	124	7	2	ƒ	10	9
Frankfurter	2, ⅞ × 7"	102	246	14	2	ƒ	20	18
Liverwurst	2 oz.	56	132	8	2	0	11	—
Sweetbreads, braised, calf	3½ oz.	100	170	32	0	0	3	—
Tongue, beef	3 oz.	85	205	18	ƒ	0	14	13
FISH AND SEAFOODS								
Clams, steamed or canned	3 oz.	85	87	12	2	0	1	—
Cod, broiled	3½ oz.	100	170	28	0	0	5	0
Codfish cakes, fried	2 small	100	175	15	9	—	8	—
Crabmeat, cooked	3 oz.	85	90	14	1	0	2	0
Fish sticks, breaded, fried	5	112	200	19	8	0	10	5
Flounder, baked	3½ oz.	100	200	30	0	0	8	0
Haddock, fried	3 oz.	85	135	16	6	0	5	4
Halibut, broiled	3½ oz.	100	182	26	0	0	8	0
Herring, kippered	1 small	100	211	22	0	0	13	0
Lobster, steamed	½ aver.	100	92	18	ƒ	0	1	0
Mackerel, canned	3 oz.	85	155	18	0	0	9	0
Oysters, raw	6-8 med. or ½ cup	120	85	8	3	0	2	0

Lino-leic acid grams	MINERALS					VITAMINS				
	Iron mg.	Cal-cium mg.	Phos-phorus mg.	Potas-sium mg.	Sodium mg.	A units	B₁ mg.	B₂ mg.	Niacin mg.	C mg.
—	2.4	20	312	219	125	0	.2	.2	4.4	0
ƒ	4.2	98	360	500	1,060	100	ƒ	.2	3.5	0
1	5.9	14	365	520	1,000	130	ƒ	.3	5.6	0
ƒ	6	14	203	190	90	30	.2	1	6.8	—
—	13.1	18	220	320	250	3,150	.5	4.8	10.7	0
2	9	8	476	380	184	53,400	.3	4.1	16.5	27
—	14.2	13	537	453	118	32,000	.2	4.2	16.5	37
—	17.9	16	572	330	85	74,000	ƒ.5	5.1	24.9	36
	29	25	539	390	111	14,000	.3	4.4	22.3	22
ƒ	1.2	4	54	110	550	0	ƒ	ƒ	1.3	0
1	1.2	6	50	215	1,100	0	.1	.2	2.5	0
—	2.8	4	120	75	450	2,860	.2	.6	2.3	0
—	.8	7	360	244	116	0	.11	.3	5	0
ƒ	2.5	7	180	240	90	0	ƒ	.3	3	0
—	5.4	74	110	230	170	100	ƒ	ƒ	.9	0
—	1	30	270	400	110	180	ƒ	.1	3	0
—	—	—	—	—	—	—	—	—	—	0
0	.8	38	170	100	900	—	ƒ	ƒ	2.1	0
3	.4	12	180	140	—	ƒ	0	ƒ	1.6	0
—	1.4	22	344	585	235	0	ƒ	ƒ	2.5	0
ƒ	.7	11	200	510	56	0	ƒ	ƒ	2.6	0
0	.8	14	267	540	56	440	ƒ	ƒ	9.2	0
0	1.4	66	254	—	—	110	ƒ	.1	3.4	0
0	.6	65	192	180	210	0	.1	ƒ	1.9	0
0	1.9	221	260	—	—	20	ƒ	.3	7.4	0
0	6.6	113	150	110	80	320	.2	.2	3.3	0

* Includes oleic acid.
— No data available.
ƒ Indicates trace only.

FOOD	Approximate Measure	Wgt. in grams	Calories	Protein grams	Carbohydrate grams	Fiber grams	Fat grams	Saturated fatty acid* grams
FISH AND SEAFOODS (*Continued*)								
Oyster stew, made with milk	1 cup	230	200	11	11	0	11	—
Salmon, canned	3 oz.	85	120	17	0	0	5	1
Sardines, canned	3 oz.	85	180	22	0	0	9	.4
Scallops, breaded, fried	3½ oz.	100	194	18	10	0	8	—
Shad, baked	3 oz.	85	170	20	0	0	10	0
Shrimp, steamed	3 oz.	85	110	23	0	0	1	0
Swordfish, broiled	1 steak	100	180	27	0	0	6	0
Tuna, canned, drained	3 oz.	85	170	25	0	0	7	3
VEGETABLES								
Artichoke, globe	1 large	100	8-44	2	10†	2	0	0
Asparagus, green	6 spears	96	18	1	3	.5	0	0
Beans, green snap	1 cup	125	25	1	6	.6	0	0
Lima, green	1 cup	160	140	8	24	3	0	0
Lima, dry, cooked	1 cup	192	260	16	48	2	0	0
Navy, baked with pork	¾ cup	200	250	11	37	2	6	6
Red kidney, canned	1 cup	260	230	15	42	2.5	1	0
Bean sprouts, uncooked	1 cup	50	17	1	3	.3	0	0
Beet greens, steamed	1 cup	100	27	2	6	1.4	0	0
Beetroots, boiled	1 cup	165	68	1	12	.8	0	0
Broccoli, steamed	1 cup	150	45	5	8	1.9	0	0
Brussels sprouts, steamed	1 cup	130	60	6	12	1.7	0	0
Cabbage, as coleslaw‡	1 cup	120	140	1	9	1	14	4
Sauerkraut, canned	1 cup	150	32	1	7	1.5	0	0
Steamed cabbage	1 cup	170	40	2	9	1.3	0	0
Carrots, cooked, diced	1 cup	150	45	1	10	.9	0	0
Raw, grated	1 cup	110	45	1	10	1.2	0	0
Strips, from raw	1 med.	50	20	0	5	.5	0	0
Cauliflower, steamed	1 cup	120	30	3	6	1	0	0
Celery, cooked, diced	1 cup	100	20	1	4	1	0	0
Stalk, raw	1 large	40	5	1	1	.3	0	0
Chard, steamed, leaves and stalks	1 cup	150	30	2	7	1.4	0	0
Collards, steamed leaves	1 cup	150	51	5	8	2	0	0
Corn, steamed	1 ear	100	92	3	21	.8	1	0
Cooked or canned	1 cup	200	170	5	41	1.6	0	0

Lino-leic acid grams	Iron mg.	Cal-cium mg.	Phos-phorus mg.	Potas-sium mg.	Sodium mg.	A units	B₁ mg.	B₂ mg.	Niacin mg.	C mg.
		MINERALS						**VITAMINS**		
—	3.3	269	230	310	940	640	.1	.4	1.7	0
0	.7	160	280	340	45	60	ƒ	.2	6.8	0
4	2.5	367	490	540	480	190	ƒ	.2	4.6	0
—	1.4	110	338	470	265	0	ƒ	.1	1.4	0
0	.5	20	300	350	75	20	.1	ƒ	7.3	0
0	2.6	98	250	205	130	50	ƒ	ƒ	1.9	0
0	1.1	20	250	780	51	2,000	ƒ	ƒ	10.3	0
4	1.2	7	300	240	700	70	ƒ	.1	10.9	0
0	1.3	50	69	300	30	150	ƒ	ƒ	.7	8
0	1.7	18	43	130	3	700	ƒ	ƒ	.9	18
0	.9	45	20	204	2	830	ƒ	.1	.6	16
0	2.5	44	105	320	2	290	.2	.1	1.9	15
0	1.5	15	75	306	1	ƒ	.3	.1	1.3	0
0	4.2	112	226	420	960	ƒ	.1	.1	1.3	ƒ
0	4.6	74	350	750	6	0	.1	.1	1.5	0
*	3.8	19	170	514	3	40	.2	.1	1.3	*
*	3.2	118	45	332	76	5,100	ƒ	.1	.3	30
*	1	24	44	324	64	30	ƒ	ƒ	.5	10
*	2.1	190	100	405	15	5,100	ƒ	.2	1.2	105
*	1.7	44	95	400	14	520	ƒ	.1	.6	60
9	.5	47	30	240	130	80	ƒ	ƒ	.3	50
*	.8	54	45	210	915	0	ƒ	.1	.2	24
*	.8	78	50	240	23	150	ƒ	ƒ	.3	53
*	.9	38	55	600	75	18,130	ƒ	ƒ	.7	6
*	.9	43	29	410	51	13,000	ƒ	ƒ	.7	7
*	.4	20	19	205	25	5,000	ƒ	ƒ	.3	3
*	1.2	26	84	220	11	100	ƒ	.1	.6	34
*	.5	54	40	300	80	0	ƒ	ƒ	.4	7
*	.2	20	18	130	30	0	ƒ	ƒ	.2	3
*	3.6	155	54	475	120	8,100	ƒ	.1	.1	17
*	1.2	282	75	393	40	11,700	ƒ	.2	1.6	75
*	.5	4	120	300	ƒ	300	ƒ	ƒ	1.1	12
*	1.3	10	102	400	472§	520	ƒ	.1	2.4	14

* Includes oleic acid.

— No data available.

† Largely inulin, which is not utilized in the body.

ƒ Indicates trace only.

‡ With mayonnaise.

§ Salted.

FOOD	Approximate Measure	Wgt. in grams	Calories	Protein grams	Carbohydrate grams	Fiber grams	Fat grams	Saturated fatty acid* grams
VEGETABLES (*Continued*)								
Cucumbers, ⅛" slices	6	50	6	8	1	.2	0	0
Dandelion greens, steamed	1 cup	180	80	5	16	3.2	1	0
Eggplant, steamed	1 cup	180	30	2	9	1.2	8	0
Endive (escarole)	2 oz.	57	10	1	2	.6	8	—
Kale, steamed	1 cup	110	45	4	8	.9	1	—
Kohlrabi, raw, sliced	1 cup	140	40	2	9	1.5	8	—
Lambs' quarters, steamed	1 cup	150	48	5	7	3.2	8	—
Lentils	1 cup	200	212	15	38	2.4	8	—
Lettuce, loose leaf, green	½ head	100	14	1	2	.5	8	—
Iceberg	½ head	100	13	8	3	.5	8	—
Mushrooms, cooked or canned	⅔ cup	120	12	2	4	8	8	—
Mustard greens, steamed	1 cup	140	30	3	6	1.2	8	—
Okra, diced, steamed	1½ cup	100	32	1	7	1	8	—
Onions, mature, cooked	1 cup	210	80	2	18	1.6	8	—
Raw, green	6 small	50	22	8	5	1	8	—
Parsley, chopped, raw	2 T.	7	2	8	8	8	8	—
Parsnips, steamed	1 cup	155	95	2	22	3	1	—
Peas, green, canned	1 cup	100	68	3	13	1.4	8	—
Fresh, steamed	1 cup	100	70	5	12	2.2	8	—
Frozen, heated	1 cup	100	68	5	12	1.8	8	—
Split, cooked	½ cup	100	115	8	21	.4	8	—
With carrots, frozen, heated	1 cup	200	53	3	10	1	8	—
Peppers, pimientos, canned	1 pod	38	10	8	2	8	8	—
Raw, green, sweet	1 large	100	25	1	6	1.4	8	—
Stuffed with beef and crumbs	1 med.	150	255	19	24	1	9	8
Potatoes, baked	1 med.	100	100	2	22	.5	8	—
French-fried	10 pieces	60	155	1	20	.4	7	3
Mashed with milk and butter	1 cup	200	230	4	28	.7	12	11

Lino-leic acid grams	MINERALS					VITAMINS				
	Iron mg.	Cal-cium mg.	Phos-phorus mg.	Potas-sium mg.	Sodium mg.	A units	B₁ mg.	B₂ mg.	Niacin mg.	C mg.
0	.2	5	9	80	3	0	ƀ	ƀ	.2	4
ƀ	5.6	337	126	760	230	27,300	.3	.2	2.3	29
ƀ	.9	17	60	390	2	10	ƀ	ƀ	.9	8
—	2	45	28	215	9	1,700	ƀ	ƀ	.1	6
—	2.3	230	57	260	29	8,000	ƀ	.2	.8	60
—	.8	66	70	520	10	ƀ	ƀ	ƀ	.3	85
—	2	460	100	—	—	14,650	.1	.4	1.4	120
—	4.2	50	238	505	15	40	ƀ	ƀ	1.2	0
—	2	35	26	260	9	1,900	ƀ	ƀ	.3	18
—	.5	20	22	175	9	300	ƀ	ƀ	.3	6
—	.9	8	105	180	400†	0	ƀ	.3	3	3
—	4.2	308	60	510	68	10,050	.2	.2	2	60
—	.7	82	62	370	2	740	ƀ	ƀ	.8	20
—	2	67	88	315	24	0	ƀ	ƀ	.4	10
—	.4	65	22	115	2	500	ƀ	ƀ	.2	16
—	.4	14	7	80	2	580	ƀ	ƀ	.2	14
—	2.2	88	120	570	22	0	ƀ	.2	.3	19
—	2.8	23	67	96	270	500	.1	ƀ	1	8
—	2.9	22	122	200	2	960	.3	.2	2.3	24
—	2.8	19	86	135	225	600	.2	ƀ	1.7	13
—	2.7	22	89	296	23	40	.2	ƀ	.9	0
—	2.2	25	57	260	84	9,000	.2	ƀ	2.3	20
—	.7	9	20	50	ƀ	800	.2	ƀ	2.7	20
—	.4	22	25	170	ƀ	370	ƀ	ƀ	.4	120
ƀ	3	60	180	387	420	420	.2	.2	3.5	60
—	.7	13	66	500	4	10	.2	ƀ	2.2	25
4‡	.7	9	6	510	6	0	ƀ	ƀ	2.8	8
ƀ	2	45	150	654	660	470	.2	.2	2.6	16

* Includes oleic acid.
ƀ Indicates trace only.
— No data available.
† Salted.
‡ If fried in oil.

FOOD	Approximate Measure	Wgt. in grams	Calories	Protein grams	Carbohydrate grams	Fiber grams	Fat grams	Saturated fatty acid* grams
VEGETABLES (*Continued*)								
Potatoes, pan-fried	½ cup	100	268	4	33	.4	14	6
Scalloped with cheese	½ cup	100	145	6	14	.4	8	7
Steamed before peeling	1 med.	100	80	2	19	.4	‡	—
Potato chips	10	20	110	1	10	‡	7	4
Radishes, raw	5 small	50	10	‡	2	.3	0	—
Rutabagas, diced	¾ cup	100	32	‡	8	1.4	0	0
Soybeans, unseasoned	1 cup	200	260	22	20	3.2	11	0
Spinach, steamed	1 cup	100	26	3	3	1	‡	—
Squash, summer	1 cup	210	35	1	8	.6	‡	—
Winter, mashed	1 cup	200	95	4	23	2.6	‡	—
Sweet potatoes, baked	1 med.	110	155	2	36	1	1	—
Candied	1 med.	175	235	2	60	1.5	6	5
Tomatoes, canned whole	1 cup	240	50	2	9	1	‡	—
Raw, 2 by 2½″	1 med.	150	30	1	6	.6	‡	—
Tomato juice, canned	1 cup	240	50	2	10	.6	‡	—
Tomato catsup	1 T.	17	15	‡	4	‡	‡	—
Turnip greens, steamed	1 cup	145	45	4	8	1.8	1	—
Turnips, steamed, sliced	1 cup	155	40	1	9	1.8	‡	—
Watercress, leaves and stems, raw	1 cup	50	9	1	1	.3	‡	—
FRUITS								
Apple juice, fresh or canned	1 cup	250	125	‡	34	—	0	0
Apple vinegar	½ cup	100	14	‡	3	0	0	0
Apples, raw	1 med.	130	70	‡	18	1	‡	—
Stewed or canned	1 cup	240	100‡	‡	26	2	‡	—
Apricots, canned in syrup	1 cup	250	220	2	57	1	‡	—
Dried, uncooked	½ cup	75	220	4	50	2	‡	—
Fresh	3 med.	114	55	1	14	.7	‡	—
Nectar, or juice	1 cup	250	140	1	36	2	‡	—
Avocado	½ large	108	185	2	6	1.8	18	12
Banana	1 med.	150	85	1	23	.9	‡	—
Blackberries, fresh	1 cup	144	85	2	19	6.6	1	—
Blueberries, canned	1 cup	250	245	1	65	2	‡	—
Cantaloupe	½ med.	380	40	1	9	2.2	‡	—

Linoleic acid grams	MINERALS					VITAMINS				
	Iron mg.	Calcium mg.	Phosphorus mg.	Potassium mg.	Sodium mg.	A units	B₁ mg.	B₂ mg.	Niacin mg.	C mg.
8†	1.1	15	100	775	225	0	.1	ƒ	2.8	20
ƒ	.5	127	112	310	450	320	ƒ	.1	.9	10
—	.8	11	56	407	3	10	.1	ƒ	1.2	15
3†	.4	6	38	210	200	ƒ	ƒ	ƒ	.6	0
—	.5	5	53	130	4	15	ƒ	ƒ	.1	11
0	.4	40	35	170	4	350	ƒ	ƒ	.7	21
7	5.4	150	360	1,080	4	60	.4	.1	1.2	0
—	.2	114	33	470	74	11,800	.1	.2	.6	30
—	.8	8	32	480	8	700	ƒ	.1	1.3	24
—	1.6	23	49	510	2	6,100	.1	.1	.6	7
—	1	36	58	300	12	8,900	.1	ƒ	.7	24
1	1.6	50	70	360	18	11,600	.1	.1	1.1	30
—	1.5	27	44	552	28	2,500	.1	ƒ	1.7	40
—	.9	16	40	360	5	2,600	ƒ	ƒ	.8	35
—	1	17	80	540	36	2,500	.1	ƒ	1.8	38
—	.1	2	3	160	260	300	ƒ	ƒ	.4	2
—	3.5	375	75	—	—	15,300	.1	.6	1	90
—	.8	62	51	345	87	ƒ	ƒ	ƒ	.6	28
—	.8	75	27	140	25	2,500	ƒ	1	.4	80
0	1.2	15	22	200	5	90	ƒ	ƒ	ƒ	2
0	.6	6	9	100	1	0	0	0	0	0
—	.4	8	13	130	1	50	ƒ	ƒ	ƒ	3
—	1	10	11	210	4	80	ƒ	ƒ	.1	3
—	8	28	37	600	2	4,500	ƒ	ƒ	.9	10
—	4.1	50	75	780	19	8,000	ƒ	.1	3	9
—	.5	18	30	280	1	2,900	ƒ	ƒ	.7	10
—	.5	22	30	440	ƒ	2,300	ƒ	ƒ	.5	7
2	.6	11	42	600	4	310	.1	.2	1.7	15
—	.7	8	44	390	1	190	ƒ	ƒ	.7	10
—	1.3	46	46	210	ƒ	290	ƒ	ƒ	.5	30
—	.5	100	15	200	2	100	ƒ	ƒ	.2	30
—	.8	33	64	910	40	6,000	ƒ	ƒ	1	65

* Includes oleic acid.
† If fried in oil.
ƒ Indicates trace only.

— No data available.
‡ Unsweetened.

FOOD	Approximate Measure	Wgt. in grams	Calories	Protein grams	Carbohydrate grams	Fiber grams	Fat grams	Saturated fatty acid* grams
FRUITS (Continued)								
Cherries, canned, pitted†	1 cup	257	100	2	26	2	1	—
Fresh, raw	1 cup	114	65	1	15	.3	∫	—
Cranberry sauce, sweetened	1 cup	277	530	∫	142	1.2	∫	—
Dates, dried	1 cup	178	505	4	134	3.6	∫	—
Figs, dried, large, 2 by 1"	2	42	120	2	30	1.9	∫	—
Fresh, raw	3 med.	114	90	2	22	2	∫	—
Stewed or canned, with syrup	3	115	130	1	32	2	∫	—
Fruit cocktail, canned	1 cup	256	195	1	50	.5	∫	—
Grapefruit, canned sections	1 cup	250	170	2	44	.5	∫	—
Grapefruit, fresh, 5" diameter	½	285	50	1	14	1	∫	∫
Grapefruit juice†	1 cup	250	100	1	24	1	∫	—
Grapes, American, as Concord	1 cup	153	70	1	16	.8	∫	—
European, as Muscat, Tokay	1 cup	160	100	1	26	.7	∫	—
Grape juice, bottled	1 cup	250	160	1	42	∫	∫	—
Lemon juice, fresh	½ cup	125	30	∫	10	∫	∫	—
Lemonade concentrate, frozen	6-oz. can	220	430	∫	112	∫	∫	—
Limeade concentrate, frozen	6-oz. can	218	405	∫	108	∫	∫	—
Olives, green, canned, large	10	65	72	1	3	.8	10	9
Ripe, canned, large	10	65	105	1	2	1	13	11
Oranges, fresh, 3" diameter	1 med.	180	60	2	16	1	∫	∫
Orange juice, fresh	8 oz. or 1 glass	250	111	2	25	.2	∫	—
Juice, frozen concentrate	6-oz. can	210	330	2	78	.4	∫	∫

Lino-leic acid grams	MINERALS					VITAMINS				
	Iron mg.	Cal-cium mg.	Phos-phorus mg.	Potas-sium mg.	Sodium mg.	A units	B₁ mg.	B₂ mg.	Niacin mg.	C mg.
—	.7	37	30	135	8	2,680	ſ	ſ	.4	13
—	.4	18	20	270	8	620	ſ	ſ	.4	10
—	.8	34	27	150	3	80	ſ	ſ	.3	5
—	5.7	105	110	1,300	1	100	.1	.2	3.9	0
—	1.7	80	55	390	15	40	.1	ſ	.8	0
—	.4	35	20	110	8	90	ſ	ſ	.6	2
—	.4	36	21	105	8	50	ſ	ſ	.4	0
—	1	23	30	350	12	360	ſ	ſ	1	5
—	.7	32	35	237	2	20	ſ	ſ	.5	75
0	.5	21	54	290	4	10	ſ	ſ	.3	72
—	1	20	40	280	2	20	ſ	ſ	.4	84
—	.4	13	30	120	5	100	ſ	ſ	.3	4
—	.6	18	30	240	6	110	ſ	ſ	.4	7
—	.8	28	33.	450	1	ſ	.1	ſ	.6	ſ
—	.2	8	13	80	4	20	ſ	ſ	.1	50
—	.4	9	15	170	5	40	ſ	ſ	.7	66
—	.7	11	12	118	ſ	ſ	ſ	ſ	.2	160
ſ	1.2	65	13	45	1,400	200	ſ	0	0	0
ſ	1.1	56	11	23	650	60	ſ	ſ	0	0
—	.5	50	40	300	ſ	240	1	ſ	.3	75
—	.5	27	42	500	2	500	.2	ſ	1	129
—	.8	69	115	1,315	4	1,490	.6	.1	2.4	330

° Includes oleic acid.
† Unsweetened.

— No data available.
ſ Indicates trace only.

FOOD	Approximate Measure	Wgt. in grams	Calories	Protein grams	Carbohydrate grams	Fiber grams	Fat grams	Saturated fatty acid grams
FRUITS (*Continued*)								
Papaya, fresh	½ med.	200	75	1	18	2.8	8	—
Peaches, canned, sliced	1 cup	257	200	1	52	1	8	—
Fresh, raw	1 med.	114	35	1	10	.6	8	—
Pears, canned, sweetened	1 cup	255	195	1	50	2	8	—
Raw, 3 by 2½"	1 med.	182	100	1	25	2	1	—
Persimmons, Japanese	1 med.	125	75	1	20		8	—
Pineapple, canned, sliced	1 large slice	122	95	8	26	.4	8	—
Crushed	1 cup	260	205	1	55	.7	8	—
Raw, diced	1 cup	140	75	1	19	.6	8	—
Pineapple juice, canned‡	1 cup	250	120	1	32	.2	8	—
Plums, canned in syrup	1 cup	256	185	.1	50	.7	8	—
Raw, 2" diameter	1	60	30	8	7	.2	8	—
Prunes, cooked‡	1 cup	270	300	3	81	.8	1	—
Prune juice, canned‡	1 cup	240	170	1	45	.7	8	—
Raisins, dried	½ cup	80	230	2	61	.7	8	—
Raspberries, frozen	½ cup	100	100	8	25	2	8	—
Raw,‡ red	¾ cup	100	57	8	14	5	8	—
Rhubarb, cooked, sweetened	1 cup	270	385	1	98	1.9	8	—
Strawberries, frozen	1 cup	227	242	1	60	1.3	8	—
Raw‡	1 cup	149	54	8	12	1.9	8	—
Tangerines, fresh	1 med.	114	40	1	10	1	8	—
Watermelon, 4 by 8"	1 wedge	925	120	2	29	3.6	1	—
BREADS, CEREALS, GRAINS, AND GRAIN PRODUCTS								
Biscuits, 2½" diameter§	1	38	130	3	18	8	4	3
Bran flakes	1 cup	25	117	3	32	1.3	8	—
Bread, cracked wheat	1 slice	23	60	2	12	.1	1	1
Rye	1 slice	23	55	2	12	.1	8	8
White,‖ 20 slices, or a	1-lb. loaf¶	454	1,225	39	229	9	15	11
Whole-wheat	1-lb. loaf	454	1,100	48	216	67.5	14	10
Whole-wheat	1 slice	23	55	2	11	.3	1	—
Corn bread of whole-ground meal	1 serving	50	100	3	15	.3	4	2

Lino-leic acid grams	MINERALS					VITAMINS				
	Iron mg.	Cal-cium mg.	Phos-phorus mg.	Potas-sium mg.	Sodium mg.	A units	B₁ mg.	B₂ mg.	Niacin mg.	C mg.
—	.5	40	32	470	6	3,500	≠	≠	.6	112
—	.8	11	35	310	6	1,100	≠	≠	1.4	7
—	.5	9	22	31	5	1,320†	≠	≠	1	7
—	.5	13	30	75	12	≠	≠	≠	.3	4
—	.5	13	29	182	3	30	≠	≠	.2	7
—	.4	7	28	310	1	2,710	≠	≠	.1	11
—	.7	26	9	150	1	100	.1	≠	.2	11
—	2.6	75	15	140	2	210	.2	≠	.4	23
—	.4	22	12	210	1	180	.1	≠	.3	33
—	1.2	37	22	370	2	200	.1	≠	.4	22
—	2.7	20	25	213	2	260	≠	≠	.9	3
—	.3	10	10	100	≠	200	≠	≠	.3	3
—	4.5	60	100	810	10	2,800	≠	.2	1.8	3
—	9.8	34	100	625	5	—	≠	≠	1.1	4
—	2.8	50	112	575	19	15	.1	≠	.4	0
—	.6	12	17	95	≠	80	≠	≠	.6	20
—	.9	40	37	190	≠	130	≠	≠	.3	24
—	1.1	112	39	510	15	70	≠	0	.2	17
—	1.3	50	34	220	3	80	≠	.1	.4	93
—	1.2	20	24	157	2	50	≠	≠	.5	60
—	.4	33	23	110	2	420	≠	≠	.2	30
—	1.2	63	96	600	2	520	≠	≠	.2	6
≠	.7	61	58	40	208	0	≠	≠	.7	0
—	2	25	248	480	960	0	.1	.1	3.4	0
0	.4	16	25	50	115	0	≠	≠	.3	0
0	.4	17	29	52	120	0	≠	≠	.3	0
2	10.9	318	662	720	2,655	0	1.1	.7	10.4	0
4	10.4	449	1,083	810	2,880	0	1.2	1	11.9	0
—	.5	23	54	40	144	0	≠	≠	.7	0
2	1.1	60	205	75	314	100	≠	≠	.3	0

* Includes oleic acid.
— No data available.
† If yellow only.
‡ Unsweetened.

≠ Indicates trace only.
§ Made with refined flour.
|| "Enriched" with vitamins B₁, B₂, niacin, and iron.
¶ Contains 4% milk solids.

FOOD	Approximate Measure	Wgt. in grams	Calories	Protein grams	Carbohydrate grams	Fiber grams	Fat grams	Saturated fatty acid* grams

BREADS, CEREALS, GRAINS, AND GRAIN PRODUCTS (*Continued*)

FOOD	Approximate Measure	Wgt. in grams	Calories	Protein grams	Carbohydrate grams	Fiber grams	Fat grams	Saturated fatty acid* grams
Cornflakes†	1 cup	25	110	2	25	.1	ß	—
Corn grits, refined, cooked	1 cup	242	120	3	27	.2	ß	—
Corn meal, yellow	1 cup	118	360	9	74	1.6	4	2
Crackers, graham	2 med.	14	55	1	10	ß	1	—
Soda, 2½" square	2	11	45	1	8	ß	ß	—
Farina†	1 cup	238	105	3	22	0	ß	—
Flour, soy, full fat	1 cup	110	460	39	33	2.9	22	0
Wheat, all purpose†	1 cup	110	400	12	84	.3	1	—
Wheat, whole	1 cup	120	390	13	79	2.8	2	—
Macaroni, cooked	1 cup	140	155	5	32	.1	1	—
Baked with cheese	1 cup	220	475	18	44	ß	25	24
Muffins of refined flour†	1	48	135	4	19	ß	5	4
Noodles	1 cup	160	200	7	37	.1	2	2
Oatmeal, or rolled oats	1 cup	236	150	5	26	4.6	3	2
Pancakes, buckwheat, 4" diam.	4	108	192	7	21	.5	8	—
Wheat, refined flour,† 4" diam.	4	108	250	7	28	.2	9	—
Pizza, cheese, ⅛ of 14" diam.	1 section	75	180	8	23	ß	6	5
Popcorn, with oil and salt	2 cups	28	152	3	20	.6	7	2
Puffed rice†	1 cup	14	55	ß	12	ß	ß	—
Puffed wheat,† presweetened	1 cup	28	105	1	26	.6	ß	—
Rice, brown	1 cup	208	748	15	154	1.2	3	—
Converted	1 cup	187	677	14	142	.4	ß	—
White†	1 cup	191	692	14	150	.3	ß	—
Rice flakes†	1 cup	30	115	2	26	.1	ß	—
Rice polish	½ cup	50	132	6	28	1.2	6	—
Rolls, breakfast, sweet	1 large	50	411	3	23	.1	12	11
Of refined flour†	1	38	115	3	20	ß	2	2
Whole-wheat	1	40	102	4	20	.1	1	—

Lino- leic acid grams	MINERALS					VITAMINS				
	Iron mg.	Calcium mg.	Phosphorus mg.	Potassium mg.	Sodium mg.	A units	B_1 mg.	B_2 mg.	Niacin mg.	C mg.
—	1.2	6	23	40	265	0	.1	ƒ	.6	0
—	.7	2	24	200	2	ƒ	ƒ	ƒ	.4	0
2	1.8	6	178	284	1	500	.4	.1	2	0
—	.3	3	56	45	90	0	ƒ	ƒ	.2	0
—	.1	2	19	12	110	0	ƒ	ƒ	.1	0
—	.8	31	29	20	33	0	.1	ƒ	1	0
11	8.8	218	613	1,826	1	221	.9	.3	2.3	0
—	3.2	18	87	86	1	0	.4	.2	3.2	0
—	3.9	49	464	445	3	0	.6	.2	5.1	0
—	.6	11	82	276	1	0	ƒ	ƒ	.4	0
1	2	394	363	132	1,192	970	.2	.5	1.9	0
8	.7	74	80	62	221	60	ƒ	.1	.7	0
8	1	16	52	—	—	60	ƒ	ƒ	.7	0
1	1.7	21	140	142	508	0	.2	ƒ	.4	0
—	1.2	249	360	245	464	230	.1	.2	.7	0
—	1.3	258	159	135	470	110	.1	.1	.9	0
ƒ	.7	257	147	96	525	570	ƒ	.1	.8	8
.4	.8	4	90	—	646	0	ƒ	ƒ	.7	0
—	.3	2	82	57	8	0	ƒ	ƒ	.6	0
—	.5	4	38	110	180	0	.1	ƒ	1.4	0
—	4	78	608	310	18	0	.6	.1	9.2	0
—	1.6	53	214	300	6	0	.3	ƒ	7.6	0
—	1.6	46	258	247	4	0	ƒ	ƒ	7.6	0
—	.5	9	44	60	329	0	.1	ƒ	1.7	0
—	8	35	553	357	ƒ	0	.9	.2	14	0
ƒ	.4	42	54	56	185	70	ƒ	ƒ	.8	.0
0	.7	28	39	34	202	ƒ	.1	ƒ	.8	0
	1	46	112	100	225	0	.1		1.5	0

° Includes oleic acid.
† "Enriched" with vitamins B_1, B_2, niacin, and iron.
ƒ Indicates trace only.
— No data available.

FOOD	Approximate Measure	Wgt. in grams	Calories	Protein grams	Carbohydrate grams	Fiber grams	Fat grams	Saturated fatty acid* gram
BREADS, CEREALS, GRAINS, AND GRAIN PRODUCTS (*Continued*)								
Spaghetti with meat sauce†	1 cup	250	285	13	35	.5	10	6
With tomatoes and cheese	1 cup	250	210	6	36	.5	5	3
Spanish rice with meat†	1 cup	250	217	4	40	1.2	4	—
Shredded wheat, biscuit	1	28	100	3	23	.7	1	—
Waffles, ½ by 4½ by 5½″‡	1	75	240	8	30	.1	9	8
Wheat germ	1 cup	104	245	26	34	2.5	7	3
Wheat-germ cereal, toasted§	1 cup	65	260	20	36	2.5	7	3
Wheat-meal cereal, unrefined	⅔ cup‖	30	103	4	25	.7	1	—
Wheat, unground, cooked	¾ cup	200	275	11	35	4.4	1	—
SOUPS, CANNED, AND DILUTED¶								
Bean soups	1 cup	250	190	8	30	.6	5	4
Beef and vegetable	1 cup	250	100	6	11	.5	4	4
Bouillon, broth, consommé	1 cup	240	24	5	0	0	—	—
Chicken or turkey	1 cup	250	75	4	10	0	2	2
Clam chowder, without milk	1 cup	255	85	5	11	.5	2	0
Cream soups (asparagus, celery, etc.)	1 cup	255	200	7	18	1.2	12	12
Noodle, rice, barley soups	1 cup	250	115	6	13	.2	4	3
Split-pea soup	1 cup	250	147	8	25	.5	3	3
Tomato soup, diluted with milk	1 cup	245	175	6	22	.5	7	6
Vegetable (vegetarian)	1 cup	250	80	4	14	—	2	2
DESSERTS AND SWEETS								
Apple betty	1 serving	100	150	1	29	.5	4	—
Bread pudding with raisins	¾ cup	200	374	11	56	.1	11	11

Mucus, covering stomach walls, 83   Myocardial infarction, 61

Lino-leic acid grams	MINERALS					VITAMINS				
	Iron mg.	Cal-cium mg.	Phos-phorus mg.	Potas-sium mg.	Sodium mg.	A units	B₁ mg.	B₂ mg.	Niacin mg.	C mg.
3	2	25	262	670	2,017	690	ƒ	.1	2.1	33
2	2	45	235	407	955	830	ƒ	ƒ	1	15
—	1.5	35	98	577	790	2,260	ƒ	ƒ	1.7	15
—	1	13	122	116	1	0	ƒ	ƒ	1.3	0
1	1.4	124	150	114	327	310	.1	.2	1.1	0
3	5.5	57	744	550	5	0	1.4	.5	3.1	0
3	4.9	32	722	630	1	110	1.6	.9	4.1	0
—	1.1	15	130	126	1	0	.2	.1	1.4	0
—	1.6	40	400	174	1	0	.1	.1	4.8	0
ƒ	2.8	95	254	445	1,007	260	ƒ	ƒ	1	2
ƒ	.8	12	50	265	1,067	2,100	ƒ	ƒ	1	—
—	1	2	32	129	780	0	ƒ	ƒ	1	0
ƒ	.5	20	75	—	751	0	ƒ	.1	1.5	0
1	1	36	49	225	1,099	1,070	ƒ	ƒ	1	0
ƒ	.5	217	157	295	1,058	200	ƒ	.2	.1	0
1	.2	81	45	69	2,224	30	ƒ	ƒ	.7	0
ƒ	1.4	31	152	275	959	450	.2	.2	1.4	0
ƒ	.7	267	155	417	1,055	2,200	ƒ	.2	1.2	0
ƒ	.8	32	40	170	855	2,900	ƒ		1	8
—	.7	24	36	100	152	100	ƒ	ƒ	.4	1
ƒ	2.2	218	228	430	400	600#	.1	.3	.2	0

FOOD	Approximate Measure	Wgt. in grams	Calories	Protein grams	Carbohydrate grams	Fiber grams	Fat grams	Saturated fatty acid° grams
DESSERTS AND SWEETS (*Continued*)								
Cakes, angelfood	1 slice	40	110	3	23	0	8	—
Chocolate cake, fudge icing	1 slice	120	420	5	70	.3	14	11
Cupcake with icing	1	50	160	3	31	8	3	2
Fruit cake, 2 by 2 by ½"	1 slice	30	105	2	17	.2	4	3
Gingerbread, 2" cube	1 piece	55	180	2	28	8	7	6
Plain cake, without icing	1 slice	55	180	4	31	8	5	4
Sponge cake, without icing	1 slice	40	115	3	22	0	2	2
Candy, caramels	5	25	104	8	19	0	3	3
Chocolate creams	2	30	130	8	24	0	4	4
Fudge, plain, 1" square	2 pieces	90	370	8	80	.1	12	11
Hard candies	1 oz.	28	90	8	28	0	0	0
Marshmallows, large	5	30	98	1	23	0	0	0
Milk chocolate	2-oz. bar	56	290	2	44	.2	6.	6
Chocolate syrup	2 T.	40	80	8	22	0	8	8
Doughnuts, cake type	1	33	135	2	17	8	7	4
Gelatin, made with water	1 cup	239	155	4	36	0	8	8
Honey, strained	2 T.	42	120	8	30	0	0	0
Ice cream, custard, see Dairy products								
Ices, lime, orange, etc.	1 cup	150	117	0	48	0	0	0
Jams, marmalades, preserves	1 T.	20	55	0	14	8	0	0
Jellies	1 T.	20	50	0	13	0	0	0
Molasses, blackstrap	1 T.	20	45	0	11	0	0	0
Cane, refined	1 T.	20	50	0	13	0	0	0
Pie,§ apple, ⅐ of 9"-diam. pie	1 slice	135	330	3	53	.1	13	11
Cherry	1 slice	135	340	3	55	.1	13	11
Custard	1 slice	130	265	7	34	0	11	10
Lemon meringue	1 slice	120	300	4	45	.1	12	10
Mince	1 slice	135	340	3	62	.7	9	8
Pumpkin	1 slice	130	265	5	34	.8	11	11

Linoleic acid grams	MINERALS					VITAMINS				
	Iron mg.	Calcium mg.	Phosphorus mg.	Potassium mg.	Sodium mg.	A units	B₁ mg.	B₂ mg.	Niacin mg.	C mg.
—	.1	2	40	40	113	0	∫	∫	.1	0
∫	.5	118	162	184	282	140†	∫	.1	.3	0
∫	.2	58	54	72	150	50	∫	∫	.1	∫
∫	.8	29	38	165	52	50†	∫	∫	.3	∫
∫	1.4	63	33	222	119	50†	∫	∫	.6	0
∫	.2	85	50	40	150.	70	∫	∫	.2	0
∫	.6	11	49	32	70	210	∫	∫	.1	0
∫	.8	40	22	48	55	40	∫	∫	∫	0
∫	.2	18	16	30	63	∫	0	0	∫	0
∫	.1	13	72	132	180	50	∫	∫	∫	0
0	0	0	0	0	8	0	0	0	0	0
0	0	0	2	2	13	0	0	0	0	0
0	.6	72	115	192	47	100	0	0	0	0
0	.5	0	36	120	20	0	0	0	0	0
3‡	.4	23	63	26	80	40	∫	∫	.4	0
0	0	0	0	0	122	0	0	0	0	0
0	.4	2	2	22	2	0	∫	∫	∫	2
0	0	∫	∫	5	∫	0	0	0	0	∫
0	.1	14	∫	19	3	∫	∫	∫	∫	1
0	.1	13	∫	15	3	∫	∫	∫	∫	1
0	2.3	116	14	585	19	0	∫	∫	∫	0
0	.9	30	9	185	3	0	0	0	0	0
∫	.5	9	29	106	400	220	∫	∫	.3	1
∫	.5	14	33	140	405	520	∫	∫	.3	2
∫	1.6	162	151	182	382	300	∫	.2	.4	0
∫	.6	24	65	66	337	210	∫	.1	.2	1
∫	3	22	50	236	600	10	∫	∫	.5	0
∫	1	70	92	219	285	2,480	∫	.1	.4	8

* Includes oleic acid.   † If made with butter or fortified margarine.
∫ Indicates trace only   ‡ If fried in oil.

FOOD	Approximate Measure	Wgt. in grams	Calories	Protein grams	Carbohydrate grams	Fiber grams	Fat grams	Saturated fatty acid° grams
DESSERTS AND SWEETS (*Continued*)								
Puddings, milk,† rice and bread‡								
Sugar, beet or cane	1 cup	200	770	0	199	0	0	0
3 teaspoons or	1 T.	12	50	0	12	0	0	0
Brown, firm-packed, dark	1 cup	220	815	0	210	0	0	0
Syrup, maple	2 T.	40	100	0	25	0	0	0
Table blends	2 T.	40	110	0	29	0	0	0
Tapioca cream pudding	1 cup	250	335	10	42	0	10	9
NUTS, NUT PRODUCTS, AND SEEDS								
Almonds, dried	½ cup	70	425	13	13	1.8	38	28
Roasted and salted	½ cup	70	439	13	13	1.8	40	31
Brazil nuts, unsalted	½ cup	70	457	10	7	2	47	31
Cashews, unsalted	½ cup	70	392	12	20	.9	32	18
Coconut, shredded, sweetened	½ cup	50	274	1	26	2	20	19
Peanut butter, commercial‖	½ cup	50	300	12	9	.9	25	17
Peanut butter, natural	½ cup	50	284	13	8	.9	24	10
Peanuts, roasted	½ cup	50	290	13	9	1.2	25	16
Pecans, raw, halves	½ cup	52	343	5	7	1.1	35	25
Sesame seeds, dry	½ cup	50	280	9	10	3.1	24	13
Sunflower seeds	½ cup	50	280	12	10	1.9	26	7
Walnuts, English, raw	½ cup	50	325	7	8	1	32	7
BEVERAGES								
Alcoholic, beer (4% alcohol)	2 cups	480	228	8	8	0	0	0
Gin, rum, vodka, whiskey (86 proof)	1 oz.	28	70	0	8	0	0	0
Wines, dessert (18.8% alcohol)	½ cup	120	164	8	9	0	0	0
Table (12.2% alcohol)	½ cup	120	100	8	5	0	0	0

Linoleic acid grams	MINERALS					VITAMINS				
	Iron mg.	Calcium mg.	Phosphorus mg.	Potassium mg.	Sodium mg.	A units	B₁ mg.	B₂ mg.	Niacin mg.	C mg.
0	0	0	0	0	0	0	0	0	0	0
0	0	0	0	0	0	0	0	0	0	0
0	5.7	167	38	688	60*	0	0	0	0	0
0	.6	41	3	70	4	0	ƒ	ƒ	ƒ	0
0	.3	2	1	10	1	0	0	0	0	0
1	1	262	265	337	390	580	.1	.4	.2	0
8	3.3	163	353	541	2	0	.2	.6	2.4	0
8	3.3	163	353	541	140	0	ƒ	.6	2.4	0
11	2.3	114	464	476	1	ƒ	.6	.1	1	0
1	2.9	29	242	325	40§	70	.3	.1	1.2	0
0	1	8	56	176	0	0	ƒ	ƒ	.4	1
7	.9	29	154	309	300	0	.3	.1	6.2	0
7	1	30	204	337	2	0	.5	.1	7.9	0
7	1	37	200	337	2§	0	.2	.1	8.6	0
7	1.2	36	144	300	1§	60	.4	.1	.4	1
10	5.2	580	308	360	30	15	.4	.1	2.7	.0
15	3.5	60	418	460	15	0	1.8	.2	13.6	0
20	1.5	50	190	225	1	15	.1	.1	.4	1
0	ƒ	10	60	50	14	0	ƒ	ƒ	1	0
0	0	0	0	ƒ	ƒ	0	0	0	0	0
0	ƒ	4	ƒ	37	2	0	ƒ	ƒ	.1	0
0	.5	10	11	100	6	0	ƒ	ƒ	.1	0

* Includes oleic acid.
† See Dairy products.
‡ See Grain products.

ƒ Indicates trace only.
§ Add 200 mg. for salted nuts.
‖ Sugar and hydrogenated fat added.

FOOD	Approximate Measure	Wgt. in grams	Calories	Protein grams	Carbohydrate grams	Fiber grams	Fat grams	Saturated fatty acid* grams
BEVERAGES (Continued)								
Carbonated drinks								
Artificially sweetened	12 oz.	346	0	0	0	0	0	0
Club soda	12 oz.	346	0	0	0	0	0	0
Cola drinks, sweetened	12 oz.	346	137	0	38	0	0	0
Fruit-flavored soda	12 oz.	346	161	0	42	0	0	0
Ginger ale	12 oz.	346	105	0	28	0	0	0
Root beer	12 oz.	346	140	0	35	0	0	0
Coffee, black, unsweetened	1 cup	230	3	‡	1	0	0	0
Tea, clear, unsweetened	1 cup	230	4	0	1	0	‡	0
SUPPLEMENTARY FOODS								
Bone meal or powder	½ t.	2.5	0	0	0	0	0	0
Calcium gluconate	7½ t.	11	—	0	0	0	0	0
Calcium lactate	3½ t.	5	—	0 ·	0	0	0	0
Dicalcium phosphate	1 t.	4	0	0	0	0	0	0
Desiccated liver, defatted†	¼ cup	37	120	28	3	1.6	‡	—
Lecithin, granular	2 T.	15	105	0	0	—	11	9
Powdered yeast, brewer's debittered	¼ cup	33	91	13	12	.6	‡	‡
Primary, grown on molasses‡	¼ cup	33	115	16	11	2.3	4	—
Torula	¼ cup	40	148	20	10	.2	3	‡
Torula, calcium fortified‖	¼ cup	40	148	20	10	.2	3	‡

Lino-leic acid grams	MINERALS					VITAMINS				
	Iron mg.	Cal-cium mg.	Phos-phorus mg.	Potas-sium mg.	Sodium mg.	A units	B₁ mg.	B₂ mg.	Niacin mg.	C mg.
◦	◦	◦	—	—	—	◦	◦	◦	◦	◦
◦	◦	◦	—	—	—	◦	◦	◦	◦	◦
◦	◦	◦	—	—	—	◦	◦	◦	◦	◦
◦	◦	◦	—	—	—	◦	◦	◦	◦	◦
◦	◦	◦	—	—	—	◦	◦	◦	◦	◦
◦	◦	◦	—	—	—	◦	◦	◦	◦	◦
◦	.2	9	9	40	2	◦	◦	ƒ	.6	◦
◦	ƒ	ƒ	ƒ	58	ƒ	◦	◦	ƒ	ƒ	◦
◦	1.8	1,000	516	ƒ	ƒ	◦	◦	◦	◦	◦
◦	0	1,000	0	0	0	◦	◦	◦	◦	◦
◦	0	1,000	0	0	0	◦	◦	◦	◦	◦
◦	0	1,000	778	0	0	◦	◦	◦	◦	◦
—	6	10	600	480	140	0	.2	4.4	11.3	70
1.1	ƒ	ƒ	500	ƒ	ƒ	—	—	—	—	—
ƒ	5	70	584	631	40	ƒ	5.2	1	12.9	0
—	2.5	81	231	600	165	0	8	8	33	0
2	7	90	600	800	6	0	6	6	40	0
2	7	600	600	800	6	0	10	10	100	0

◦ Includes oleic acid.

— No data available.

ƒ Indicates trace only.

† Supplies 370 milligrams of cholin, 74 of inositol, 5.5 of pantothenic acid, and 18.5 micrograms of vitamin B₁₂ as well as other B vitamins.

‡ One-half cup of flake yeast has the same nutrients as ¼ cup powdered.

§ Fortified with calcium, as directed on page 320.

Index

Abdomen, water blisters, on, 134-135
Abdominal cramps, vitamin B₈ and, 141
Abscesses, 134
in stomach, 151
Absorption, effect on, of diarrhea, 152; drugs, 36
Accidents, adrenal exhaustion and, 262
diet for, 269
stress induced by, 23-24
Acetylcholin, 240-241
Achilles' tendon, shortening of, 303
Acetone, 97-98
Acetone acidosis, after surgery, 267
symptoms of, 98
Acid, neutralization of, 88
"Acid stomach," 146
Acid urine, 192
Acidophilus culture, 315
bacteria supplied by, 144; concentration of, 144
effect of, on constipation, 147; histamine, 89; monilia albicans, 36; putrefactive bacteria, 140; ulcers, 89
laxative nature of, 147
Acidophilus milk, biotin deficiencies and, 132
calcium absorbed from, 261
effect of, on allergies, 167; intestinal bacteria, 37; putrefactive bacteria, 157
value of, in gout, 190
Acidosis, acetone, 97-98
as stress, 100
diabetic, vitamin B₁ and, 100
potassium deficiency and, 101
prevention of, 123
symptoms of, 123
Acidulated milk, for allergies, 167
Acne, adolescent, 135
vitamin A for, 313
x-ray treatments for, 301
Acne rosacea, 135
ACTH, 23, 26

ACTH therapy, decreasing toxicity of, 30
effect of, 29
effect of, on allergies, 159; blood potassium, 236; blood pressure, 213, 217; body protein, 108; pantothenic acid, 30, 110-111; sodium, 164; sprue, 154
pancreatic damage from, 157, 293
Acute illness, incidence of, 335
Addis, Dr. Thomas, 200
Addison's disease, adrenal exhaustion and, 237-238
relation of, to muscular weakness, 238; scleroderma, 293; skin pigmentation, 130-131; stress, 237-238
Adenoids, enlargement of, 119, 127
infection of, 126
removal of, 267
Adequate diet, intestinal parasites and, 156
requirements of, 309-321, 406-407
Adequate meals, planning of, 346
Adhesions, as scar tissue, 41-42, 46
in eyes, 284
prevention of, 264
Adolescence, deficient diets during, 333, 336
Adolescent girls, anemia and, 231
Adolescents, acne of, 135
effect on, of sweets, 259
high requirements of, 247
inadequate diets of, 333, 336
vitamin E for, 317
Adrenal cortex, degeneration of, 25
faulty diet and, 25
hormones produced by, 23
Adrenal damage, from ACTH therapy, 110; deficiencies of linoleic acid, 25, pantothenic acid, 25, potassium, 110, vitamin A, 25, vitamin B₂, 25, vitamin C, 25-26, vitamin E, 25
Adrenal exhaustion, characteristics of, 26

439

Carotene, absorption of, 180, 312
  effect on, of iron salts, 33; mineral oil, 148
  sources of, 312
Carrots, 145
Car sickness, 141
Cashew nuts, saturated fat in, 77
Cataracts, associated with diabetes, 101-102
  effect on, of faulty circulation, 48
  emotionally induced, 287
  experimental production of, 115, 282-283
Cathartics, harm of, 148
Celiac disease, factors triggering onset of, 155
  relation to, of folic acid, 155; gluten, 154; salt intake, 155; vitamin B₆, 156
  symptoms of, 154
Cell damage, vitamin E and, 264
Cell nucleus, vitamin E essential for, 236-237, 244
Cells, breakdown of, 229
  permeability of, 118, 162
Cellulose, effect of, on intestinal bacteria, 145, 157
  lacking in roughness, 322
  sources of, as fiber, 408-434
Cephalin, 51
Cereals, fortified, misrepresentation of, 338; nutrients discarded from, 337-338
  unrefined, nutrients supplied by, 328
Cerebral atherosclerosis, effect on, of lecithin, 52
  strokes associated with, 212
  symptoms of, 48
Cerebral palsy, 296, 318
Cheese, calcium content of, 320
  emphasis on, during illness, 327
  low-sodium, 201
  processed, 53
Chemical fertilizers, 319, 321, 341-342
Chemicals, cancer induced by, 300, 302
  detoxification of, 34, 171, 173, 343
  effect on stomach, 83
  relation of toxicity, to cataracts, 283; gall-bladder inflammation, 183; hepatitis, 176; kidney damage, 196; liver damage, 170, 173; pancreatitis, 189; tissue damage, 115-116
  use of, in food processing, 343
Children, American, muscular fitness of, 336
  bone mineralization of, 253
  character problems of, 168
  effect on, of sweets, 259

incidence of cancer among, 335
massive doses of vitamin E given to, 237, 294
pantothenic-acid requirements of, 161
suffering from anemia, 229; celiac disease, 154; cirrhosis, 176; congenital errors of metabolism, 296; cystic fibrosis, 294; kidney stones, 195; leukemia, 306-307; liver damage, 170; mental retardation, 237; muscle weakness, 236; muscular dystrophy, 244; nearsightedness, 284; nephritis, 194; slow muscular development, 244
value to, of whole grains, 338; vitamin A, 313; vitamin E, 317
Choking, muscular weakness and, 239
Cholesterol, absorption of, 52
  amount of, in brain, 49
  as bile constituent, 179
  deposition of, around eyes, 48; in arterial walls, 48-59; kidneys, 217; tumors, 131-132; over scars, 55; under skin, 48
  faulty utilization of, 50
  functions of, 49
  relation of, to essential fatty acids, 49-50; gallstones, 181-182; psoriasis, 131-132
  sources of, 49
  synthesis of, 49, 51; effect on, of vitamin C, 56
  see also Blood cholesterol
Cholin, amounts given, 54, 58, 103, 194
  deficiencies of, and anemia, 230; fatty liver, 173-174; hemorrhage, 198; kidney damage, 194; liver damage, 173-174; ulcers, 84-85
  deficiencies of, in children's diets, 67; in infant formulas, 66
  detoxifying action of, 173
  effect of, on bile acids, 53; blood cholesterol, 53-54; cholesterol excretion, 54; constipation, 214; coronary patients, 53; dropsy, 214; fatty liver, 173-174; high blood pressure, 213-214; insomnia, 214; lecithin synthesis, 53, 174; muscles, 240; salt toxicity, 215
  effect on, of alcohol, 65
  intake of, 241
  lecithin as source of, 174
  relation of, to betain, 299; blood pressure, 213; experimental cancer, 299, 302; fat intake, 176; kidney diseases, 193-194; kidney stones, 206; lecithin synthesis, 51;

refined, 323-324, 337-338
relation of soil to mineral content of, 341-342
symbolic meanings of, 146, 323
to emphasize, during illness, 322, 326-329
undigested, bacteria and, 143
unrefined, as source of nutrients, 32, 51, 338
Foot spasms, 222
Forgetfulness, 48, 474
Formula diet, for reducing, 78
Formulas, *see* Infants' formulas
Fortified milk, advantage of, 31, 89, 329
preparation of, 329
variations of, for reducing diets, 78; ulcer diets, 89
Fortified yeast, 327
4-H garden clubs, as potential food producers, 342-343
Fowl, 323, 327
Fractures, 179, 255-256
Fried foods, 58, 90, 322, 323
Fruits, 328
Fungus infestations, 36, 136, 151

Galactose, cataracts and, 282
Gall bladder, abnormalities of, 179-186
diet suggestions for, 184-186
importance of emptying, 182
inflammation of, 183-184
Gallstones, 181-182
Gamma globulin, injections of, 122
Gangrene, 48, 55, 101-102
Gardens, home, 342
Gas, distention, 87, 158, 185, 322
see also Intestinal gas
Gastric fistula, 82-83
Gastric juice, 142
Gastritis, 151
Gelatin, amino acids lacking from, 189, 310
glycine content of, 205
Gelatin desserts, 323
Gels, phosphorus absorption and, 208
Girls, inadequate diets of, 336
Glaucoma, 284-286
Globulins, 230
Glomeruli, 192
Glucose, calcium absorption and, 259
Glutamic acid hydrochloride, 142
Gluten, and celiac disease, 154-156
Gluten enteropathy, 154
Gluten-free diet, 154-155
Glycine, excess of, 310
relation of, to oxalic acid, 205; uric acid, 189

Glycogen, formation of, 23, 170, 171
relation to, of fatigue, 171; insulin, 94
storage of, 267
Goats' milk, 167
Goiter, 45, 278, 279
toxic, 287
Gonadotropin, 272
Gout, causes of, 188-190
effect on, of emotional upsets, 190; rancid fats, 189; scarring, 46-47; stress, 188; uric acid injections, 189; vitamin E, 188-189
prevention of, 191
Grains, unrefined, value of, 155, 336-338
Grand mal, 221-222
Granular lecithin, *see* Lecithin, granular
Green leafy vegetables, antistress factor in, 28, 31
potassium in, 216
Growth, high requirements during, 161
Gums, bleeding of, 124, 141
infection of, 141

Hair, color, restoration of, 138-139
folic-acid deficiency and, 307
graying of, 138-139
growth of, 138; on face, 172
Halitosis, causes of, 140
relation of, to bile flow, 180; vitamin-B₆ deficiency, 274
Hands, cold, 273, 278
cracked skin of, 133-134
numbness in, 225
swelling of, 247
tingling of, 225
trembling of, 223
twitching of, 223
water blisters on, 134-135
Hangnails, 138
Hay fever, effect on, of emotions, 112, 128, 165; vitamin A, 162; vitamin C, 162-163
Headaches, as allergic manifestation, 159, 160
associated with acidosis, 98; anemia, 227; emotional problems, 117, 165-166; high blood pressure, 212-213, 214; infrequent meals, 311; iron deficiency, 230; kidney damage, 193; low blood sugar, 74, 97, 165, 277; menopause, 250; menstruation, 246-247, 277; nearsightedness, 284; pantothenic-acid deficiency, 160; stress, 278; vitamin-A toxicity, 313; vitamin-B₁

Mucus, covering stomach walls, 83
  effect on, of chemicals, drugs, herbs, **83**
  production of, 87
  relation to, of vitamin A, 87
Multiple sclerosis, 241-243
  early symptoms of, 235
Mumps, 121
Muscle cells, destruction of, 237
Muscle cramps, associated with adrenal exhaustion, 238; low calcium intake, 247; magnesium deficiency, 149, 223; pantothenic-acid deficiency, 238; salt deficiency, 176, 199-200
  calcium for, 247
Muscle damage, vitamin E and, 236-237
Muscles, abnormalities of, 235-245
  breakdown of, 236, 238, 243
  calcium deposits in, 237
  effect on, of cholin deficiency, 240-241; cortisone, 239; potassium deficiency, 236; prolonged stress, 237-238; protein deficiency, 244; vitamin-A deficiency, 244; vitamin-B₆ deficiency, 244
  flabbiness of, 236
  inflammation of, 238
  lack of elasticity of, 237
  longitudinal splits in, 243
  partial paralysis of, 236, 238
  relation to, of creatine, 241; essential fatty acids, 243; potassium, 236; vitamin E, 236-237
  scarring of, 236-237, 239, 241, 243, 244
  sluggishness of, 236
  spasms of, 223, 256
  weakness of, 236, 237
Muscle sheaths, inflammation of, 238
Muscle spasms, magnesium deficiency and, 149, 223
  prevention of, 277
Muscle weakness, recovery from, 236, 237
  relation of, to adrenal exhaustion, 237-238; pantothenic-acid deficiency, 27, 238; potassium deficiency, 236; vitamin-E deficiency, 236-237
Muscular atrophy, 243-244
Muscular dystrophy, 243-245
  early symptoms of, 235
Mustard, 323
Mustard gas, 305
Myasthenia gravis, diet suggestions for, 241
  recovery from, 239-240
  relation of, to stress, 242
  symptoms of, 239

Myocardial infarction, 61
Myoglobin, 230, 231
Myositis, 238-239, 292

Natural vitamins vs. synthetic, 318
Nausea, 98, 141, 145
Nearsightedness, 283-284
Neck, muscular weakness of, 239
  rigidity of, 222
Nephritis, diet suggestions for, 200-201
  effect on, of cholin, 194; lecithin, 194; vitamin C, 198; vitamin E, 126, 195-196
  experimental production of, 193-195
  inadequacies of diets given for, 199-200
  relation to, of cholin deficiency, 194; essential-fatty-acids deficiency, 195; high blood pressure, 214; magnesium deficiency, 195; protein deficiency, 193-194; scar tissue, 126; strep throat, 196; stress, 197; toxic drugs, 196
  supplements for, 201
  susceptibility to, 193
  symptoms of, 193, 194
Nephrosis, associated with anemia, 197; atherosclerosis, 48; heart disease, 197
  diet suggestions for, 200-201
  effect on, of cholin, 194; vitamin E, 195-196
  relation of, to salt intake, 198
  supplements for, 201
Nerve damage, 232, 234, 243
Nervous tension, associated with acidosis, 98; calcium deficiency, 246, 249-250, 275; low blood sugar, 97; magnesium deficiency, 219; menopause, 250; menstruation, 246
Neuritis, 101, 227
New diseases, 335
Niacin, 149
Niacin amide, recovery from deficiency of, 289
  relation of, to anemia, 230; brittle diabetes, 110; diarrhea, 148-149; canker sores, 127; eczema, 133, mental health, 274; skin pigmentation, 130-131; sore mouth, 140-141; tongue abnormalities, 140, 288-289; Vincent's disease, 127
  sources of, 408-435
Nicotine, effect on circulation, 225
Nicotinic acid, toxicity to, 34
Night sweats, menopausal, 250
Night vision, vitamin A and, 281